Helping Women Keep Well

*A Guide to Health Promotion and Illness Prevention
for the Health Professional*

Helping Women Keep Well

*A Guide to Health Promotion and Illness Prevention
for the Health Professional*

Richard H. Blum, Ph.D.
W. LeRoy Heinrichs, M.D., Ph.D.

Stanford University School of Medicine

Irvington Publishers, Inc.
New York

Copyright ©1988by Irvington Publishers, Inc.

All rights reserved. No part of this book may be reproduced in any manner whatever, including information storage or retrieval, in whole or in part (except for brief quotations in critical articles or reviews), without written permission from the publisher. For information, write to Irvington Publishers, Inc., 740 Broadway, New York, New York 10003.

Library of Congress Cataloging-in-Publication Data

```
Blum, Richard H.
   Helping women keep well
                                             Richard H. Blum, W.
   LeRoy Heinrichs.
         p.    cm.
      Bibliography: p.
      Includes index.
      ISBN 0-8290-1793-3 : $44.50 (est.)
      1. Women--Health and hygiene.  2. Women--Diseases.  3. Health
   promotion.  4. Medicine, Preventive.  5. Physician and patient.
   I. Heinrichs, W. LeRoy.  II. Title.
      [DNLM: 1. Health Promotion.  2. Health Services.  3. Primary
   Prevention.  4. Women--psychology.   WA 108 B658h]
   RA564.85.B58 1988
   613'.0424--dc19
   DNLM/DLC
   for Library of Congress                                   88-2752
                                                                CIP
```

IRVINGTON PUBLISHERS, INC.
740 Broadway
New York, New York 10003

DEDICATION

To David Williams and the Fellows and Scholars of
Wolfson College, Cambridge.

RHB

My thanks to Phyllis, Stephen and Lynn

WLH

Contents

Acknowledgements		*xv*
Foreword		*xvii*
Prologue		*xix*
About the Authors		*xxiii*
Section I	An Introduction to Health Promotion: The Psychobiological Context	*xxv*
Chapter 1	Health Promotion for Women *Introduction* *Health Promotion: What is it?* *The Health Professional's Role* *Historical Development*	1
Chapter 2	Converging Trends: The New (Re)emphasis *U.S. Federal Initiatives* *Work In Psychobiology* *Changes In Population Health Status*	17

Rising Costs For Illness Care
Early Findings From Cigarette Smoking Studies
Individual Health Attitudes Are Responsive
Combatting Toxins And Poverty Is Expensive
Is It Victim Blaming?
More Options For Self Health Care
Expansion
Medical-Legal Signs Of Changing Times
Feminism, The Women's Health Movement, And Conflict
Women Want Women's Problem-Oriented Centers
Shifting Responsibilities Should Bring Better Health
New Roles and Well-being

Section II	*Illness and Unwellness: Psychosocial–Behavioral Factors*	47
Chapter 3	Health Complaints of Women "Out There" in their World	49

          Introduction
          A Preview With Health Promotion Implications
          Fallible Statistics
          Morbidity As Measured By Self-Reports In Health Surveys In Populations At Large
          Medical Visits Relation And Experienced Unwellness

            Self-Rated Overall Health Status
            That Ubiquitous "Stress"
            Common Risk Factors Qua "Stress"
            The Socio-Economic Data Paradox
            Other High Symptom Level Correlates
            Emotional And Personality Disorder
            Symptoms As Self-Appraisal: Two Systems In Conflict
            Same Words, Different Meanings
            Cultural-Ethnic Variations
            Situational Roles, Troubles, And Complaints
            Summary Comment

Chapter 4   Prevalence of Diagnosed Conditions Among Women: Behavioral Considerations   87
            Comment
            Summary

Chapter 5   Mortality, Diagnosed Morbidity, and Psychosocial–Behavioral Risk: Longitudinal Studies
            The Work Done
            Summary

Chapter 6   Obstetrical Risk   127
            Caution
            Obstetrical Risk Prediction
            Comment

                  On Methodological Matters:
                      Risk Prediction
                  Allowable Conclusions
                  Summary

Chapter 7	Women's Conditions Linked to Psychosocial–Behavioral Factors	175

                  Comment and Caution
                  Thinking About Costs
                  Summary comment

Section III   *Case Examples*   *213*

Chapter 8	The Experiences of Six Women	215

                  One Woman's Fiery Vulvo-
                      Vaginitis
                  A Girl's Painful Sexual
                      Maturation
                  Cyclic Symptoms as a
                      Manifestation of Metabolic
                      Endocrinopathy
                  Just a "Touch" of Pregnancy
                  "Self-Induced" High Risk
                      Pregnancy
                  Prematurity—A Legacy of
                      Socio-Economic
                      Deprivation
                  Conclusion

Section IV   *Office Based Health Promotion Activities*   *225*

Chapter 9	From Poor Compliance to Good Cooperation	227

                  Regarding Instructions
                  Wise Anticipation and
                      Informational Pre-treatment

          Creating the Right Atmosphere
          Incompatible Outcomes
          Time Dose-Effect Relationships
          Women's Sexual Problems: A Special Case of the Incomplete Medical Visit
          Communications and Assuring Support
          The Contrary Case: The Professional as Saboteur
          Genetic Counseling: When Is It Not? A Case in Point
          Powerlessness Is Bad News
          Summary

Chapter 10   More on Getting Cooperation: Securing Long Term Change in Health Behaviors   247
          Kinds of Social Supports
          The Illusion of Control and Spontaneous Change
          Continuing Contact and Other Essentials
          When Is Success Not Enough? And When Is Knowledge Not Enough?
          The Problem Patient: Her Number Is Legion
          To Repeat, Reach Out!
          The Whole Woman and Whole Programs
          Finding Your Alter Ego
          Summary

Chapter 11   Evaluating and Targeting for Change   273
          Getting the Information

        Psychosocial Behavioral Risk
          Profile Inquiry: A History
          Taking and Evaluation
          Reminder List
        The Professionals Themselves
        The Hospital Where One
          Practices
        In Obstetrics Particularly
        In the Hospital or Medical School
        Summary

Chapter 12   Negotiating Diagnoses Through Referral: A Simple Health Behavior   299
        A New, Simple Health Behavior
          for Somatizers
        Summary comment

Chapter 13   Referral for Serious Biopsychological Concomitants of Reproductive System Conditions   309
        Cancer: Sexual Dysfunction
          and Depression
        Drug Regimes
        Infertility
        Pelvic Pain
        Hysterectomy
        Surgical Abortion, Perinatal
          Loss
        PMS
        Other Precipitating States:
          The Woman's
          Reproductive System As
          An Illness Site Particularly
          Sensitive to Emotion
        Misery without Referral
        Resistance
        Networks Again

        Legitimizing A Holistic
          Approach
        Summary

Chapter 14   Future Directions   331
        Systematization in Obstetrical
          Risk Prediction
        Search for Underlying
          Covariance in Gynecological
          Illness
        Working on "Best Test"
          Consensus
        Etiological Mechanisms
        Locating and Learning
          Acceptable Complaints
        Too Much Medication: Is There a
          Way Out?
        More Attention to Sleep Disorder
        Mother-Daughter Pairs and
          Prediction
        Not Yet a Whole Picture
        Placebo Main Effect
        Fatigue or Low Energy
        Classifying Somatizers
        Reexamining Roles and
          Institutions
        Reexamining Values Affecting
          Concept Choices for Research:
          Is There, Should There Be, a
          Perfect Low-Risk Woman?
        Research on Diversity for
          Wellness Is Needed
        Testing Interventions
        Needed: Nourishment
        Summary

List of Tables

Table I	The Ten Leading Causes of Death in the United States: 1900–1980	21
Table II	U.S. National Prevalence Data from Records	89
Table III	Psychosocial and Behavioral Features Implicated in Obstetrical Complications and Adverse Perinatal Outcomes	133
Table IV	Diseases of Women, and Men, Associated with Psychosocial and Behavioral Risk Components	177
Table V	Conditions and Diseases of the Female Reproductive Tract	188
Table VI	Psychological Tests Used in Risk Assessment, Self-Report Health Status, Psychosomatic Research, and Illness Impact Studies	334

Bibliography   *359*

Author Index   *427*

Subject Index   *443*

Acknowledgements

The first phase in the work leading to this book, research concerned with women's behavior and the improvement of obstetrical risk prediction, owes much to the contribution of and collaboration with Suzanne Arms, Professor James Bush (Department of Community and Family Medicine, University of California, San Diego), Professor Philip Darney (Department of Obstetrics-Gynecology, University of California Medical Center, San Francisco), Dr. Pamela Eakins (Center for Research on Women, Stanford University), Professor Calvin Hobel (Department of Obstetrics-Gynecology, University of California Medical Center, Los Angeles), Warren Pearse (Director, American College of Obstetricians and Gynecologists) and Judith Rooks.

Phase two, initial drafting and issue identification, centered on work with colleagues in Cambridge and London. There, one enjoyed the wisdom and encouragement of Dr. Beulah Bewley (President, UK Medical Women's Federation), Martin Richards (Director, Child Care and Development Unit, University of Cambridge), Professor Geoffrey Chamberlain, (Department of Obstetrics and Gynecology, St. Georges Hospital Medical School, London), and Vivienne Speller (Director of Education, Wandsworth Health District, London).

For phase three, the final development of the manuscript, we owe much to the constructive editorial comments of Professor Nancy Adler (Health Psychology, University of California Medical Center, San Francisco), Dr. Warren Pearse of ACOG, and Professor Paul Weinberg (Department of Obstetrics-Gynecology & Reproductive Sciences, University of Texas Medical School, Austin).

Foreword

"Helping Women Keep Well" addresses the issues of the contemporary woman. The term "preventive medicine" has had little appeal in the past, but for now and in the future, prevention—not disease—is the byword.

A number of themes emerge from this book. The core consists of *Health Promotion; Disease Prevention; Wellness*, and the blending of psychosocial and psychosomatic aspects of disease and wellness.

Those members of the health care team that care for women, especially those in obstetrics and gynecology, are afforded an important arena and opportunity for health promotion and disease prevention. The first few chapters underscore the fact that practitioners are poorly prepared and unorganized for this new responsibility. In all aspects of education, whether for the health care team or the patient, it is important that wellness and patient responsibility for this wellness be emphasized. It is imperative in our medical schools and postgraduate training programs that this theme become an integral part of the educational process. The vehicle for modeling this process is continuity of patient care so that health care providers appreciate changes across time in wellness, disease and psychosocial events. Wellness as a major issue in women's health care for family physicians and obstetrician-gynecologists has not as yet focused on the inner conflicts and discomforts that are related to illness in the woman.

The authors present convincing epidemiological evidence that primary care providers fail to focus on the behavioral and emotional aspects of disease. They also show that morbidity and mortality may be related to behavior and psychosocial circumstances in a given patient. These findings require action on the part of health professionals.

If health care providers are to promote wellness and the woman's independent responsibility for health, these professional interactions must begin in the office practice setting. Educating and gaining the woman's participation are essential. Women must come to understand their own psychosocial realities as these affect their health, wellness and bodily functions. For success, each woman will want to delineate and adopt a workable plan for her own problem identification and control that stresses prevention of disease, both physical and emotional.

Practitioners often tend to be too busy or otherwise unable to communicate with the inner feelings and attitudes of patients. Yet we know that there is no substitute for taking time to talk to your patient and to demonstrate genuine concern for her physical and emotional welfare. For intervention beyond that, the availability in the health care team of a health psychologist or other professional oriented toward wellness and assumption of patient responsibility is essential.

The book has an extensive 1200 item bibliography, many valuable tables, and documentation cited from leading medical science organizations, all of which emphasize its thrust.

The authors are to be commended for their forward thinking in assembling this much needed information with its perspective for the essential future health care for the woman.

> Frederick P. Zuspan, M.D.
> The R.L. Meiling Professor and Chairman
> Department of Obstetrics and Gynecology
> The Ohio State University

Prologue

Shortly after the end of World War II it became customary for physicians to work collaboratively with social workers and psychologists in caring for patients. Soon nurses and other health professionals were participating in the coordinated process of planning and administering medical care. With such dispersion of activities coupled with the rapid proliferation of medical technology, physicians began to spend less and less time with their patients, tending mainly to technical and administrative functions such as operating endoscopes, ordering tests and prescribing.

Recently, since the patient more and more has been included as a member of his or her "health care team," there is again a need for the full participation of the ultimately responsible physician whose scientific training and clinical experience must be applied fully to understand the patient and her problem. No longer can a physician's diagnosis consist merely of correctly labeling an illness. The word diagnosis, taken from the Greek, means to know thoroughly, to understand the patient as well as the disease. The treatment, too, must be appropriate not only to the disease but to the individual characteristics of the patient as well.

The authors of the book, a health psychologist and gynecologist-obstetrician, have reminded the physician of his obligation thoroughly to understand his or her patient. In so doing they have made a monumental contribution to sane comprehensive medical care with the emphasis on prevention— keeping well.

While concerns for the special medical problems of women have their roots in the pre-Christian era, modern gynecology, as a surgical specialty, had its beginnings in the United States with Ephraim McDowell (1771-1830) of Kentucky and James Marion Sims (1813-1883) of South Carolina. When Johns Hopkins Hospital opened in

1886, there were no facilities for obstetrics but a gynecologist in chief was appointed as one of the initial staff and medical school faculty. He was Howard A. Kelly, a 31 year old surgical virtuoso who had established a gynecological clinic in Philadelphia. Obstetrics came along at Hopkins, first as a sub-department under Dr. Kelly, and later as a separate department headed by Dr. John Whitridge Williams.

While pediatrics, the care of children, is classified as a primary care specialty, obstetrics-gynecology usually is not, although some physicians practice as if it were. The concept of a specialty for the total care of women is envisioned in this comprehensive book by Blum and Heinrichs, the major emphasis on staying well. Thus, instead of serving as a textbook of women's diseases, it is a treatise on prevention.

The introductory historical sketch that describes how, over the years, important medical innovations have been resisted by the "establishment" is especially telling. New landmark contributions, most significant for gynecologists-obstetricians, antisepsis and anesthesia, were ignored and even scorned for years by many prominent and well established practitioners. So it was with the detrimental effects of cigarette smoking that were recognized more than 40 years ago by Alton Oschsner in New Orleans and Evarts Graham in St. Louis. So it has been with the psychosocial approach to bodily disorders and diseases, despite 40 years of clear experimental evidence of measurable changes in visceral function resulting from emotionally stressful circumstances.

The authors have assembled an impressive collection of data on the behavior of patients and physicians in the actual practice situation. They have shown convincingly that health cannot be defined as the absence of disease. Indeed, it is common to encounter women who are sick in the absence of definable disease. Disease may make a late appearance, however, depending on special features of a woman's personality, beliefs, optimism, coping strategies and so forth, as shown by Carol Thomas and her colleagues at Johns Hopkins. James J. Lynch, of the University of Maryland, has pointed out in his two books, THE BROKEN HEART and THE LANGUAGE OF THE HEART, that there may be serious pathogenic effects of loneliness and dejection. On the other hand, he identified a salutary effect of human dialogue, companionship and social support. The psychosocial approach, applied as a preventive in gynecological practice, may eventually assume an importance comparable to antisepsis or modern sepsis.

A strong feature of the book is the authors' emphasis on cooperative planning between patient and physician in the whole medical care process. They show how such strategy not only makes the recommended therapeutic measures more acceptable but helps the physician better understand the patient and the patient better understand herself. Commendably, the authors do not preach a dogma based on the availability of present knowledge, but call for intensification of further careful scientific inquiry. They are even cautious about accepting answers from current research, especially in interpreting data from surveys and epidemiological studies that involve larger numbers and large opportunities for errors of inclusion and exclusion. They point out the potential hazards of drawing inferences from groupings of people that do not have clear limits, or even uniform characteristics: socio-economic class, for example, educational level, or various psychological states and traits. The authors do not scorn such studies, but neither do they view them as conclusive. Rather, they accept the inferences drawn as provisional until further evidence is adduced.

What of the future? The comprehensive approach proposed in this book will certainly promote a broader understanding of obstetrics and gynecology, of what is involved in being a woman's doctor. When the time comes, physicians will realize and act upon the knowledge that the practice of medicine is not merely treating disease, but caring for people—an old idea whose time may finally have come.

STEWART WOLF, M.D.
Director, Totts Gap Research Institute

About the Authors

Richard H. Blum, Ph.D. and LeRoy Heinrichs, M.D., Ph.D. are co-directors of the Health Promotion Unit (clinic) and Professors of Gynecology and Obstetrics in the Stanford University School of Medicine. Dr. Heinrichs is Emeritus Chairman of that department, in which he has for nine years maintained a large clinical practice of obstetrics and gynecology with emphasis on gynecologic endocrinology and infertility. A Fellow of the American College of Obstetricians and Gynecologists, The Endocrine Society and The Pacific Coast Fertility Society, he is an internationally recognized authority on environmental factors that disturb female reproductive processes. An associate editor of Gynecologic and Obstetrical Investigation, an international journal of reproduction, Dr. Heinrichs has contributed extensively to modern practice concepts.

Dr. Blum has been Consulting Professor of Psychology at Stanford, and Director of Research for the Medical Review and Advisory Board of the California Medical Association. A Fellow of the American Psychological Association and American Public Health Association and a member of the American Society for Psychosomatic Obstetrics and Gynecology, his earlier books include *Management of the Doctor-Patient Relationship, Health and Healing and Rural Greece, Alcoholism: Modern Psychological Approaches and Treatment, Horatio Alger's Children: The Role of the Family in the Origin and Prevention of Drug Risk, Controlling Drugs: International Handbook for Psychoactive Drug Classification, Drug Education: Results and Recommendations, Pharmaceuticals and Health Policy*, and, for patients, *A Commonsense Guide to Doctors, Hospitals and Medical Care*.

Professors Blum and Heinrichs have been working since 1981 on women's beliefs, choices and conduct as it affects their illness risk. The development of their Health Promotion Unit at Stanford is one of the first such "whole woman" medical school programs in the nation for disease prevention and enhanced wellness for women.

SECTION I

An Introduction to Health Promotion: The Psychobiological Context

1

Health Promotion for Women

Introduction

"Health promotion" and "health behaviors" are terms now in widespread use reflecting important concepts for those engaged in health education, research, prevention, and policy. With the advent of new clinical sub-specialties and with disease prevention optimistically encompassing new goals, considerable media and professional attention is directed to individuals and their health practices and to the environmental, psychological, and sociological variables determining these practices. Interest is high for tests of effective methods that are applicable by communities, institutions, groups, or individuals to reduce illness risk. Considerable progress is also being made in research on psychophysiological response patterns and on the neuroendocrine and immune system processes which act as final pathways mediating individual reactions such as stress and coping, which frequently function to increase or diminish risks of disease expression and the course of illness.

These developments are such that the women's health specialist is well advised to keep pace with major trends and findings, and to incorporate them into clinical practice. The data are persuasive as to the vital role that health practices and associated psychosomatic variables play as risk factors for a variety of important gynecological and maternal conditions and general health status. Public campaigns directed at smoking, obesity, Type A conduct, alcoholism and drug abuse do stimulate patient inquiries while personal experience with such efforts may occasionally lead to unanticipated health consequences that confront the physician, as for example: toxicity of health foods and vitamins/minerals, crash diets, or distressing withdrawal symptoms from nicotine or other substance abuse.

The health professional whose adequate history-taking reveals a patient with undesirable health practices or situations who appears at illness risk will want to know what new treatments may work, what are appropriate referrals, how is adherence to remedial programs better to be secured? The conscientious professional will wish to examine how effectively he/she communicates so as to optimize his/her own role as health educator, to better reach immediate goals with respect to regimen cooperation/compliance, and for understanding and facilitating changes in health practices. One also recognizes that new emphasis on patient responsibility for self-care implies yet further changes in the doctor-patient relationship, in health care delivery, and in community standards for defining quality of medical care. Some caregivers with an interest in these issues will want to adopt facilitory professional behaviors in order to remain competitive in the health care market.

It is our intent here to provide an overview of major findings, and of related trends and issues, for the women's physician and to others treating or advising women in health matters. Our presentation, while thorough, cannot be complete, for the fields to be embraced are multiple, and the literature is "vast," as the Carnegie Foundation Subcommittee on Modification of Patient Behavior for Health Maintenance and Disease Control reported back in 1977. We seek to build a bridge between behavioral health and specialists in obstetrics-gynecology, and family and community medicine as well as between other physicians, nurse practitioners, midwives, psychologists, nurses, and educators responsible for important aspects of women's health. We offer practical suggestions so that the women's specialist can properly develop his or her interest in health maintenance so as to be more effective in facilitating better health practices. For the woman, enhanced "wellness" can thereby be achieved.[1]

Health Promotion: What Is It?

"Health promotion" describes at one level the intent of policy makers to inform the public about health issues, and initiate programs designed to reduce health risk conduct through increased citizen knowledge and responsibility. Examples of major policy implementation are the 1984 U.S. legislation establishing a new Office of Disease Prevention and Health Promotion in DHHS, the 1985 report from the Institute of Medicine (Science, 1985) recommending massive new funding for behavioral research (it notes that behavioral disorders are implicated in 50% of all morbidity and mortality), the United Kingdom's Health Education Council's 1983 recommendations for a "national strategy for health education and promotion" and the Canadian "Operation Lifestyle" (Lelonde 1976) which, at the provincial governmental level, passed seat belt laws, engaged industry in health education and sent to governmental family allowance recipients a self-health behavior test, the "lifestyle profile." Canadian data indicates that 18% of all deaths and 18% of all years of life lost prematurely are attributable to cigarette and alcohol use alone. Detels and Breslow (1984) accurately summarized such findings by stating that "the way people live largely determines their health."

An expert committee of the Institute of Medicine (1985) has called for increased governmental responsibility to reduce low birth weights (such babies are forty times more likely to die in the first weeks of life and constitute up to two-thirds of all newborn deaths). The recommendation proposed a new range of Medicaid or other insurance paid nontraditional preventive services to pregnant women, including psychosocial counseling and efforts to combat specific health risk behaviors. Somewhat improved reimbursement schemes followed in late 1985 when the American Cancer Society, in a commitment to cancer control through self-help, introduced a 10 step "Taking Control" public educational program, with five habits to be adopted and five, when present, to be curtailed.

At the level of implementation, health promotion involves several disciplines. Health educators seek better planned, executed and evaluated (usually more complex and long-lasting) educational programs. These now can report success, as opposed to the prior record in health education where, when looked at on a study by study basis, failure was usual. The work of Farquhar (1984) and his colleagues at Stanford on risk reduction for cardiovascular disease in the three and five community studies is notable; also conducted at Stanford was the in-school five year (successful and unsuccessful) illegal drugs - alcohol-tobacco reduction educational experiment (Blum et al. 1976, Blum et al. 1978).

Herd (1983) in offering a biobehavioral perspective on coronary arteriosclerosis describes the two major health promoting interventions with the greatest apparent success. In North Karelia, Finland, a government-supported community-wide program used mass media, health education, and service provision. While control counties also showed reductions, risk factors in the experimental county were markedly reduced such that the incidence rate of acute myocardial infarction among men fell by almost 17%, and women about 10%, and cerebrovascular accidents declined among women 35.5% and among men by almost 13% over the five year period. In the second study in Oslo, small groups rather than community wide methods were employed; here counseling and instruction were targetted on smoking and diet. Over five years risk factors decreased markedly with 45% of high risk men reducing smoking and 25% ceasing it altogether. By the end of the five year trial the incidence of myocardial infarction and sudden death was reduced 47% over that experienced by controls. Such growing knowledge about risk, better prediction, and such intervention models, whether community wide, group, individual, or combined, provide the best basis for the optimism underlying today's health promotional thrust.

Within communities, the workplace proves an exceptional setting for inducing conduct change, since incentives and disincentives can stringently be applied at the same time that group norms and supports are made available as resources and reinforcements. The work situation is one where emotional commitments of workers and self-esteem are components to be developed. Some of the first demonstrations of success came in required alcoholism counseling (see Blum and Blum, 1967). Now one sees workplace-provided programs for occupational safety, substance abuse control, stress management, exercise, weight control, type A behavior change, counseling for the accident prone, and more "upbeat," based on some data linking life satisfaction and felt personal efficacy with health levels, programs for creativity, educational growth, and life enhancement.

Within the community are voluntary structured groups (sometimes offered commercially as classes or "treatments") whose members face common life-style and the often associated personality and situational problems. These health promotion activities can involve education, task training and rewards, group support, the "buddy system," helpful social networks, the imposition of authoritative value systems and norms, member "contractual" commitments, new integrating personal perspectives, and group psychotherapeutic components. Alcoholics Anonymous is probably the oldest and best known of these. There are also involuntary programs, court imposed or part of probation, for driver safety, alcoholism, or illicit substance abuse.

Today one finds such groups organized as "support" or "self-help" groups (see Hamburg and Killilea, 1979) to address obesity, exercise, substance abuse, cigarette smoking, diabetes and other chronic disease care, PMS, infertility, post-mastectomy and post-abortion adjustment, physical handicap, sexual dysfunction, arthritis and many other difficulties. Groups are also organized for education and training in health habits, typically as classes in clinics or hospitals, for example antenatal preparation and breast self-examination, or in school, nutrition and meal planning, sexuality, driver and drug education or meditation/yoga for tension reduction. In some instances support and/or educational groups are part of industrial or neighborhood programs, or are community college or church adult education offerings.

Health promotion is also attentive to behavior other than that identified epidemiologically as a risk factor in the etiology or outcome prediction of either the major chronic life-style diseases typically studied, or of morbidity/mortality prevalence rates generally. The field concerns itself with conduct and with associated beliefs, thought processes and feelings, which are important features of self and family care. Individual decision making is one such area, coping with illness another, and compliance a third. For example, there are large numbers of people who may require medical care but do not seek it, even when it is readily available. Conversely, there is another large group, those "worried well" or "somatizers" who make visits that the physician and third party payers consider unnecessary. Can education improve the faulty decision making process (if and when that is the nub of it) and do so without adverse consequences? And for those "beyond" education, where social marginality or as yet undefined emotional distress contribute strongly to under or over utilization (respectively), can one mobilize correcting resources? For example, do under-utilizers gain easier access via new neighborhood medical or nutrition centers, or does instruction for self-care involvement via local, lay, home visitors make a difference? (Yes, it does.) Or, for "over-users," are they constructively influenced by care focusing on those human-problem or "concern" components which may underlie medical visits? (Again, yes.)

Mental health treatments are known (Budman 1984, Mumford, 1984) to reduce medical service over-utilization not simply for the "worried well" but for seriously ill patients too. And one expects that those women treated by counseling for gynecological illness and intervention-related depression are better able to be "in charge" of their family life and emotions. In both these instances the line is blurred between health promotion that is typically conceived as focusing on people as they live in the community, emphasizing health maintenance through responsible lifestyles, as opposed to the familiar medical model of specialist responsibility for recognition and treatment of disease, and for primary care itself. In health promotion, the methods are ordinarily those already noted, support-for-change groups, or classes to build skills or confidence (see Brown and Lewinsohn, 1984) or media campaigns coupled with community norm-setting, group activation and perhaps individual counseling as well.

Yet one finds that conventional treatment in the form of professional-patient (or client) interaction is also implicit in that health promotion which relies on behavioral medicine, or health psychology to change either bad habits or chronic problems, some of which are themselves health risk features. Biofeedback and relaxation methods are used, for example, in the treatment of hypertension. Presurgical psychological preparation is also useful to "innoculate" against adverse post-operative emotional responses, which, distressing in themselves, also delay recovery. And there are one-to-one, couple or group treatments for the so common sexual dysfunctions occurring de novo in women following reproductive organ surgery or x-ray therapy for malignant diseases. The successfully-treated, moderate hypertensive reduces her risk of hospitalization during pregnancy for eclampsia. A woman's depression associated with hysterectomy, despair upon selective abortion following genetic counseling, or colostomy, in themselves require attention as disabling, painful conditions that put the women at risk of social isolation and sexual dysfunction, both of which erode interpersonal intimacy and social resources which appear necessary for maintaining future overall good health status. The technical assurance of survival without also securing the patient's gladness that she is alive is professionally and humanely an inadequte achievement. Quality of life, and "wellness," must be simultaneous medical goals.

Whether or not health promotion and disease prevention should be considered part of "behavioral medicine" is a matter not yet resolved. Within behavioral medicine, Gentry (1984) would include all health and behavior-related work from sociology through pharmacy, from psychotherapy through dentistry, and research and practice that addresses etiology, host resistance, disease mechanisms (i.e., stress altered physiology), patient decision making, compliance, and health education and behavioral treatments as interventions at individual and community levels. Matarrazo (1984), on the other hand, following the new thrust on "wellness," prefers "behavioral health" as that interdisciplinary field stressing responsible, self-initiated individual or shared activities for health and well-being maintenance.

The Health Professional's Role

Implicit in the optimism of renewed interest in health promotion and on wellness is the expectation that it is readily possible for the physician, nurse, midwife, and others to enlarge their contributions to the woman's health status and felt well being. These contributions would not be radically new ventures in obstetrical-gynecological practice, but rather are an expansion of the normal goals of the women's physician and his or her patient. What is required, we believe, is an open perspective ready to take advantage of what has been recently learned, including, for example, in practice, how to achieve a more effective and, perhaps, less personally stressful interpersonal role for the physician than that offered by the traditional one-way communication approach. What is necessary generally is a willingness to be guided by that empirical evidence which demonstrates environmental-personal-biological interactions in the evolution of disease, in the somatic expression of distress, and in disease management. As Eisenberg (1984) has said, "all disease is psychosomatic in the sense that social and somatic forces enter into the genesis of clinical conditions."

Health education at the traditional level is still common in the old-fashioned way, as in making written or didactic classroom lecture information available in isolation, passively, without regard to the context of the life and resources of a possible reader, without the opportunity for interpersonal exchange and feedback as to the student's (or patient's) understanding of the material and in relation to his/her own health practices. Library shelves with home medical advisor texts thereon, office tables with pamphlets of advice, the bored hygiene teacher reciting her notes, or the physician's hurried words of instruction are examples. The endorsement of health promotion is hardly an advocacy for these tired approaches for which the efficacy judgment is pessimistic. Although cumulatively in concert with other sources and events, possibly there has been an effect; the reduction in cigarette smoking over expected rates of increase over the last decades may be an example (Warner, 1981). What is likely is that health education, when suitably intensive and multifaceted, and always aiming for audience (patient, consumer) active involvement will have long term possible effects (Green et al. 1980).

The current thrust suggested for office and clinic-based innovative, expanded efforts for cooperation in new kinds of adherence envisions the physician as comfortable and effective as a health educator. The physician is not seeking to impose adherence or change, but to facilitate conditions compatible with a patient's wishes for self-control and self-confidence which are directed to the patient's own understanding of the importance of responsibility for and the practice of self-help for self-health. This is an office version of the proposal for innovation in obstetrical hospitals in antenatal care offered by Parboosing and Kerr (1983). They consider the period of maternity contact as an "opportunity to consolidate a doctor's relationship with the family and to capitalize on a unique opportunity for health education." It is innovation which recognizes that given the dramatic decline in perinatal mortality/morbidity that "much of the residue of death and damage is less influenced by traditional obstetrical skills than by socioeconomic determinants." To this statement must be added, "and psychosomatic-behavioral determinants." We cannot find statistical evidence for Labarba's statement (1984) that, of present, perinatal mortality/morbidity, 75% can be attributed to environmental factors or agents (he includes drug use and biosocial status). Nevertheless, anyone responsive to the data on etiology of chronic disease and heretofore obstetrically "not avoidable" deaths (see Russell, 1983) is likely to come to the same conclusion that the business of the women's specialist includes the obligation to study and seek to influence these "external" variables.

Let us give a concrete example of the importance of one of these "external" factors, an example drawn from a developing country where one can compare a sanitation effort against change in a psychosocial variable. Brazil suffers a high rate of poverty and poor sanitation, both in turn related to the risk of neonatal and infant death. We cite Merrick (1983) to the effect that the probability of an infant dying by age of two ranges from 10% to 21% depending upon socioeconomic class (SEC), region, or urban vs. rural locale. Gastrointestinal disease reduces nutrient absorption up to 30% and risk of GI infection is associated with contaminated drinking water. Very poor maternal nutrition can also be associated with duration of breast feeding[2] and in Brazil breast feeding duration is short. Inadequate food preparation hygiene is also common.

It would be easy to assume that under these conditions the best single remedial step to be taken is the mainstay of public health sanitation, cleaning up the water supply, i.e., providing clean piped water. That is what happened over the period 1970-1976. But at the same time other social changes were also occurring, for example, expanding public education. Merrick examines the relative effects of these changes as a cause of the observed subsequent decline in neonatal infant mortality. Getting clean piped water to a residence accounted for 20% of the observed reduction in deaths. But improving the mother's education accounted for 34% of the reduction, independent of water supply change.

Historical Development

The clinical and scientific evolution of obstetrics and gynecology has played, and is playing, a central role in today's interest in promotion and prevention. Some of the very earliest observations, for example those of Galen on the role of emotion in predisposing to illness, and the most recent calls for expanded efforts toward prevention, focus on the health of women and babies and its relationship to environmental, psychosocial, and behavioral risk factors and their reduction. In the early development of modern medicine, for example, work on puerperal sepsis by John Leake (1772) first suggested environmental causal factors, with an evolving focus on contagion by Alexander Hamilton (1781), Alexander Gordon (1795), Oliver Wendell Holmes

(1855), Ignaz Semmelweis (1861) and Lister in 1867. The suggestion and then the confirmation that attendants of women were transmitting infection led to proposals for prevention, as Pritchard, MacDonald and Gant (1985) and Barron and Thomson (1983) in their history of obstetrical epidemiology note, much before bacterial infection per se was understood. Equally consequential, resistance among physicians to improved practice based on sound observation of contagion continued nevertheless, with subsequent unnecessary loss of life. This history serves to remind us of the resistance in practice to the implications of major discoveries, including those associated with psychosocial-behavioral influence on illness, and also that the astute clinician may be the one making great discoveries, as for example Oshner and Graham with their insight into the impact of cigarette smoking as a causal risk in cancer.

James Blondel in 1729 evidenced (See Oakley et al. (1982)) a quite modern obstetrical comprehension of the interrelationship among environmental events, maternal response and status, and fetal outcome. Blondel wrote, "The prosperity of the fetus does depend on the welfare of the mother . . . whatever is detrimental to her is directly, or indirectly, prejudicial to the other;" and, in understanding the negative role of stress, "Tis very necessary to gratify the longing of a pregnant woman, if it be possible and safe." The identification of factors in risk prediction to guide clinical strategies can be attributed to W.J. Little (see the Lancet, 1843-44) who not only observed that prenatal and perinatal events affected infant health status and developmental prospects, but that these latter could also be strongly affected by the kind of ensuing environmental (education) experiences.

The next signal development was with Ballentyne (see Oakley, 1982) who, in 1902, referring to antenatal care as a "new department of medicine," insisted on the need to understand the causes of maternal and fetal death, and associated physiology with preventive endeavors as the clinical focus. Then, in the early 1930's Munroe Kerr reported on the relationship of maternal mortality to occupation (socioeconomic class, or SEC), age, and parity. His work was followed by Baird in Aberdeen who, founding a group which brought epidemiology and social science systematically to obstetrics, concluded that psychosocial characteristics were contributing as much to morbidity — or its absence— as was medical care.

The 1985 report on Preventive Health Care in Obstetrics-Gynecology Training (ACOG 1985), sponsored by the Department of Health and Human Services brings one up-to-date with respect to recognition of the importance of preventive and educational interventions on the part of the physician engaged in women's health care - that in relationship to the expanding array of known external risk elements and within-patient and family emotional and behavioral factors. The report reminds us of the kinds of doctor-patient contacts or shared objectives which are, or should be, focused on prevention and promotion strategies for women, as for example those identified by the Surgeon General's report, Healthy People (1979), which are for family planning, pregnancy and infant health, immunization, sexually transmitted diseases, smoking and health, misuse of alcohol and drugs, nutrition, and physical fitness and exercise. The women's health specialist is also concerned with other priority areas identified by the Surgeon General, for example the detection and control of high blood pressure, toxic agent control and education—crucial for teratogenic prevention in pregnancy, occupational health, accident prevention education, fluoridation education (emphasized in pregnancy), education for the control of infectious diseases, and stress coping techniques.

The ACOG report, drawing from the USPHS National Ambulatory Medical Care Survey (1980-81), observes that about 62% of all office visits to ob-gyn specialists are for "non illness" care (diagnosis, screening, prevention). For three-fourths of women, such office visits include a request for another appointment, i.e., repeat visits—the implication of which is that a continuing doctor-patient relationship is implicit in the ordinary practice of women's medicine. The report, citing unpublished practice studies by Mendenhall (1977, 1981), observes that over one-fourth of all doctor-patient encounters include counseling and education, while almost one-fifth of all gynecological visits are specifically focused on prevention. These figures are to be compared with a 9% preventive focus rate for encounters in internal medicine, family/general practice, and general surgery. The implication is clear that much of the care of women occurs in a continuing relationship where wellness, prevention, safety, are central matters.

It is unlikely that anyone engaged in the health care of women would disagree - not with Blondel in 1729, Ballentyne in 1902 or ACOG in 1985. But agreeing to and trying to engage in health promotion/

disease prevention, and doing well as judged by the current state of the art based on available knowledge and resources are not the same. As women themselves, and ACOG also tells us, there is much progress in individual practice yet to be made. In later chapters we discuss the discrepancies which exist between how women and their physicians perceive what has transpired between them by way of information exchange, or understanding as such, including the counseling women desire but may fear to request and do not receive. ACOG, for example, reports findings of a physician administered survey of patient attitude (a method fraught with methodological pitfalls) showing that while overall care satisfaction was reportedly high, 44% of women indicated their information needs are not adequately being met.

The ACOG residency training report attends to a major source of inadequacy; physicians in training do not receive sufficient education or institutional experience and support. Consider that:

> "Formal education in preventative medicine was either absent from the resident's past, or described as ineffectual when it existed" (p72) (Residents) seldom volunteered the usefulness of patient contacts to support . . . general health maintenance (p73)
> There was distinctly less interest and evident ability . . . in the management of symptoms of emotional origin, in social problems as they impact on symptom generation and medical treatment, and on issues of diet and nutrition. Few . . . adopt a position appropriate to primary health care for women, preferring to refer . . ." (p73)

Given a short list of health maintenance behaviors, less than half of the residents being assessed (a small sample drawn from five settings) considered as important to health the following: excessive alcohol use, annual health or periodic screening examinations, adequate sleep, stress avoidance or automobile seat belt use. Not even for smoking, exercise, weight control or diet, were all of the residents convinced that these were important to health maintenance. And, when it came to spontaneous mention of behaviors consequential for health, in assessment discussions held with the visiting faculty study team, with respect to obesity, drug use, smoking or poor diet observed in patients, residents "rarely" suggested that patient self-control efforts were desirable. In regard to levels of information, residents proved relatively well informed about contraception management and drugs affecting pregnancy, but poorly informed on psychological and behavioral risk factors affecting maternal mortality (including those set forth in patient records as clinical variables), or on demographic-cultural factors affecting reproduction and family planning effectiveness. Evident was the lack of structured teaching within the training centers, sometimes the absence of faculty there with interests in prevention, and in some cases institutional pressures so great with "a crushing patient load," that there was no chance at all for working toward long-term health goals. Also found absent in training was instruction and experience in primary care of the sort which would encourage much that is valuable, as for example continuity of care, ready availability of care, attention to the family as well as to the patient, and broad interests across the range of medical specialties. Such inadequacies in training and institutional interest illustrate Tilson's (1984) conclusion, after a broad review of preventive medical and public health efforts, to the effect that, "One of the great barriers to establishing programs directed...at health promotion has been the world-wide failure of such efforts to gain the support of physicians...." (p. 162)

Given these current medical educational deficiencies in orientation, knowledge, teaching, institutional support, and the opportunity for those who are to become women's health specialists, one must infer that the natural evolution of women's health care, for all of its great historical achievements and current standards, is not a smooth developmental course. At the very least, care-givers must be assured encouragement and training for health promotion. Insofar as these are known to be lacking, one acknowledges an insufficient current competence among practitioners, and widespread felt needs among women for more sensitive professional assistance in those self care matters involving emotions, knowledge, life styles and habits, problems in living,[3] and environmental contexts.

It is no doubt the case, as the Scientific Council of the American Medical Association (1983) concluded, "Physicians need to improve their skills in fostering patients' good health and in dealing with long recognized problems such as hypertension, obesity, anxiety, and depression, as well as the excessive use of alcohol,[4] tobacco and drugs" this as part of instruction to patients "about healthful living." Reports such as that of the AMA Council are, of course, part of the thrust toward health promotion in medicine, just as is the ACOG evaluation of physician training which, after concluding that residents "do not understand broader principles of prevention or the . . . concepts of preventive health care" proposes that "it is necessary for the specialty to clarify its concern and responsibilities for prevention . . . that "undergraduate and particularly graduate medical education need to be changed to reflect the realities of present and future practice," that "reimbursement plans should reflect the importance of preventive care" and, that "demonstration projects in women's preventive care are important." (p.3)

What is happening today? Health promotion/disease prevention as a psychobiological effort is but an extension of historical progress and awareness in medicine, including awareness of deficiencies in knowledge, training, and practice. It is apparent that both awareness and deficiency exist within specialties such as obstetrics-gynecology, and in medicine generally, as noted in the AMA report. The psychobiological thrust necessary for preventive medicine as such, and for adequate care as an embracing value, applies to primary care physicians with women patients, typically family and community practitioners, internists, general surgeons, and to obstetricians-gynecologists. It also applies to other specialists as well, for as we will see in later chapters, the well-being of the cancer patient, for example, is very much dependent upon the oncologist's sensitivity and sophistication in matters psychobiological, in promoting well being as well as survival.

We believe that neither the generalist nor the specialist in medicine, nor the allied practicing professions such as nursing, health psychology, or midwifery, would disdain, knowingly, the major tasks of disease prevention and enhanced well being, for, and shared responsibility with the women. Be that so, the physician and allied care-givers are already committed to the perspective and practice of health promotion.

FOOTNOTES

1. For reviews, programs, handbooks see: *Stress, Health and Social Environment: Psychobiological Approaches to Medicine*, Henry, J.P. and Stephans, P.M. (1977), The Surgeon General's Report, *Healthy People* (1979); Hamburg, D.A. Elliot, G.R., and Parson, D., *Health and Behavior Frontiers of Research in the Behavioral Sciences*, National Institute of Medicine; Taylor, R.B., Ureda, J.R. and Denham J.W. *Health Promotion: Principles and Clinical Applications*, 1982, Matarazzo, J.D. *Behavioral Health: A Handbook of Health Enhancement and*

Disease Prevention, 1984; Gentry W.D. *Handbook of Behavioral Medicine*; (1984) Stone G.C., Cohen, F. and Adler, N., *Health Psychology* (1982). P.H.S. Task Force, *Women's Health* 1985. For short seminal articles overview; see Knowles, J.H., (1977) "Doing better and feeling worse: Health in the United States", Cassell, J. (1976), "The contribution of the social environment to host resistance," and Eisenberg, L. (1984) "The ambiguities of psychosomatic medicine."

2. A nutrition and antibody effect, but possibly also a body contact cerebellar-mediated stress and mirasmus buffering variable.

3. The inadequacy of obstetrics-gynecology residents' training, interests, and skills serves as an illustration of widespread deficiencies in the attention and skills of those in the health professions when facing behavior with potentially dire health consequences. Take alcoholism, certainly an important risk factor in obstetrics and, according to a 1985 report (The Neglected Disease in Medical Education, *Science*, 229, 741-742), the third leading cause of death in the U.S. ("Cause" here implies a necessary but also "perhaps" not sufficient role in the context and etiological chain of events, since death certificates will read across a range of entities from vehicular or industrial accidents through homicide to cardiovascular incidents to cirrhosis). It is a condition consuming 15% of all health care dollars, and one implicated in 20% of general hospital admissions (up to 50% of admissions to all types of hospitals including psychiatric). Estimates are that alcoholism is diagnosed in less than 5% of all cases where it is present. Obviously diagnostic acumen, beginning with case history adequacy, is absent and, further, so is physicians' treatment confidence—for even though improvement and/or recovery rates run from 60% to 95%, only 27% of physicians polled stated they felt competent in treatment. Indeed that confidence is likely misplaced and overstated since overall curriculum time devoted to substance abuse—including alcoholism—in medical schools is less than 1% (*Science* cites a study by Pokorny 1976 through 1981). About one quarter of all schools offer no education for treatment at all.

4. Ibid.

2

Converging Trends: The New (Re)emphasis

In this chapter we will describe other developments which, converging, account for the current thrust for health promotion and related disease prevention, or as is sometimes said, toward "wellness," to which the work of the women's health professional is joined.

U.S. Federal Initiatives

The commitment of the woman's physician to preventive medicine as such is consistent with the longstanding national commitment to public health as such. McGinnis (1985) in a brief history of the Federal role in prevention notes that in 1796, Congress authorized President George Washington to establish a quarantine system. In 1798 an act was passed creating the Marine Hospital Service which was the predecessor to the U.S. Public Health Service. In 1930 the National Institutes for Health were created. In 1958, a U.S. Public Health Service group set to work in prospective medicine as an approach to primary care medical practice (see Robbins and Blankerbaker, 1982). McGinnis attributes the recent preventive initiatives to work such as the 1964 Surgeon General's report on smoking and health, the 1971 President's Committee on Health Education, the 1973 Health Maintenance Organization (HMO) Act mandating Federally certified HMO's to have preventive and educational services, the 1976 HEW Forward Plan for Health, and in 1977, the establishment of an HEW Task Force on Disease Prevention and Health Promotion. In 1977-79 the childhood immunization initiative occurred with a target of 90% immunized for childhood vaccine-preventable diseases. Ninety-five percent are now adequately immunized. The next stage, the Surgeon General's Report, Healthy People (1979) is part and the origin of much that is being done today. As goals for 1990 the Report calls for, among others, a 35% reduction in infant mortality and a 25% reduction in deaths for adults.

Work In Psychobiology

A dramatic recent expansion has occurred in the field of psychobiology which investigates person-environmental interactions and identifies and describes responding and mediating internal pathways and effects. Begin with Galen, the preeminent philosopher-physician who, Greer and Morris (1975) remind us, observed that cancer occurred more often in melancholic than in sanguine women. His were the first medical observations linking mood and temperament to disease etiology. Guy in 1759 proposed that depression and life stress were factors in cancer etiology. Work exploring the possibility of such relationships continues today (Riley et al. 1981, Anisman and Sklar 1984).

Henry and Stephens (1977) in their presentation of research, and evolving theory based on animal laboratory, field primate, anthropological, epidemiological, and experimental studies in humans, employ the concept of a "biogrammar" (citing Tiger and Fox) as well as their own "cultural canon" compatible with Jung's work. They trace the work of Cannon on stress and Seyle on distress and note that Donnison in 1938, comparing the absence of hypertension in his local African patients with blood pressure readings in urban Europe, conceptualized chronic disease as a response to stressful environments. Page (1949) is credited with the appreciation of the role of the brain as a regulatory center in hypertension as the classic psychosomatic case demonstration of the mosaic multifactorial disease process occurring over a long period of time. The work was continued by Kurtsin, Weiner, and now many others. Henry and Stephens discuss Halliday's psychosomatic concerns. His observation that peptic ulcer, hypertension, diabetes, and heart disease are affected by the milieu and changes in that, and by emotional factors arising from personal, social, and work situations. Evidence for environmental psychophysiological effects was being put forward in the United Kingdom when Baird in obstetrics, and Morris (1957) in epidemiology were addressing closely related matters.

At the same time, Harold Wolff in the US, was making his great contributions to the direct study of emotionally induced stress on migraine, asthma exacerbation and gastric secretions and hyperremia. In his work he was joined by Stewart Wolf and that partnership produced seminal books on headache, gastric function and pain. Wolf and Goodell in turn wrote about Harold's work, and further investigated stress and disease. Much later, they wrote on how to integrate behavioral science data and perspective with clinical medicine. Hinkle, a Wolff associate, moved such work from the laboratory to natural groups. By studying large numbers of employees, he showed relationships between personality as a mediator of work and other life situations which could be stressful, and illness risk. Hinkle was also able to show how the perception of the situation as an attitudinal feature of personality (or as susceptibility or stress vulnerability) operates to affect health. Hinkle, so Henry and Stephens remind us, also gave attention to personality-perception variables as discrete, i.e., while many people might respond to bereavement, isolation, and other extreme human loss as devastating life events with implicit illness stress risk, some individuals are inured to loss. This was the same period, the 1950s, in which for psychology, the role of learning and personality structure as influences on perception, and perception itself as a way of understanding environmental reactions, was becoming a dominant topic. At the same time, the psychophysiological research given impetus by John Lacey led to discrimination among quite specific response patterns. That was fundamental to work today seeking to identify high versus low risk ways of responding to stressors, as in the development of hypertension, tumors, or gastrointestinal pathology.

We will find that the present work on which health promotion is based and the research to which it leads ranges from neuroendocrinologically measured, differentiated stress patterns to quite broad social and ethical issues. We shall encounter a number of specific variables, and broader psychosocial constructs as items identified in obstetrical risk, gynecological disease, pain, symptom levels and diagnosed morbidity or recorded mortality. This monograph, however, does not address the chain of events from inherited behavioral patterns, critical early experience and behavior programming, role of the neocortex and limbic system, or neuroendocrine responses to social interaction to disease triggerings. For that schema refer initially to Henry and Stephens (1977).

The field is in a transitional period. Given a multiplicity of findings and considerable debate about the replicability of many of them. Gynecology and obstetrics do not yet enjoy sufficient data to allow formulation of a satisfying consistent, integrating, psychobiological etiological theory. There exists, however, a series of integrating conceptions for subsets of data, for example, how social support and belongingness, personality assets and perceived control may be protective. Conversely, one can understand how socially disorganized, resource limited poor coping and learning styles, and personality deficient conditions may exacerbate risk. Selye's concept of imposed and experienced stress as altering risk, either in facilitating adaption (psychologically and physiologically), or producing maladaptive responses which with repetition can become pathogenic and then disease, is central. The regulatory model of the brain as an information processing, subsystem moderating, feedback dependent integrator whose competence depends on functional intactness and which in fact may itself be seen as *the* health maintenance system (see Schwartz, 1979) is useful as well.

Contributions from sub-disciplines in psychology have been considerable as evidenced by the wide use of terms such as "behavioral medicine" and "health psychology" as rubrics for the field. To this latter field, Feuerstein, Labbe, and Kuczmierczyk (1985) offer a thorough introduction and overview. "Behavioral" psychology, while generating optimism about improved capabilities for teaching by manipulation of rewards and punishments to shape behavior, and through feedback, provides an important but insufficient history to account for today's health promotion efforts. Nevertheless, optimism about health maintenance and disease/distress coping is central to health promotion and behavioral medicine.

Changes In Population Health Status

There have been dramatic changes in health status of the U.S. population with respect to the major causes of death, and subsequent life expectancies. (See Table I).

Table I[1]
The Ten Leading Causes of Death in the United States: 1900-1980*

	1900	1940	1980
Pneumonia and Influenza	1	5	6
Tuberculosis (all forms)	2	7	-
Diarrhea, Enteritis & Ulceration of the Intestines	3	-	-
Diseases of the Heart	4	1	1
Intracranial Lesions of Vascular Origin	5	3	-
Nephritis (all forms)	6	4	-
All Accidents**	7	6	4
Cancer***	8	2	2
Diphtheria	10	-	-
Diabetes Mellitus	-	8	7
Motor Vehicle Accidents	-	9	-
Premature Birth	-	10	-
Cardiovascular Diseases	-	-	3
Chronic Obstructive Pulmonary Diseases	-	-	5
Cirrhosis of the Liver	-	-	8
Atherosclerosis	-	-	9
Suicide	-	-	10

Consider that life expectancy in ancient Greece (Angel 1954) in 1200 BC was about 36 years, in 400 BC about 41, in the U.S. in 1900 47 years, in 1950 68 years, in 1977 73 years and in 1977 for someone already age 65, it was 80 years. As Berkman and Breslow (1983) comment, these changes represent "one of the most spectacular health advances in the history of humanity." It has been a result primarily of reduction in infant mortality, and communicable disease affecting children. In Japan where life expectancy at birth for women is 80, diet also plays an eminent role.

Increasing in prevalence in the U.S. since 1900 have been lung cancer, drug and alcohol addition, vehicular deaths and cardiovascular disease and for youth, violent deaths (Surgeon General's Report, 1979). By 1965, mortality for some of these was improving in the U.S. as, for example, a coronary heart disease (CHD) mortality drop, 1965-79, or 30%. This is not the case in the United Kingdom where upward trends for CHD prevail. Among older adults, mortality today is primarily attributable to cancer, diabetes, coronary heart disease, and among youth, vehicular accidents, violence and suicide (Berkman and Breslow, 1983, citing Erhardt and Berlin).

These national figures should not obscure our awareness of widespread geographical, age, race or sex differences. In some counties, homicide will be the leading cause of death for young men. In some cities, acquired immune defiency (AIDS) as in 1985, is the leading cause of death among all males age 21-40. Death certificates may read cancer or pneumonia, just as with a heroin addict the certificate may read bacterial endocarditis. These conventions, or delicacies, remind us that "causes" of death listed in tables are conventions, sometimes arbitrary choices from among the available mass of pathology. For the purposes of health promotion the research question is whether or not the risk of dying from this particular, or general class of processes, depended upon the behavior of the person, or his or her psychosocial attributes. The public health and clinical question, the immediately practical one, is whether or not interventions— at a mass or individual level— are known and proven which could reduce the risk. The public policy economic question is whether the interventions produce enough greater well days to be justified public, industrial, or insurance program expenditures. The citizen's question is whether or not the risk derived from behavior, setting, or trait is consequential enough to matter in terms of quality of life and longevity.

One can follow the wisdom of Paykel (1978) in discriminating among "relative risk"— the chances of developing morbid or mortal outcome among those exposed to X or doing Y or being Z as opposed to those absent risks X, Y, or Z, "attributable risk" which is, statistically, how much of the occurrence (variance) of a multidetermined disorder can be laid on the doorstep of a particular risk factor present be it X or Y or Z, versus "brought forward time" which is, if the calculation is possible, how much faster one would experience onset of, or death from that disorder which is in any event in the cards or in process. "Consequential" for the citizen means the question— is the increased probability great enough to persuade one to take the trouble to change? For an excellent discussion, with tables for age groups and risk calculation data for individuals, see the work of Robbins and Blankenbaker (1982) on "prospective medicine."

The Surgeon General's 1979 report, and the report of the National Institute of Medicine propose that half the mortality from the ten leading causes of death is attributable to unhealthy life styles, including health practices. The Surgeon General's two volumes identify as areas for disease prevention and health promotion: infant and child health, injuries, dental care and periodontal disease, mental disorders, cancer, cardiovascular and coronary heart disease, tobacco-alcohol- other drug abuse, and more generally, improving workplace environments, and reducing the functional dependence of the elderly. Hamburg (1982), summarizing major risk factors, identifies cigarette smoking, excessive alcohol intake, substance abuse, adverse dietary habits, sedentary living, reckless driving, non-compliance in medication regimens, and maladaptive social pressure responses as targets. Health and Human Services secretary Harris, in 1980, set forth fifteen measurable objectives for better health by 1990: (a) As preventive health services, control of high blood pressure, family planning, pregnancy and infant health, sexually transmitted diseases. (b) As health protection, control of toxic agents, occcupational safety and health, accident prevention and injury control,[2] fluoridation and dental health, surveillance and control of infectious diseases. (c) As health promotion, smoking, misuse of alcohol and drugs, nutrition, physical fitness and exercise, control of stress and violent behavior.

The contribution of daily living risks to chances of dying vary immensely by type of practice. Hatcher et al. (1986), presenting data developed by Cates and others, illustrates that while a cigarette smoker's relative death risk in one year is 1/200, a motorcyclist's is 1/1000, a non-legal abortion is 1/3000, a non-smoking oral contraceptive user's is 1/63,000. Such risk statistics may guide money allocations to public policy for prevention, whereas for the clinician any reducible risk will be worth presenting to patients as a realm for awareness in decision-making and possible change.

There is overlap among the categories in the Federal reports, and a considerable range with regard to specificity or generality. Regardless of that, one sees that the women's specialist in ordinary practice is concerned with most of these areas, and as health specialist, is clinically responsible for primary work in several of them. What the women's physician now needs is more specific information as to particular items that are possible, and sometimes common and powerful influences on obstetrical and maternal conduct, reproductive disease and behavior, that lack of wellness which is brought to the physician's attention as organically unsubstantiated symptomatology, fatigue, pain, or as complaints about sexuality, and sometimes, as problems in living. What the physician also needs are specific suggestions to be applied to practice or, if he or she is interested in research, suggestions as to some of the interesting problems to pursue. In this monograph we begin to address these needs. We must say, however, that not only is the psychosocial, biobehavioral context of reproductive conduct, feeling, and illness more complex than may first be appreciated by newcomers, but that the optimism for quick effectiveness via those preventive, protecting, or health promoting efforts advocated may be misplaced. We suspect events here will be like those characterizing other developments in our field: a few remarkable interventions discovered and capable of dramatic effects, a few early heralded methods which, upon application, will prove at least too costly if not sometimes disastrous, and for the rest, reasonable rather than exponential progress.

Rising Costs For Illness Care

There are economic pressures to contain ever-inflating professional-institutional illness and care costs. President Rogers of the Robert Wood Johnson Foundation forecasts that by 1990 health care costs could account for up to 14% of the gross national product. In 1984 it was 10% (Matarazzo, 1984, citing Waldo). These arise at least in part from (a) a larger population living longer but experiencing a variety of illness conditions including serious chronic ailments, (b) high public expectations of greater freedom from pain, illness and disability, (c) the growth of medical knowledge and technology with associated higher costs, (d) a tendency to use new expensive technology or to advocate surgery (e.g., microsurgery of fallopian tubes and coronary artery bypass surgery) even when efficacy for many cases operated is not demonstrated (see Chard and Richards, 1977) (Cyr et al., 1984) and (e) the presence of profit motivation, expansion of activities for their own sake, and management inefficiencies in the health services, including among materials suppliers, administrators, insurers, regulators, and providers. Overuse by "worried well" insured patients is also a kind of inefficiency. Insofar as health promotion is seen as restraining costs by preventing illness, programs will be supported on cost effectiveness grounds. Insurers, whether of personal health or automobile liability, are now rewarding the nonabuser with lower premium costs.

Several components in the public reaction, mediated legislatively, may be recognized. There is the rising visible prevalence of illnesses and injuries where individual behavior plays a strong role in causation, and the public knows it. Such behaviors include cigarette smoking, alcoholism, heroin injection, careless exposure to sexually transmitted diseases, failure to use seat belts, and unplanned pregnancies among those not equipped to be responsible parents (the same group at high risk of obstetrical complications with subsequent more expensive care). Another component is the felt burden of taxation with increasingly restricted national growth in disposable income. Taxpayers hurt. A third component is the shift over the last half century from individual payments for own family health care to either insurance (including employer) or government, i.e., third party payers. Whether paying an insurance premium or a tax bill, the working taxpayer can recognize that he is paying for the treatment of others whose conduct, seen as avoidable through being responsible, brought on the illness, injury, or welfare pregnancy.

Knowles in 1977 spoke of the public duty, a "moral obligation" to preserve one's own health insofar as one could. Matarazzo (1984) is one who has pointed out that this "irresponsibility," when paid for by those who at least see themselves as more responsible, can generate the public demand for health responsibility as public duty. A health matter is becoming a moral, public policy, and indeed "criminal" issue as states pass laws requiring motorcyclists to wear helmets, passengers to wear seat belts, employers to provide safe workplaces, manufacturers to prevent toxic exposures, drinkers to avoid driving or smokers not to smoke in enclosed public places. Another set of costs is not directly medical but associated with the inability of the ill to work—thus increasing social support payment requirements and reducing contributions to the state from taxable income. The 1985 Report of the Board on Mental Health and Behavioral Medicine, of the Institute of Medicine notes that "More that one third of the Americans who report that they are unable to pursue their major activity because of poor health attibute their disability to hypertension, heart condition, or diabetes—all of which have heavy behavioral components."

Other economic forces arise from institutional responses to cost control efforts by Federal and private insurers, or by health care corporations whose members are simultaneously their patients and insured clients. An example are those in health maintenance organizations (HMO) or other comprehensive health care plans where payment is by advance premium (capitation). It is certainly to the advantage of an HMO receiving a set fee from employers, patients, or both, to minimize the costs of care provided. Disease as well as over utilization are enemies of cost containment for non profit and for-profit institutions being prepaid. In the same way, preferred provider organization (PPOs) plans and those being paid under Federal diagnosis-related fixed pay schemes (DRG) have incentives to reduce higher costs associated with severity and duration of acute or chronically disabling illnesses. To the extent that illness incidence, severity, duration, disability, or complications can be moderated by less costly services rendered by way of preventive schemes or early intervention, and the the extent health promotion is viewed as such an approach, that promotion will be endorsed.

The reader is referred to the timely discussion by Eisenberg (1986) with regard to the risks of the profit motive to ethical scientific and community obligations. Insofar as programs of health promotion may be substituted for, or provide an institutional excuse for delaying access to needed care, the cost-containment motive for preventive efforts must be examined critically.

One must recognize further complexities here. For example, where competition among capitation provides for the healthiest patients, defined in terms of statistical risk, there may be incentive to humor the "worried well" whose frequent but inexpensive-to-render office visit may be seen as necessary for their retention in a program. Similarly the struggling practitioner in a highly competitive area may not have an incentive to reduce services to his or her patients, and so may be less than enthusiastic about that health promotion perceived, over optimistically, as thoroughly effective.

Early Findings From Cigarette Smoking Studies

Epidemiological studies implicating cigarettes in lung cancer were the first in general medicine dramatically to call attention to potentially self-controllable behavior as capable of improving health. Robbins and Blankenbaker (1982) remind us that the surgeons, Ochsner and Graham, concerned about epidemic lung cancer in the 1930s, found in retrospective analysis, a preponderance of smokers among their lung disease cases. This prompted prospective studies reported in the mid 1950s by Hammond and Horn in the U.S. and Doll and Hill in the United Kingdom. These showed that smokers were at ten times greater risk of lung cancer than non-smokers. Such findings became part of initiatives in medicine, for example, by the American Academy of General Practice which argued the need for primary care physicians who could concern themselves with such non-specialty concerns as general health conduct. These findings in turn contributed to Federal initiatives earlier discussed.

Individual Health Attitudes Are Responsive

Health promotion, or something working along with it, is having an effect. Matarazzo (1984) reviews opinion poll data showing that Americans do recognize a number of the environmental-behavioral items which are threats to health, and further, that 60% believe the individual must work actively at being healthy, with about half also seeing themselves as able to be in charge (to have control over) their future health. Nationwide, a very important, worrisome, one person in ten, however, believes that he or she has no control at all over his/her health.

There are efforts to change lifestyles. One sees smoking reduction, weight and cholesterol control, jogging and health club growth and the like. But such efforts can be difficult and for some perhaps impossible without assistance. Yet Matarazzo cites survey data showing that in 1978 at least, the majority of city dwellers were not aware of important locally available programs and resources. The women's health professional must educate himself or herself so as to be able to impart to patients information on trustworthy local resources.

Combatting Toxins And Poverty Is Expensive

There are economic pressures, felt alike by taxpayers and their representatives, to restrain costs associated with efforts to correct social conditions and environmental hazards even though those are shown to be associated with, and sometimes causal for, morbidity/mortality risk. Most notable costs have been incurred in efforts to overcome poverty and its associated disadvantages, for of all of the gross factors (categories) predictive of general morbidity/mortality, low socio-economic status (SEC) (which correlates with education, work, physique, neighborhood, knowledge) is one of the most abiding. There is an interrelationship here with public health cost control efforts, for tax paid programs to assure access to nutrition, sanitation, prenatal prevention, medical care and rehabilitation are directed primarily to the poor. Yet there are other expensive programs such as those to clean up toxic wastes, and reduce other environmental exposure to carcinogens or other pathogens (asbestos, PCBs, etc.). The preventive part of this effort also imposes regulatory costs as well as derived higher passed-on consumer costs arising from industry conformity to regulation. An analogue is the cost of FDA control of pharmaceuticals. Regulatory policy is here blurred since most household/industrial chemicals may not be thoroughly screened for pathogenicity or teratogenicity arising from non-ingestive exposure (see Mehlman et al., 1978, Hayes et al., 1984), nor are health foods or bottled waters always monitored for their possible dangers. In any event, there can be an appeal in focusing low-cost health promotion efforts on individuals, as opposed to high cost clean up, environmental quality control, and related research and regulation. Perhaps it is part of the political movement to private sector responsibility, i.e., as an individual rather than community responsibility and burden. Eisenberg (1984) has, however, warned against substituting exhortation to individuals for the needed regulatory intervention by government to reduce environmental risks.

Is It Victim Blaming?

In a related vein, where the political and ideological implications are strong, those advocating health promotion can be accused of "victim blaming." The term implies not only the presumed inability of those most at risk of illness to change themselves—those who are nevertheless asked to do just that—but also that health promotional ideology represents a self-interested effort to shift responsibility and costs from the well, wise, and wealthy to the poor, puzzled, and pathological. These critics, and they include many in community medicine and public health, are aware of the powerful adverse effects of poverty and marginality on health but also they claim similar detrimental effects on self-help competence and confidence. They also have in mind the prior failures of health education, the continuing results of which are with us in current rates for lung disease, STD, drug use, vehicular accidents, alcoholism, death by violence, and unwanted pregnancies.

There are several kinds of data which might throw a light on at least the empirical side of the dispute. To what extent is health behavior, incompetence, and paralyzing hopelessness/helplessness more prevalent in lowest income classes, and beyond remedy at the individual level? A related question is to what extent is membership in the disadvantaged frozen? In the U.S., studies on class mobility indicate that over decades, while some number of people always stay below the poverty line, membership in that group is quite fluid. Although one in four American lived in a family that received some welfare source income once or more over 10 years, only 8% of all those recipients were dependent on welfare for more than 7 years out of 10 (Duncan, 1984). In the U.S. at least it is most of the poor who get richer and some of the rich who get poorer. In the U.K. there is also class mobility. As Illsley (1983) has shown, the poorest class has been getting smaller and contributing less, however consistently disproportionate, to total morbidity/ mortality in obstetrics. Its membership and reproductive disadvantage are not frozen by class boundary impermeability but instead continued by selective recruitment through marriage where the less healthy and less apt marry one another. With the rise of class-linked unmarried motherhood, especially in the U.S., lower class perpetuation may no longer require marriage to transmit selective disadvantage.

There is another side of "victim blaming" which touches deeply on the emotions of the seriously ill and those close to them. It may affect what researchers feel they dare do, and how they present their findings. Poignant examples derive from the increasingly widespread reports that personality features may be associated with cancer risk. Consider the plight of the women with breast cancer, surely devastating enough by way of fear for life and abhorrence of mutilation should there have been radical mastectomy, when she reads in the popular magazines that emotional repression is suspected, via immune suppression processes, to be etiological. She stands charged by herself and her family with a personal defect, however mutedly "objective" the trait characterization may be written. The victim is to blame. Another case of widespread blame is heard with respect to acquired immune deficiency syndrome (AIDS) victims. "The sin of homosexuality," say the healthy righteousness, when the victim is "being punished by God."

The essayist Susan Sontag (1979) argues that our society views the cancer victim as a pariah, "morally contagious." Research workers who claim, as wrongly today she believes as were earlier observers who characterized tuberculosis as arising from character, make the tragedy worse for the patient. "... there is mostly shame attached to a disease thought to stem from repression of emotion ..." (p. 46), and "The cancer personality is regarded...with condescension...as one of life's losers" (p. 48) and, "Psychological theories of illness are a powerful means of placing the blame on the ill. Patients who are instructed that they have, unwittingly, caused their disease are also being made to feel that they have deserved it" (pp. 55-56). Sontag indicts most of that which constitutes either psychosomatic theory or health promotion efforts. She writes, "Theories that diseases are caused by mental states and can be cured by will power are always an index of how much is not understood about the physical terrain of a disease...psychologizing seems to provide control over the experiences and events...over which people have in fact little or no control...(it is) sublimated spiritualism...affirming the primacy of 'spirit' over matter." She goes on to say, "The promise of a temporary triumph over death is implicit in much of the psychological thinking..." (pp. 54-55). She insists instead upon single cause theories for all illness, arguing that a multi cause theory of disease is only a metaphor for its being mysterious, that is, being not at all understood. Current views of cancer are, according to Sontag, metaphors for a paranoid, fearful view of malignant energies in the cosmos, of demonical possession, or corruption in society and mismanagement of the environment. The metaphor is, she believes, in the service of antagonism to the urban world and an expression of a philosophical-political premise, a false one, that disease arises from imbalance in nature, in society, in persons. She does not deny that imbalance, i.e., human dissatisfaction and failure, but contends that it is wrong. To have illness stand for something it is not is to damage its victims, she says, and to fail to address the economic and political defects which give rise to the metaphor. Sontag offers some of the most vociferous criticisms of health promotion as a concept. Certainly the disrepute into which earlier subjective psychodynamic characterizations of psychosomatic illness sufferers fell reinforces her position whereas the cancer of work has today yielded only tentative personality findings. Furthermore, the disease group which Sontag primarily considers for her diatribe, cancer, does not yet show benefits from health promoting efforts which are part of the multicausality theory of risk which she, we believe gravely erroneously, denounces. With all the effort against smoking, toxins, pollutants, and for screening and in new treatments, the age adjusted cancer rates in the U.S. are higher now than 20 years ago (1962 at 170.2/100,000 prevalence and in 1982 at 185/100,000).

Brandt (1985) considers the recent history of venereal disease and affirms not simply widespread victim blaming but argues that as a corollary medical control has been adversely affected, since medicine is embedded in society's values. He quotes from Time Magazine derogatory characterizations of herpes sufferers said to be (one presumes on the basis of someone's research) excessively angry, promiscuous hedonists. Like Sontag, Brandt sees illness—here VD in the U.S.—as a symbol for a corrupted, polluted society. As long as there is moral satisfaction that VD exists as a revenge against promiscuity, and thereby reducing it, efforts at its medical control are said to be diminished as an implicit moral policy. In spite of the general success of medicine to control infectious disease, STD has not been targetted (herpes, AIDS are changing that in fact), and are growing in prevalence and kind. Brandt argues that it is the thrust of American medicine to emphasize individual responsibility, trying to change behavior, that in contrast to assigning responsibility to social and external forces not under individual control. He deems this effort a failure, and appears to call for at least a diversified model relying much more heavily on infectious disease single vector vaccine only or by-quarantine control.

For Brandt then, health promotion is a dominant motif which has failed. He would, it seems, return to Ehrlich, Flemmings, and microbial models. As for the current thrust on probability in multiple causality, be that differential competence in immune systems, genetic liability, or stress vulnerability, Sontag would have us abandon these. Such advocacy is, we believe, materialism most bold, with the mind-body dichotomy embraced whole-hog with the "spirit," as psychobiology set aside in favor of material causes single and microbial. There is no credit given either to wise ancients— Empedocles wrote about 450 BC considering ideas, sensations, flesh, and blood all as equally active realities (Smith 1976), or to workers today striving for psychobiological synthesis and realistic complexity.

Medicine today is itself strongly materialistic and too often singular because of the appropriateness of microbial and surgical models. In medicine are many who are indifferent to the approaches of public health and preventive medicine. And there are in medicine those who may well be what Brandt says, moralists about sexuality. But it is difficult to show that in their medical practice they also practice disdain and the failure to medicate infectious disease. As for personality features in cancer, it seems unlikely that the average technically oriented oncologist is so biased by those data as to derogate his patients. Indeed if there is a failing, we believe it is that suitable responsibility is denied the average patient. Her potential for self-control of risk is discounted. For example, patients with recurring sexually transmitted diseases are treated pharmacotherapeutically and routinely, with no efforts made to induce prophylaxis or alter contact choice patterns, for patients are assumed, in this worst case, to be beyond responsibility.

There is an evident tension between promises associated with health promotion and other ideologies, political or medical. The issue of "victim blaming" becomes a touchstone about which are distributed various perspectives about psychobiology versus the mind-body dichotomy, about singly determined or probabilistic multiple causation in disease, and about choice, will, responsibility, and human malleability in having a role in life's course; these opposed to theories either of external determinism or sheer randomness. When and to what extent human control does exist, and when so in whose hands, or in what portions allocated to person versus community are indeed fundamental points at issue. These will not be resolved here.

Enter at this point; conflict about the domain and power properly those of the physician or other healers. Is he or she to work authoritatively by "doing" surgery, examination, prescribing with the patient always in the passive mode, or are there realms for shared evaluation and endeavour? Is there room for a kind of medicine which not only deals with the woman qua patient in office or surgery or family centered delivery room, but also looks with her at her world "out there," outside, where she lives? These are themes which recur in health promotion. It is well to note in the "victim blaming" controversy their many manifestations.

In the meantime, day to day, one does ask how should one handle the obvious relationship of disapproved behavior— homosexuality, promiscuity, alcoholism, or even not "hanging loose" emotionally in contrast to "neurotic" repression— which may be reported as consequential elements in the multiple determinants of a range of illnesses? Is there a "best" way of presenting data on personality components which appear to play a role in illness vulnerability whether that is stress reactivity in ulcers or early onset delinquency among heroin users? Health promotion does presume, fundamentally, a philosophical view of humans as responsible for what they do, as rational and self-determining powers. It faces the same problems as does the law or psychiatry or sociology in identifying both the limits of that power and those conditions associated with its being expanded or diminished. When personality traits are suggested as etiological, i.e., repression as a cancer "culprit," is there a way to speak of this— assuming the present tentative data were to become a valid statement of probability— without increasing the anguish of the ill patient? We believe there is. It is by the same objectivity and compassion which has been, over time and in as many situations as it can be summoned, the rule of the healer.

More Options For Self Health Care

Another trend in support of health promotion is its compatibility with a growing "pluralism" in the U.S. with respect to the ways people seek to maintain health, and the providers or facilitators they rely upon. This is compatible in the UK with Klein's (1983) view of the National Health Service as an instrument paradoxically effective for limiting demands on health services, with a subsequent trend in the public toward "less deference to professional expertise, more self help, more consumer participation, and more tolerance of diversity" (in providers, sources, health status). In the U.S. one is familiar with older established and institutionalized non-medical or non-medicalized ways of maintaining health, as for example Christian Science, lay-midwives, ethnic curanderas, and faith healers. Now one sees a variety of practitioners of "wholistic medicine," health food faddists, and particularly in the mental and behavioral health arena, such as EST, Ekankar, and "scream therapy."

Each of these choices for health outside the "medicalized" system, and in obstetrics the popularity of home birth with midwife is one, implies recognition that ways of staying healthy, or choosing care rely on individual competence to choose and act. That thrust is in keeping with McKeown's (1976) observation "the determinants of health are largely outside the medical care system." Or, to follow Antonovsky (1980), most of us stay alive on our own in spite of a lot of toxic, stress, and microbial reasons not to. However, one cannot forget that once an illness episode self-defined as consequential occurs, or an event of importance such as pregnancy arises, almost everyone will become a patient. And once a patient, determinants of health are surely also within the system.

Expansion

The medical system is itself expanding via health promotion for disease prevention and wellness. As medicine moves to concern itself with lifestyles and how to work with individuals or small groups to change them, there is a "medicalization" of the approach to self care (see Antonovsky, 1980) at the same time that biological medicine is becoming "psychosocialized." As Eisenberg (1984) said in his address on psychosomatics in obstetrics and gynecology (included in his scheme: behavior - environmental interaction), it is essential in the task of doctoring "to ascertain the events in the patient's life which bring her to the office now . . . and to evaluate mental status, cultural background, and what patient and family expect from care." He concludes, "psychosomatic medicine is too important to be left to specialists. It is the medicine all physicians and surgeons must learn to practice."

Medical-Legal Signs Of Changing Times

One may interpret pluralism and diversity in terms of a trend to redefine health responsibilities. One sees this redefinition in concepts of the doctor-patient relationship and malpractice suit incidence. Beginning in the 1950s, and first in California, there occurred a dramatic rise in the incidence of medical malpractice suits. These actions demonstrated that patients were becoming actively more critical of their doctors, taking aggressive steps to protect their own interests, these arising from new expectations and demands. Physicians in response spoke of "lack of gratitude" on the patient's part, as well as growing litigiousness in the society and blamed attorneys for their patient's reactions. Studies of malpractice origins (Blum, 1956, 1958a, 1958b, 1958c) observed that the immediate (proximal) "cause" of suits was to be found in deteriorating interpersonal relationships between physician and patient following an incident (whether or not defined by the jury or insurance carrier as "real" malpractice) about which the patient was dissatisfied and to which the physician responded with defensiveness and either righteousness or being noncommunicative.

The broader phenomenon implicated, however, was increasing public dissatisfaction with traditional medical roles and conduct. Many citizens no longer wanted their doctors to play God— though paradoxically it was just those wanting a God who were more likely to sue during the 1950s when their unrealistic expectations were "let down." Physicians' practice, both in terms of quality of care and of the nature of the doctor-patient relationship, was measured against increasingly high standards. Respect, information flow, informed consent, and empathy were all becoming conditions for defining a good relationship. The courts agreed; "informed consent" is now a required standard of practice.[3]

Developments during this period, from the 1950s on, are summarized in John Burnham's 1982 article aptly entitled, "American Medicine's Golden Age: What Happened to It?" Burnham tells us that as Americans came to expect from physicians comfort and happiness, as well as health, disillusionment set in. Dissatisfaction with hospitals and "the system" arose as unreasonable expectations were not met, especially as chronic diseases stayed chronic. As patients' sophistication as consumers increased, so too did popular psychological explanations for illness. These, embracing psychosomatics, did not always accord the physician competence for diagnosis or treatment.

Nonmedical reformers set to work. Burnham cites Carter's 1958 book *The Doctors Business* as one of the first works, followed in 1961 by Sanders, *The Crisis in American Medicine*. These and other works were critical of quality of care, of patient-doctor status differences, of the economic motives in medicine, and of the operation of "the system" itself. One thinks of Szasz (1963) and Illich (1976) as outstanding contemporary iconoclasts.

As Burnham observes, there grew a demand for more patient participation and control, i.e., for greater responsibility and less status differential. He writes, "the entire society was moving toward social leveling, the high status necessary for professional authority was being eroded." Coincidental was the growth of "romantic individualism," seen not simply in the exaltation of person vis-a-vis authority, anti-materialistic, anti-technology "flower children," and student rebels. Some of the trends were toward irresponsibility, as in expanding drug use, and, in our view, out-of-wedlock adolescent births.

What we earlier noted in terms of common practice—people taking care of themselves outside of the medical system—now may be seen as having strong cultural value and belief components as well. For the "yuppies" (young, upwardly mobile professionals) self help for health is "right." The health promotion thrust may be interpreted then as an appeal to what at least more fortunate citizens—those with capacity for "controlling their lives"—already believe is in their best interest. Lifestyle management becomes one of the duties of living that is acknowledged by competent and educated people. Nevertheless, for those still not in control of their lives, or not caring, the goal of health promotion for greater individual future oriented disciplined responsibility will be very difficult to achieve and maintain.

Feminism, The Women's Health Movement, And Conflict

Feminism as a movement, and its associated insistence that women "be in charge of their bodies," including "taking back birth, away from doctors, to the woman," advocates an individual health responsibility and is an aspect of egalitarian, democratic ideology which would further reduce, or do away with status differentials. It is part of changing times. Here the emphasis is the right of equality and self-direction for women with men generally, and, in health matters women versus physicians, most of whom are men. It is by no means a cordial disagreement, as reference to the work of critical commentaries such as Susan Arms (1975) shows.

Notman and Nadelson (1978) describe the current medical care structure as hierarchical. The physician is the authority and the woman is expected to conform to traditional social role expectations that she be compliant and uninformed: a "childlike" position with a "paternalistic" professional. Insofar as illness induces regression to dependency—a normal phenomenon—it may invite paternalism, and feed the physician's sense of being omnipotent. Note that it is just the physician who plays God, is paternalistic, encourages passivity, who is most at risk of a breakdown in the doctor-patient relationship which engenders malpractice litigation (Blum, 1958).

Notman and Nadelson observe that the woman herself may further encourage male physician vanity by using seductive coping mechanisms, and sometimes overt sexual transactions will occur. These events should not obscure the general discomfort which, they contend, the average male physician may have about his women patients' sexuality. Notman and Nadelson remind us that very little is taught about sex in medical school, nor in ob-gyn residency, so no wonder that women, given also their often greater emotional expressiveness, make the male physician ill-at-ease. That can become worse if what the woman requires is counseling for collaboration, an activity which the physician had hardly intended to be the thrust of his practice.

Yet the modern woman does require counseling to guide her management of her body because of reasons such as the following. She wants fewer or no children than women in earlier generations, and requires therefore contraception and sometimes abortion. She may be active sexually with many partners and will require surveillance, instruction in how to avoid, and treatment for STD. She may be engaged in highly competitive stressful work associated with possibly with Type A coronary heart disease risk. She needs monitoring and stress management. Breaking into a man's world, her stress-related alcohol and cigarette consumption increases, recognition and treatment for which will be sorely needed. She may be actively lesbian, wanting a physician who can accept that and, when necessary, help or provide artificial insemination so she may have a baby without contact with a man (Olesker and Walsh, 1984). She may want advice on natural or home birth and will want a cooperative physician and setting. If she does want a large family and is pregnant, say for the fourth time, she may face the hostility of her anti-large-family friends. Absence of social supports could mean greater obstetrical complication risk, because at least minimal support is a stress buffer. She will want her physician to appreciate her needs and himself be supportive. The feminist may elect to be a single mother, wanting a baby but not a husband. She expects her physician to understand her independence and instinct, and to help her in planning. As a modern woman she will also accept her own sexuality and want in her relationships— with husband or others— sexual pleasure. She can need counseling or psychological treatments to assure this.

All of the foregoing needs of the modern woman are real, but none (but for STD), including pregnancy, is an illness. The illness model which the conventional physician applies is inappropriate, and poses dilemmas for the traditional physician. Notman and Nadelson make the further observation that women's health professionals have often been accused of insensitivity to their patients' needs, new roles, new demands. They propose that this insensitivity may be particularly widespread among those whose primary interests are surgical, and after all ob-gyn is a surgical specialty. Surgery is a specialty minimizing communication, one, Notman and Nadelson contend, that has values that are antithetical to facing, dealing satisfactorily with, problems and needs that are not organic pathology. They cite Pasnau (1975) to the effect that women's health specialists are particularly ill at ease with situations requiring commmunication or engendering the expression by a woman of her feelings. Yet her feelings are bound to be at the core of her view of herself as competent, responsible, a man's equal, and of her sexuality, assertive motherhood, and occupational commitment.

The surgeon's limitations will mean that primary care, preventive interventions, are likely to suffer. Notman and Nadelson write, "The potential for a preventive approach in both physical and mental health is important. It requires complex skills and psychological understanding that have not been part of the traditional training in obstetrics-gynecology" (p.6). Effective prevention depends upon the physician, or nurse, encouraging self help and collaborative responsibility.

A feminist, Elkin (1980) contends that "...self help and the basic issue of shared responsibility is not settled nor yet generally accepted in the medical world" (p. 86). That involves, says Elkin, demystification of their bodies, being informed consumers, setting up knowledge and problems sharing groups, and heartfelt opposition to the derogatory implication that women's health problems and complaints are neurotic, the latter as a thrust in treatment and training where there is "blatent sexism in medical school textbooks." The modern women is as active, in demanding her right to a respectful medical concern for her feelings of unwellness, her opposition to being dosed with tranquilizers or estrogen, as she is now assertive in her other "her body is her own" rights, in sexuality, motherhood, abortion, wage and occupational status, and Constitutional (the Equal Rights Amendment) demands. Elkin writes, "We can no longer ignore an illness simply because the patient's experience cannot be validated by a laboratory report" (p. 91).

Heide (1978) extends the feminist criticism of medicine, invoking racist and socio-economic ideological criticisms as well, for the American medical structure is denounced for being "white" and "capitalist" as well as "patriarchal." She denounces medical condescension, and its expenditures on technology in lieu of social programs with potential for disease prevention, as for example better nutrition and housing. She sees women's self help groups as essential, as "assertive nurturance" one woman to another. Desirable are women's health centers, consumerism, and intuitive and holistic approaches to care. She speaks of the abuse of the powerless by the powerful, offers psychosurgery on women as an example, insists on improvements in insurance reimbursement schemes in support of preventive health care, and states that what is fundamental is "...control of our bodies and for self- determined reproductive choices." This is one feminist's obstetrical manifesto.

Guzinski (1978), an obstetrical-gynecological specialist, offers more moderate observations. She refers to findings to the effect that more than half of obstetrical-gynecological specialists do care for women's other-than-reproductive system needs and conditions, but that these professionals are hardly trained for such primary care (recall Chapter 1). It is historically understandable that the emphasis is surgical, but as corollary, the professional may well resent that which takes time away from the preferred activity of surgery and takes away the income from that as well. From this conflict, women's needs versus the professional's training and preference, may come unnecessary prescribing, rejection of the woman by referring her out, and doing that which one knows how best to do, and is paid best for, even when that is not appropriate, i.e., surgery for which there is insufficient or no indication. Self-justifications associated with the conflict, and its undesirable resolutions in favor of patient rejection, other prescribing and surgery, in any event can lead, warns Guzinski, to the distortion of the professional's self-view, exaggerating the surgical capacity to heal and his/her powers as healer in that realm.

We would add, with respect to the possibility of the resentment on the part of the professional, if that is joined by a predictable resentment on the part of the woman as well, one can surely understand how any surgical or obstetrical bad result could lead to malpractice-suit-generating confrontations. That is compatible with our own findings on malpractice litigation (Blum, 1958). Given the frequency of such suits today directed against practitioners of ob-gyn, one's reflection is spurred as to the role of mutual resentment and inappropriate technological interventions as contributory. And given the broad nature of the conflict between technical, hierarchical, paternalistic medicine—as the feminists view this battle ground between the sexes—as opposed to the feminist assertiveness over women's rights and needs—one sees a ground fertile for planting the idea of litigation as retaliation and reform as well as redress of grievance and compensation for injuries perceived as unnecessarily, wrongly inflicted.[4]

The women's health movement is part of the thrust to preventive medicine via responsible self help. In its demands for information, collaboration, it is compatible with what we shall later discuss as empirically demonstrated elements for gaining better compliance and assisting patients to better self help. The present conflict, so visible in the "obstetrical battleground" over birth settings, methods, and who is "in charge," is not immediately conducive to the spirit of respectful cooperation in care. While the strident tone of earlier feminism is receding, the attitudinal and related conventions of medical training and practice which the women's health movement addresses remain.

Women Want Women's Problem-Oriented Centers

A study by a healthcare marketing firm (Jensen, 1986) finds an unmet demand among women for "their" kind of service. Among a national sample, 60% spoke of their unmet needs for specialized "women's center" hospital services. Foremost mentioned, by one-third of women, were expanded obstetrical/gynecological and maternal care activities.

Forty percent said they would be willing to pay more to have a female-related problem or need treated in a special women's service, with younger women expressing the greatest willingness to pay more to get what they wanted.

Some women interviewed lived in areas already served by programs advertised by hospitals as special women's services. Among women aware of these programs (one does not know what the programs really offered), more had learned of program center existence from media advertising, 38%, than any other source. Another one-third had learned by word of mouth from friends, acquaintances. Only 15% of women knowledgeable about available special services/centers had been told about them by their physicians.

One concludes that the Women's Movement reflects felt needs on the part of women for kinds of care not presently offered by their regular physicians, in particular, care for problems and needs associated with being a woman. When such specialized centers/services do exist regular physicians appear either not to be knowledgeable or interested in them, or are, perhaps, unwilling to "lose" their patient by referral. One anticipates that unless the practitioner, clinic, and hospital do become sensitive to what their patients want, do catch up to felt needs not presently met, do begin to work to establish and collaborate with such centers, centers necessarily involving "wellness" care, the physician and his/her organizations will be the losers. As will women themselves.

Shifting Responsibilities Should Bring Better Health

The move away from health "dependence" or "passivity" has positive implications for health status. Pratt (1976) found that submissiveness, in interaction with physicians, yielded poorer health care service. Families effectively asserting their own interests in encounters with the care system, received more satisfying service. Glasgow (1973) found that the "good" patients were characterized by physicians as cooperative and uncomplaining, and the "bad" ones as uncooperative, assertive, demanding, but Dunbar (1947), Calder et al. (1960), Daniels and Davidoff (1950), all studying tubercular patients, found these good or "model" patients had higher mortality and relapse rates, while those who were openly aggressive recovered more quickly. Langer and Roden (1976) report that among the elderly in a nursing home, those allowed to assume more responsibility for decisions about living had a mortality rate one-half of those institutionally passive. And Haan (1982), reviewing genetic counseling, argues that participatory medicine, more reciprocal communication, and responsibility sharing is the role style of choice to facilitate patient coping with illness, bad news, and improved preventive health— including contraceptive behavior.

While the Dunbar or Langer and Rodin findings are provocative, it is noteworthy that demonstrated gains for morbidity/mortality are restricted to institutionalized, but usually ambulatory, chronically ill patients. Given the stultifying regressing effects of chronic institutionalization, whether or not for illness, and where in any event illness may not be the full reason for being hospitalized (as with elderly patients with no family to care for them), one may not generalize from these restricted data to other conditions. Indeed Nathanson and Becker (1985) report that contraceptive compliance for teenagers is best achieved via authoritarian staff interactions, and, they cited Davis, "friendliness" (which may or may not be egalitarianism) on the part of the physician is not associated with improved compliance. Considering findings by Becker and others on mother's compliance, Nathanson and Becker propose that compliers are more realistic about the limits and the worth of medical judgement. "Realism" implies maturity, not dependence, whereas among inexperienced teenagers seeking technical contraceptive help when personal maturity is yet to come, parent-like authority styles make age-related sense.

It is important, as one moves from generalities about social change to individual studies to health promotion endorsement, to be skeptical about very enthusiastic claims relating to health behavior change and its immediate consequences. Nevertheless, it is not unreasonable to assume in adults that passivity which arises from psychological denial and immature dependency, lack of coping skills, perhaps hopelessness, is hazardous. Janis (1958), studying maladaptive post surgical reactions, found those who were the quiet, untroublesome patients preoperatively were suppressing anxiety so that when afterwards they faced their pain, physical restraint, or mutilation, they became very upset or depressed. It was this work—not consistently replicated—which discovered the need for preoperative "innoculation" that has led to presurgical counseling (Janis, 1983). Friedson (1961), too, elaborated the dangers of being "obedient" and passive and, observing how much of health care is in fact in the hands of families and individuals, emphasized the importance of responsible self care initiatives.

New Roles and Well-being

Times continue to change. The responsibility vested in the individual and in the family by the converging trends which endorse health promotion as ideology policy and practice portend yet further egalitarianism in doctor-patient relationships. For the physician the change in roles which leads to greater sharing of responsibility may yet be welcome. Hann (1982) describes, as many have, the stress of the physician, one aspect of which induces accepting perhaps unconsciously, responsibility for the many patients who prefer passivity to maturity (see Blum, 1964). And surely it is difficult, unless especially trained, for the professional to deal with that patient distress which is either a component of illness or the response to bad news. Since responsibility needlessly taken on behalf of the passive patient is simultaneously a malpractice risk if patient hopes are disappointed, accepting inappropriate responsibility perhaps forecasts an additional stress burden for the doctor. It is surely contra-indicated for achieving maximum ambulatory patient coping, cooperation, and commitment. The physician who acts more responsibly does so by creating communication and role environments where responsibility is shared as much as possible. Certainly such steps simultaneously to reduce physician stress and facilitate disease prevention and cooperation in adherence should be welcome, given studies (cited by Haan and by Revicki and May, 1985) indicating greater than expected rates of suicide, drug abuse, alcoholism and psychiatric disorder for physicians.[5]

Revicki and May, citing their own and others' work, find that emotional distress is an occupational hazard for physicians and that many are dissatisfied with their work. Occupational stress in turn leads to depression. Good occupational health psychology for the physician appears to be much the same as one expects for patients; Revicki and May observe that debilitating stress effects are reduced when there is felt family support, and a strong optimistic sense of personal control associated with decisive coping, i.e., intervention aimed at reducing stress in constructive ways. These investigators speak in terms of Kobassa's "hardy personality" as one able to reduce depression and, one presumes, other adverse effects, through such sensible action. We propose that not only what is good for the patient is good for the physician because the same mechanisms are involved, but that sharing responsibility with patients— to the extent that it is appropriate and in a manner that is effective— may be one step forward in reducing the psychosocial-behavioral health risks experienced by physicians.

We have not seen a shred of evidence in support of this, our speculation, that just as for citizens too little responsibility is bad for health, that for the doctor too much responsibility, i.e., not encouraging the patient to assume her self-direction, is also contra-indicated for the well being of both. Yet wouldn't it be salutary if the physician who acts as health promoter is also promoting his own "wellness"?

This question, like many others raised in the following pages, must await investigation. In the meantime we believe it can be demonstrated that most— not all— of the trends which have led to current emphasis on health promotion are based on reasonable propositions. In the following pages, evidence from epidemiology and experiment is set forth in further support of that thesis, and with particular respect to the work of the women's medical specialist.

Footnotes

1. * Compiled from information in Levy and Moskowitz (1982, p.122).
   ** This category excludes motor vehicle accidents in the years 1900 and 1940, but includes them in 1980.
   *** This category encompasses cancer and other malignant tumors in the years 1900 and 1940 and changes to malignant neoplasms of all types in 1980.

Reprinted from Master Lecture Series, volume 3, Psychology and Health, "Behavioral Immunogens and Pathogens in Health and Illness," by Joseph D. Matarazzo, copyright 1980, by the American Psychological Association. Reprinted by permission of the publisher and author.

2. A simple example of how relatively easily obtained behavior change might affect health derives from data about auto seat belts. In the U.S. vehicular accidents are estimated to kill 25,000 a year and injure 500,000 (drivers, passengers, intoxicated pedestrians). (Retaches 1985, Galler 1985). Safety authorities estimate that over half of these could be prevented by the use of seat belts on every journey. In European nations, where seat belt use is required by law and is also a matter of social agreement and conformity pressures, habitual use can be by 90% of all travelers; in the U.S. it is about 32%. In the U.S. in January 1985 New York State put into effect the first seat belt law, with consequent use up to 57% (Wall Street Journal, 1985). One forecasts greater conformity to law over time.

3. Litigiousness has also become profitable, not simple for attorneys but as a last resort for patients faced with devastating costs. In obstetrics these are apparent in the care of defective children, where fault real or alleged in perinatal care may become the avenue for parental "cost sharing." As one considers the financial pressures on the American family, now for the majority a unit where both parents must work, and possible resentment over inflated hospital and medical charges (with or without iatrogenic damage as a further burden), a further impetus to litigious cost recovery can be understood.

4. Insofar as conflict as crisis represents an opportunity for and stimulus to change, insofar as consumer demands and malpractice premiums represent incentives (as do HMO and other insurance changes discussed) and insofar as feminist demands appeal to American egalitarian and decent values—whether of physicians, feminists, or others—medical and allied professions are likely to find that disease prevention and "wellness" are partly achievable goals through shared responsibility, information, agreements (call that "really informed consent") become the policy treatment of choice. The women's health movement will continue to push in that direction.

5. When we later examine prospective studies linking morbidity/mortality to early temperament or mental health status where two of the major studies were done on medical students, bear in mind that physicians are a special population under stress with this higher risk for directly behavioral illness and death outcomes.

SECTION II

Illness and Unwellness: Psychosocial-Behavioral Factors

3

Health Complaints of Women "Out There" in their World

Introduction

In this chapter we describe data on illness and self-reported felt unwellness prevalence in the population at large. For the most part, the data are drawn from the United States and the United Kingdom. Whenever possible, data particular to women are presented. We contrast "at home" morbidity with physician visit rates. After elucidating some principles fundamental to health promotion, we describe some psychosocial sources of the variability observed in general morbidity among women.

Illness reports of an epidemiological nature come, basically, by three means. One source is official, enumerated, cases drawn from medical records of practitioners and hospitals. Birth and death certificates are in this case group. Another source are special studies attending to particular groups believed to be or examined for risk or for particular illness. A third source are samples drawn from the population at large so as to seek to be representative of whole populations, whether these be of a town, county, or the nation. The latter, when the measures used encompass a range, cause symptoms and illness as are typically measured by means of women's self-reports entered on one or another of many available check lists or interview schedules. These yield general morbidity data of a particular sort; guided self-assessments reporting symptoms or self- or earlier medically diagnosed illness entities. These measures provide other indices of felt unwellness, as for example fatigue or despair. There can also be medical or laboratory examinations of samples drawn from general populations independent of treatment or risk status, but these are usually intended to screen, as for example Pap smears for cervical neoplasm or case identification studies to describe the prevalence of a particular disease. In this chapter the primary data sources are those health surveys yielding self reports.

A Preview With Health Promotion Implications

We shall see that when the amount of illness or symptoms experienced is compared with medical visits the enormous discrepancy compels the conclusion that most illness, unwellness, is not, in fact, the doctor's (or other health specialist's) business. Most care is self-determined by women themselves, some of that of course as part of family advice and cultural group folk practice. This is a critical point for health promotion, for it tells us that most of what goes on with regard to health maintenance and healing is, in fact, "out there" in women's lives, that at any one time is quite unrelated to medical attention or supervision.

When we look at proportions of illness episodes to medical visits, it will become apparent that the visit decision process is also a very important one for health promotion, for the decision occurs "out there" in a woman's life. How wise that decision process is, judged from the standpoint of the health professional, will depend in part on the extent to which the woman and her family partake of the same scientific or clinical standards as does the professional for symptom evaluation, appraising potential risk, recognizing need for professional care, and making the sometimes finely tuned judgements as to what constitutes over-utilization as well as under-utilization of services. The woman's care utilization decision is extensively determined by the psychosocial context of her life in which "common sense" matters of pain and disability count. This context includes practical matters of money, convenience, and service availability, but also conditions and traits which influence whether bodily events and sensations are interpreted as symptoms, what emotions accompany these, how her family or group define symptoms as requiring or not deserving professional care, and where one is supposed to take one's problems.

Health promotion needs to address the utilization decision and influence process, for it is concerned with building a bridge between the women's specialist and the woman as she lives her life.

At the very least the health specialist wants to bring the two worlds of care as close as possible, the one system that of the woman living "out there" in her daily world and the other that of the professional system of knowledge, values, and service. It is a two way flow; the specialist cannot expect effectively to be influential unless that health professional knows and appreciates the context of the woman's life. What does she do and believe? What factors in her personal and situation impede or facilitate her health maintaining conduct and her risk of illness or accident? Strongly implied in bringing the two systems together is communication adequacy, mutual feedback, reciprocating self-assessment. These are matters we shall address again in later chapters. Our emphasis is on recognizing fully that the practice of the women's health professional, when expanding to incorporate health promotion and related disease prevention as a necessary and routine activity, begins with caring about and learning to know what is going on daily in the woman's life that bears on health and wellness. Simultaneously, a goal of health promotion is to make that interest a partnership. For her part, the informed, self-managing woman will learn more about what is helpful to wellness and disease prevention, and take more responsibility for what occurs in her relationship with the physician or other health personnel.

At its core, practice-based health promotion aims to widen and unify the definition of health responsibilities on the part of both the physician, other health professionals or providers, and the patient—and also her intimate associates. One aims to bring these often quite disparate "health care systems" together. This move toward a closer partnership aims for greater awareness of what the other is doing, and for learning more of why and how.

Another kind of bridge building is implicit through this clinical health promotion effort. It is an interdisciplinary one joining clinical practice and public health preventive medicine including health psychology. The individual practitioner rightly concerned about what is going on "out there" in a woman's life focuses his or her attention on demonstrable risk factors, the knowledge of which is derived from special group and population studies. The practitioner working with the woman and her closest associates will establish intervention priorities—where to work with her for change—based on clinical assessment. These office and clinic evaluations yield information about settings, situations, conduct, personal attributes which have been shown epidemiologically to be dangerous to health, or subversive of wellness, impeding recovery, and which have also been shown, usually on the basis of experimental treatment evaluations, to improve following intervention. One thrust of chapters in this section it to provide that symptom and illness probability and psychosocial-behavioral risk data.

Fallible Statistics

Before presenting the data, a word about error in epidemiological statistics. Prevalence data are not necessarily reliable or exact, for estimation procedures are fallible. Participation in surveys or representation in enumerations from case logs (i.e., becoming a medical case) varies as a function of some of the same biosocial characteristics which are relevant for illness etiology and prevalence itself. For example, typically poor women in minority groups are more likely to be or to become ill. They are also less likely to be at home for or to agree to cooperate in health surveys, to attend screening programs, to return for screening call back, or to receive medical attention and subsequent recorded diagnoses in proportion to their illness episodes. Further contributing to counting errors is the often low reliability of medical diagnoses (physicians disagree with one another, and can be inconsistent themselves). There is disagreement about diagnostic concepts and entities, as in the case of premenstrual syndrome (PMS). Office or hospital records can be astonishingly poor (Blum and Ezekiel, 1962). Measuring instruments, whether for reporting symptoms, laboratory work, or other physical appraisal have their own errors, some built in, some as discrepant results between two or more approaches to measurement, and others as a function of judgement. The focus of the study, whether on records or clinician opinion, is critical. When one is looking for something, and has the case finding and case identification methods worked out, one will find it more often than when one is casting a wider net, whether it is in routine examinations or epidemiological studies. It is that sort of discrepancy which often confronts us when comparing various sources of data about a particular illness. Focus bias of course can be due to more than attention and measures; it can be due to fashion, beliefs, or values.

Morbidity As Measured By Self-Reports In Health Surveys In Populations At Large

About two-fifths of the U.S adult population report non specific acute illness conditions as having occurred during one year. Upper respiratory conditions are the most common specific complaint, with a prevalence rate of more than one incident per person annually. Injuries are reported by about one-third, non upper respiratory infective and/or parasitic diseases by one-fourth, digestive disturbances by about 10%. For women respiratory diseases are more common than for men, as are GI disorders (12.5/100 persons). Genitourinary disorders are reported by about 12%, puerperal disorders by about 4%, headache by 2.4% of women (PHS vital and health statistic, 1979). Cartwright (1984) reviewing U.K. health surveys, cites studies showing two-thirds of the population reported some ill health during one month. This prevalence rates increased with age, and women of all ages complained of more ill health than men (McKewon and Lowe, 1966). Pennebaker (1984), reviewing variables associated with differential symptom reporting rates, indicated that for the U.S. females report more symptoms than males. Women also report more symptoms associated with stress (Rosenstock and Kirsch, in Stone et al., 1979). Suchman (1965) reports that women report symptoms as more severe and "take them more seriously." In the U.K., in 1977, 56% of men and 70% of women reported chronic health problems and 32% of males but 38% of females indicated some disability over a two week period.

In the United Kingdom, Bewley, Higgs, and Jones (1984), reporting on inner city London girls, found that 30% said there was something wrong with their health (obesity, ranked first, was considered by them to be ill health, rather than a health risk) and 59% had visited a physician within the prior three months. The 1954 Baltimore study (Commission on Chronic Diseases), which included a large number of economically-racially disadvantaged persons, found 30% of those under 15 years of age had a chronic condition, as did 95% of those over 65. Substantial illness (disabling, or requiring care) averaged 44%. Blum and Kernanen (1966) proposed a national chronic disease prevalence rate of 42%. In Baltimore, at that time, the most prevalent diagnostic group were women with diseases of the female genital organs, at a prevalence rate of over 13,000 per 100,000 or 13%.

Among "normal health problems" Pennebaker (1982), reviews data showing that one-fourth of American adults use an analgesic at least once a week; another 50% will do so occasionally. Presented with a list of common symptoms, 80% of all adults will indicate that they have at least one symptom currently. The average person will recall ten days of disability per year, but if questioned about recent events, will recall disability, as some restriction on normal activity due to ailments, at a rate greater than ten days a year.

Medical Visits Relation And Experienced Unwellness

In a U.K. study, Banks et al. (1975) had women keep a diary of symptoms and medical visits. The average woman had one or more symptom over one-third of the recording month, but went to a physician only about two times a year. The investigators calculate that there is one medical visit for every 37 self-perceived illness symptom episodes. Zola (1972) finds, for the U.S., that nine out of ten of self-assessed illnesses are not brought to medical attention. Antonovsky (1980) estimates that at any one time, only from one to two percent of the U.S. population are immediate clients of the professional disease care system. It is understandable then that Clumer, Baum, and Krantz (1984), reviewing the data, emphasize the extent of self health care. They cite work indicating up to 96% of all patients who seek medical advice have first treated themselves. For the United Kingdom, Wadsworth, Butterfield, and Blaney (1971) also describe the great extent of self care over medical attention.

The contrast in prevalence rates for illness episodes versus medical visits— the latter average in the U.S. for women 5.2 per year and for men 4 (Statistical Abstract 1985), and overall are about 4 per year in the United Kingdom— might well be greater were the people aware of, and thus to report, the many illnesses which are, at least for a time, asymptomatic. White et al. (1961), reviewing U.S. and U.K. data, estimate that two-thirds of all illness conditions with physical pathology will be unnoticed at any given point in time. One thinks of neoplasms, subacute sexually transmitted chlamydia infection, (asymptomatic in about 70% of women), hypertension, early ectopic pregnancy, diabetes, osteoporosis, cardiovascular pathology, and the like. As an extreme case, consider that only 1/1,000 to 1/3,000 cases of trichinosis in the U.S. are ever diagnosed (Trichinosis, Science

1985). There are also the emotional and behavioral disorders where recognition is resisted by the person and the family, as for example, alcoholism or other psychiatric disorders including major entities with genetic-neuropharmacological etiology and expression.

The decision to make a medical visit would obviously seem associated with severity of discomfort or the self-diagnosis of the probability that symptoms may represent a serious illness not amenable to self care. That is partly the case, but by no means does such a common sense scheme account for all of what people do. In the Banks study for instance, there were 14 episodes of chest pain to each medical visit, 18 of sore throat, 184 of headache, and 456 episodes of "energy change" (which we surmise to be felt fatigue including depression and tension/anxiety) for each visit. But even great pain severity and a life threatening symptom do not assure quick decisions to visit. Clymer et al. describe research on heart attack victims who delay calling a physician, or going to emergency rooms, for four and five hours. There is no difference in the delay time between those who have had prior attacks, and who thus know exactly what the danger is, and those suffering their first one. When all the delay time is logged between attack onset and initiation of attention, 75% of it is attributable to intended patient delay— whatever the emotions associated with that. And be reminded that such studies only sample those who finally do get attention; those who do not have their delay reasons uncounted, dead or alive.

Work by Zola (1972) found that another consequential variable affecting the decision whether or not to seek medical advice was what the symptom/illness does, that is, how it affects living. If it is experienced as having direct impact on an important role, say work, child care, becoming a mother, it is more likely to prompt a visit. But there are exceptions as well, particularly for women, for example, that sexual dysfunction which is rarely discussed with doctors, or behavioral disorders where the source of even major disruption in life— alcohol or cocaine for example— is something one lies to oneself and others about. Thus self-abnegation or self-protection against the threat posed if one is to be the subject of other's efforts to change a compulsion are all visit (and compliance) influences.

Clymer et al. (1984) present findings to the effect that those persons more active in self care are both less likely to delay, but also use less care than more passive individuals. Health "responsibility" may be involved here as a consistently sensible self help delay avoiding component. Roth and Cohen (1986) consider "approach" and "avoidance" with respect to approaches to illness. It is possible that approach, as doing, seeking information, facing fears is one aspect of being "active." They cite work showing that women who were otherwise rated as active approachers to problems were quicker to bring breast lumps to medical attention. And women facing elective abortion who faced it head on were less anxious pre- and post-surgically.

Matters of money and convenience also obviously play a role. Women in lower income groups seek care less often— even though they are more often at risk and ill. The more inconvenient care is, and the fewer the resources to cope with that (think of the single head of household supporting herself and several children and having neither auto or health insurance nor sympathetic employer to allow time off), the greater the barrier to a medical visit.

Such study findings illustrate that while the nature and severity of the bodily experience do influence how women self-diagnose, self-treat, and decide on health care visits, psychosocial as well as practical economic factors play a major, sometimes overriding, role. These factors operate to affect the statistics themselves, in terms of what bodily sensations are recalled or interpreted as a symptom to be reported on a health survey, as well as the speed of decision making, the choice of healers to attend (unlicensed midwife, chiropractor, faith healer, herbalist, or physician) and, of course, which symptoms are brought to attention.

Findings of the foregoing sort led Wadsworth (1974) to generate a rule, his "iceberg principle" which states that at any time diseases presented to the physician are only the tip of the iceberg. By way of caution with respect to health promotional attainments, and consonant with the data in our Table I, Wadsworth also enunciated the corollary "onion principle" to the effect that when some major class of disease is eradicated, appearing neither in studies of natural populations nor in the physician's office, subsequent or underlying ones will be revealed. Longevity and overall quality of life may well be improved, but degeneration, disease and despair, like taxes, do not disappear. Another principle is elucidated when one compares the same disease entity as observed (always, it seems, with greater prevalence) in natural population studies as opposed to that same diagnosis when arrived at by the physician. Butterfield (1968) found, only with diabetics to be sure, that untreated cases differ clinically— as presenting entities, i.e., in the pattern of signs and symptoms from those seen for treatment. Let us call that the AINT acronym, for "it ain't the same." Diseases and their hosts differ depending on the circumstances of observation and life situation.

Beginning systematically with the work of Morris (1957), and others more recently, we designate the MARLIC principle, "most at risk, last in care." It is found for almost any condition that the people most at risk and with greatest morbidity, when characterized biopsychosocially, are the least likely to seek out available services. The MARLIC principle generates major thrusts for health promotion research: to describe and better understand those psychosocial-behavioral factors which are associated with illness risk, to learn how these factors operate psychobiologically to affect disease onset and process, how risk factors can be ameliorated by public health, including health education, mass measures and how, clinically, individuals may be evaluated for and assisted to self-awareness and self-regulation for risk control, including better health care utilization practices.

Self-Rated Overall Health Status

Symptom levels, as we have seen, need not be associated with illness as diagnosed, nor with self-rated overall health status. It is useful to conceive of a range of population groups differentiated one from another by what the relationship is between relatively high symptom reporting on a typical measurement instrument (see Table VI, Chapter 15), and other health variables, as for example psychiatric status or diagnosed morbidity severity (whether acute or chronic non psychiatric disease) or medical visits or self-rated overall health status. That sorting will yield different groups, each with its own risk status and associated psychosocial correlates.

In the case of self-perceived health status when that is an overall rating, first note that a self-rating as being in poor health is itself a predicator of higher than expected mortality risk (Singer, 1976, Mossey, 1982, Goldstein et al., 1984). This is likely to be an association, in fact, with awareness of chronic physical illness so that the morbidity risk represents the operation of real illness, and the self-rating the fact and awareness of it. As might be expected, those who rate themselves as being in poor health are older, less well educated, poorer. Compatible with the MARLIC principle, these also are people who say that health services are less readily available to them, or do not (some say "would not") use health services as readily.

In a London study (Bewley et al., 1984) one-half of the females age 16-20 saw themselves as only in "fair" health. Women in the U.S., along with the elderly, report they are more disabled, defined now as having more difficulty doing routine tasks such as shopping, housework or getting about, than are men, or younger people. Women are more worried about their health than men— this a different measure than being in poor health, and they rate themselves as having less energy than other people their age. The energy variable can be one associated with depression, although for women in general we suspect it can have other significance, perhaps as a correlate of the reproductive cycle and, we speculate, a sensitivity hazard associated with that cycle. As we shall later see, women rate themselves more than men as overeating, not getting enough exercise and being inactive. Fatigue may well interrelate with such conduct patterns, whether as attitude or in fact retarding, say, exercise, or as a result of not exercising, being fat, and thus not feeling fit.

Women then, compared to men, seem to sense a health disadvantage, that as disability, worry, low energy level, and fatigue. They will be at health disadvantage, at mortality/morbidity risk, when they are in fact suffering from chronic disease and/or giving themselves an overall poor health rating. This insight and accuracy is in turn a function of psychosocial and behavioral features as well as health history, treatment access, and treatment status.

We spoke earlier of several goals of clinical health promotion arising from the so common feeling in women of not being fully well. One goal was to bring the two worlds, the woman's and the health professional's, closer together by way of understanding. The task is in seeing, and in way, experiencing illness-labeled events, within a mutually shared framework. For the physician, nurse, and other caregiver that joining is facilitated by knowing the factors which account for variability among women, and in the same woman over time, in rates of reporting feeling bad.

That Ubiquitous "Stress"

First a word about "stress," a concept often encountered when reading about psychosocial factors whether in psychosomatics, psychophysiology, epidemiology, or examining the literature on cancer or heart disease. It may be used as a description of events or circumstances, as an inference about the interaction between a woman and either her external or internal world, or as a description of a response to the world or the product of the interaction process. It is whatever an observer says it is, whether demands on a person or organ system for adaptation, i.e., the "challenge" or "insult" as physiologists say, or it can be what a woman says of her way of viewing, and recalling the experience of, an aspect of her life. When defined as a response it implies "too much," and "too long" by way of arousal and recovery rates for organ systems, or feelings. When defined as a state it implies "too much," and vulnerability. It readily implies pathological process, sometimes erratic and destabilized, as in disregulation (see Siever and Davis, 1985, in depression and also diabetes), whether as the response to or as disregulation or vulnerability already present in a malfunctioning organ system so that anomalous deleterious responses to "stressors" occur. Thus reciprocal amplification may be understood: either organ system or personality not working "normally" so that other events, internal or external, realize their virtual potential as "stressors" to, in fact, become "stress" as measured by the short or long response. But note, a stress response can also be entirely adaptive as "normal" and survival assisting, or as the cancer literature tells us (see reviews by Campbell and Cohen (1985), and Anisman and Sklar (1984)), may even confer reduced risk, i.e., impede expected tumor growth by way of enhanced autoimmune response.

Be aware that the use of "stress" within the literature is so diverse, and often so tautological or confused, that one must be on guard. Secondly, accept its ubiquity as a focus in risk and psychophysiological response research as an interaction reminder. For most risk factors with "stress," one is examining what goes on between a woman and her world as interaction. When considering "stress" as a complaint, it signifies an inner world disturbance either expressive of how the woman's outer world is being processed and experienced, or as a sense of disregulation within the hierarchy of bodily and appraising inner systems. In any event, for clinical health promotion one is intent on when and how things can be set healthier right. For discussions of the conceptual and experimental aspects of and difficulties in regard to "stress," see Steptoe and Mathew (1984), the exchange between Lazarus et al. (1985) and Dohrenwend and Shrout (1985), further commentary by Deutsch, Green, Lazarus, and Folkman, Dohrenwend and Shrout, Cohen (all as letters, comment), discussions in Feuerstein, Labbe, and Kuczmierczyk (1985), in Van Dyke and Zegans (1982), Engel (1985) versus Schneiderman and McCabe (1985) and, very importantly, Define and Monroe (1986). But when reading the contemporaries, do not forget those masters in physiology: Bernard, Cannon, and Selye, whose genius introduced the field, nor Freud, Alexander and Dunbar, Wolff and Wolf, out of whose work there arose the further stimulus to psychosomatic stress studies.

For our purposes here, stress is provisionally understood as an interaction between person and environment, one involving dynamic interrelating effects on organ systems (cardiovascular-circulatory, neuropharmacological, immune, endocrine, etc.). Environmental change and new demands on organ systems are implied leading to arousal and either adaptation and recovery or maladaption in one or several systems as the response process. Outcomes of the process are complexly determined and may or may not be associated with acute or chronic felt distress or developing pathology. Response magnitude, reciprocal person-environmental effects, recovery time all depend upon such matters as the nature of events, their meaning to an individual, the situation and range of responses available to the person, her "theoretical" baseline and her level of functioning at times of measurement, the chronicity of exposure, and individual dispositional (including apparently genetically determined) response styles.

When stress is invoked either for explanation or research, one keeps in mind that contamination in measurement, or too singular thinking in the clinician, may occur. Consider, for example, the patient who is, rightly, asked what events prior to her developing symptoms have been upsetting to her. She may mention divorce. We are sympathetic and conclude, reasonably, that the event is itself causal or at least triggering. But if one compares that symptomatic woman with other just divorced women, one may find that those who do develop high symptom complaint levels, or, typically associated, "negative affect (depression, irritability, nervousness) followed within some weeks by physical manifestations, differ from those who don't in a number of ways. For example, in the more symptomatic women there may be a higher level of reporting a number of prior events as troublesome; for example, low income women do report more bad things happening in their lives (Craig and Brown, 1984). They simultaneously have worse, less supportive social relations which otherwise can "buffer" the ill effects of hazards, and then "stress" may be loss of such resource (see Blaney, 1985). Women in high symptomatic stress response groups may also be more likely to experience a greater range of events as esteem threatening or "too much to handle." This particularly stress vulnerable patient may also be found as earlier to have been widowed young (and if marital relationships were bad, emotional recovery is likely to take longer), is chronically depressed, is in fact poor and does not have a circle of close friends with whom to talk and by whom to be assisted. Perhaps, too, she feels helpless with things "out of control," and has always had trouble expressing her feelings, i.e., she is emotionally less competent. To top it off picture her as a long time, early onset heavy cigarette smoker, who has been compulsively promiscuous (seeking love or reassurance) after her divorce and has now contracted genital warts. Furthermore, she works as a lowly clerk under a hostile boss. These conditions put her a risk epidemiologically of both cervical cancer and cardiovascular disease.

The research worker addressing stress, say for effects on the immune system, can control experimentally or parcel out statistically such multiple and interacting variables, especially if it a matter of giving long or short, controllable or uncontrollable electric shock to densely or solitary or happily housed or well or underfed mice. But the clinical practitioner deals with the patient as she is. What about her "stress"? Stress no doubt there was and is in her life, but neither her experience of what is upsetting nor her response to it—say immediate exacerbated depression, sleeplessness, and abdominal pain over the short term and cervical neoplasm or cardiac arrhythmias over the long run—are independent of other aspects of her genetic and social history, her personality, and her immediate socio-economic situation.

A recent study by Wiebe and McCallum (1986) illustrates, further, the interplay of factors. They measured health practices and symptom severity over a two month period. They expected these to be related to "stress" as measured by notable life experiences (Life Experience Survey) and rated for felt negative to positive impact. They also measured "hardiness" by psychological tests of felt self-control, alienation (or contrariwise, commitment), and "challenge" measured by a life goal evaluation test. The sample included young women and men in college. Hardiness and health practices had a greater impact on illness reports (symptoms, not medical visits) than did "stress." Nevertheless both "stress" and "hardiness" were operative and, further, hardy people maintained better health practices when under "stress." Even though, in a study of this sort, one is on guard because "hardiness" and "stress" are whatever the investigator decides to use as a scale to measure them, one may at least conclude that aspects of personality and felt major events impinging on life (as "stress") are related both to health practices and to severity of symptoms experienced over time.

Common Risk Factors Qua "Stress"

We have, in the foregoing discussion, introduced several other factors which are currently among those widely studied and frequently identified as factors operating to affect differential expression and reporting of symptoms, and as psychosocial risks associated with morbidity and mortality. We shall run across them many times again, but by way of introduction we do here note that there is reasonable evidence for the widespread operation in personal health matters of the following: chronic emotional, negative affective states—primarily anxiety and depression, social supports (intimates, and their help, community ties—their number and nature), feelings and enduring assumptions about one's ability to comprehend and control events (helplessness, confidence, mastery), socio-economic subcultural and situational milieu and status, the number and personal significance of recent adverse events—particularly bereavement, emotional competence (as ability to both express and consciously control feelings), daily "hassles," the range and options in the repertoire of coping mechanisms (what she can do for herself and what she has available to do these with), personality and behavior, habits and style (smoking, sex, etc.) itself.

Hinkle and Wolff (1957a, 1957b), the pioneers in the field of event-related stress studies, were among the first to show, in a large longitudinal (retrospective) study of employees, the relationship of illness and work time lost to personal maladaption and reported stressful circumstances. Related work (Hinkle, 1977; Thurlow, 1967) also suggested periodicity in illness cycles, the likely wide distribution of symptoms across organ systems over time and, yet also measured by incidence over time, a pattern of vulnerability for individuals of particular organ systems. And of course some individuals are consistently more often ill than others. These investigators documented the often rather diffuse nature of expressed symptomatology incorporating both physical and emotional distress. The one-quarter of the population who accounted for more than one-half of all illness episodes over 20 years of observation also had a greater spread of etiologies, of minor and major disorders, and of disease syndromes. As part of this, chronic diversity of illness also means acute illness periodicity with a greater incidence of psychological distress. It would appear that a minority, albeit a large one, of people are more illness susceptible over a range of illnesses and experience "unhappiness"conditions over their observed working lifetimes.

The index Hinkle and Wolff used is still a widely used measure tapping a wide range of symptoms. When such an instrument— and there are many descendants from that symptom inventory— is applied to individuals selected for other health relevant attributes, or experiencing different risk situations, the results offer a correlative, but possibly not cause-demonstrating method for showing a relationship between symptom levels and such phenomena as number and adversity of life events (as challenges or stress, i.e., change requiring adaption) or daily "hassles" (De Longis et al., 1982), or negative affect (Depuis and Monroe 1986).

It is important to keep in mind that stress is not only found associated with complaints, or morbidity, as measured by self-reports of people selected independently of their treatment status, but is shown as a risk variable with an etiological role for some acute specific disease. For example, and most dramatically, stress is implied in the clustering of life changes preceding the "sudden death syndrome" (for reviews see Craig and Brown, 1984, Schneiderman and McCabe, 1985). Panchieri et al., in an unpublished paper discussed by Sarason and Sarason (1982), point to how, in the etiology of myocardial infarction, it is how events are initiated, viewed, experienced, and how one is able to cope with them that specifies the impact of change events as risk factors, that much akin to Craig and Brown's (1985) emphasis on the "meaning" of events, and also Dohrenwend and Shrout (1985), or Lazarus on stress as a person-environment interaction outcome quality. Craig and Brown (1984) report that among women under 50 years of age experienced severity is also a critical feature, for it is the severe threat which leads, as they show, first to negative mood changes and then, over some weeks, to physical illness.

The Socio-Economic Data Paradox

Pennebaker (1982, 1984) reviews work, and reports his own, on symptom levels in association with psychological situations and variables. We begin with an apparent paradox, the relationship of symptom levels to socio-economic class (SEC) to health survey symptoms reporting. SEC has as components education, occupation, residential area, household density, family size, race, social marginality, medical care accessibility, sanitary conditions, knowledge levels, nutrition, safety practices, number of severe adverse events per time period, personal resources and coping skills, quality of personal relationships, in urban settings how organized and predictable lives are, intelligence, subsequent and continuing genetic effects over the generations on physique, stature, attractiveness, and other genetic attributes. These latter are as a function of a feedback loop for assortative mating (see Buss, 1985). Socio-economic class consistently shows an inverse association with health and wellness, and also happiness (Gurin et al., 1960). Family income alone is a strong predictor of negative affect (Depue and Monroe, 1984, citing Lin). The lower SEC (with variations depending on the mix of constituent elements in the foregoing component list), the more likely people are to become ill, to stay ill, to feel unwell and unhappy, and to die early. This is a nearly universal relationship across cultures and across illnesses.

Survey data (Vital & Health Statistics, #147, 1985) show a strong relationship of income to health self-reports for household members (N = 81,000 households). The poor, as opposed to higher income people, had 3.4 times more chronic conditions limiting activity, and were 4.4 times to say their health was only fair or poor rather than good or excellent. Being poor and self-rated as healthy did not appear to limit medical visits, for those in the low income group averaged 5.9 visits compared to the (survey time 1979-80) U.S. average of 4.5 visits. However, being poor and sick was another matter. Higher income people self-rated as being in fair or poor health averaged 12.8 visits annually, poor ones 10.4. Women and men will both have their reported health status and medical visits associated with income levels.

Yet, at least in some studies, people in higher SEC brackets report more symptoms, even though these same persons have the expected lower rates— compared to the SEC low group— of diagnosed morbidity. They also, as expected, rate themselves as higher in general health than do those low in SEC. We recognize here the well-off woman with chronic minor complaints often seen in office practice.

The high SEC-high symptom level association may be a function of higher knowledge and health expectation levels, and more learned responsible self-awareness for health. That is compatible with the findings of Koos (1954) who, in a pioneer study in medical sociology, found that the importance given to symptoms varies inversely with SEC levels. Given a list of 17 symptoms, including blood in urine, excessive vaginal bleeding, blood in stool, lump in the breast, pain in the chest, shortness of breath, etc., 81% of higher SEC level people said the conditions listed needed medical attention, whereas only 31% of the lower class people so stated. One presumes such knowledge-based weightings influence health survey symptom reports as well. This is compatible with a problem— or irony— relevant for health promotion. Women least at risk on psychosocial and behavioral grounds— those high on SEC— are best able to adopt and already do show the best self health help practices. It is the MARLIC principle again.

Other High Symptom Level Correlates

Pennebaker's work indicates that a measure of a personal trait of attentiveness to one's inner states is associated with higher symptom report levels among women. That inner state awareness, qua orientation, is not associated with being more accurate about one's autonomic states (the usual measure in such experiments). Most individual's estimates of an internal state correlate only about .50 with laboratory measures of that state. Pennebaker proposes that more accurate human inner attentiveness might be counter adaptive; he cites studies by Epstein and Fentz on novice and experienced acrobatic parachutists; the former were more frightened and more correct about their accompanying reactions. The latter, it is proposed, were wise to attend to the jumping maneuvers at hand and to suppress their fear and their self-monitoring of its autonomic components. Byrne, Steinberg, and Schwartz (1968) found that people with repressive styles, as opposed to those with self-sensitive ones, report fewer illness symptoms. In Pennebaker's experimental studies on autonomic function, these sensation repressing individuals are no less accurate than "sensitives" about their non pathological bodily states including those of arousal in response to challenge.

High symptom reporters are more dependent than others on external information in their reports of physical sensations, that is, they are more readily swayed (at least in experiments on heart rate) by outside events to make inferences about what is happening inside them. Pennebaker suggests they are trying harder to know about bodily changes even though they are not, and keep in mind most people are not, very accurate about the autonomic system activities typically monitored in such experiments.

Reduced or low level environmental stimulation or the absence of engaging, challenging tasks and activities also leads to greater attentiveness to bodily states. Inferable from these psychological experiments is the role of boredom and inactivity. The work suggests a woman can feel herself to be symptom free in an active setting but she becomes more bodily state oriented in situations where she is bored and where previously subliminal signs, submerged in an array of competing stimuli, now rise above sensory threshold levels, sometimes to become matters of health concern if not preoccupation. Furthermore— Mandler et al. (1958) are cited, and again it is research on autonomic function— people who are predisposed to be most variable in their autonomic system functioning are the ones who report the most symptoms. Inherent liability is related to enhanced awareness and thus to reporting. Internal fluctuation and, one speculates, exaggerated cyclicity suggest themselves as "constitutional" characteristics of consequence for the occurrence of self-awareness, felt distress and symptom levels.

We shall not, in this book, elaborate on psychophysiological processes per se. Quite important research and concepts exist with respect to disease process, much of that associated with stress, endocrine, or immune system studies. Locke (1980), Schneiderman, and McCabe (1985), Steptoe and Mathews (1984), and Van Dyke and Zegans (1982) offer thoughtful reviews. Steptoe (1984), for example, reviewing the work of Barsky and Klerman on amplifying somatic styles, of Engle on individual response specificity and of Sternbach, and also Malmo and Shagass on individual response stereotype, allow the conclusion that psychophysiological response styles as "stress" interactions may be enduring traits from childhood on. Also, that individuals differ in their response styles including multiple patterning evoked by diverse challenge, and that some are associated with disease process. Type A hostility predisposing to coronary heart disease (see Dembrowski and MacDougal, 1985) is an example. These concepts all harken back to early postulates of psychosomatic medicine to the effect that particular psychophysiological processes, as part of personality styles, predispose the involved and "vulnerable" organ systems to dysregulation (or overload) and disease.

Either genetically programmed or developed fluctuation instability, or extreme cyclical variability should be phenomena of interest in such investigations. As we shall see in a later chapter, Betz and Thomas (1979) report that temperamental instability is, in fact, a mortality risk factor. Pennebaker, whose findings on liability are of such importance here, calls attention to the need for further work on automatic liability and symptom levels. Such work relates to the concepts of dysregulation or instability as discussed by Schwartz (1983) as part of his application of systems theory to brain regulatory and subsequent health behavior. Drawing on theoretical work by Powers (1973) on hierarchical organizing-feedback systems as control levels biopsychologically, Tapp (1985) also offers a viewpoint which could link continuing liability to feedback and "set point" control (homeostatic) failures within the CNS and related endocrine systems. Symptom levels and complaints, then, when in fact related to self-awareness of fluctuating, non stabilized, or cyclical extreme systems, may be of considerably more importance for psychophysiological investigation than is currently recognized. It may also one day move to integrate work in perceptual psychology— much of that elegant respect to awareness thresholds and pattern recognition, with self-assessment of bodily states, and perhaps that accurate self-forecasting implied in self-characterization as being in poor health.

Being employed, being married, and living in households of one to three people correlate with lower levels of symptom reporting. Among young females in Pennebaker's study, correlates of high symptom reporting include cigarette smoking, low self-esteem, concern with one's appearance to others, drug use, unhealthy eating patterns, being anxious, problematic sexual histories, and coming from conflict ridden homes. Further trait correlates of high symptom reporting include lack of close relations in marriage, the absence of what is measured on one scale as "self-actualization," and for married women and, after stress, the fact of having fewer friends of their own while being reliant on their husband's social circle. High symptom reports also occur when there is great discrepancy between the degree of control in life a woman prefers and that which is actual. One may view this as frustration over unachieved aspirations in self-directed people. Related, on a locus of control measure, sensing what happens to oneself as being outside of, beyond, one's own control (Christensen in McReynolds and Chellune, 1984) is also a high symptom correlate.

Carver and Scheier (1985) find that among students during the tense pre-examination period, a test of personal optimism as an enduring personality trait correlates negatively with physical symptoms. Over a four week period those with optimistic personalities (not test related, or as far as we can tell, grade related) were predictably lower on symptom reporting. Optimism as a "positive emotion" may, according to Lazarus (1980, cited by Carver and Scheier), buoy coping with challenge facilitating persistence, recovery, and adaptive time outs. One presumes, it is not demonstrated, that optimism is associated with confidence (what Bandura calls "self-efficacy") self-assessed coping skills, and indeed resources to disallow boredom.

Emotional And Personality Disorder

Some of the conditions just described are compatible with personality distress or disorder. Is it reasonable then to expect that neuroticism or anxiety, or depression—or, better, these groups together as "negative affect"—will be one set of variables associated with a greater probability of reporting symptoms? Yes. Costa and McCrae (1985) in a study of men show those classified as neurotics report two to three times more diffuse and nonspecific complaints than well adjusted men. One presumes a similar tendency among women. Again, one is not to set up a prejudicial dichotomy between self-reported complaints versus "real" ones validated by the physician. Steptoe and Mathews (1984) review evidence to the effect that, for example, mortality increases for severe neurosis and that there are greater than normal rates of physical illness among psychiatric patients with affective disorder. Weissman (1982) shows that depressed people are more frequent users of medical facilities, that depression increases morbidity risk, and that up to one-quarter of medical patients are depressed.

Osborne (1985), in a review of the psychological evaluation of medical patients with a Mayo Clinic of 50,000 seen in the internal medicine service, conclude that these, compared to non patients, are more depressed, have more somatic concerns, and are more likely to deny emotional problems. Implicit is that such emotional problems exist. Although somatic concern is certainly understandable in physically ill people, the denial of emotion can also be understood as a reasonable quieting defense against upset when one is ill, and depression is also a natural response (it functions to conserve energy and lower expectations according to the adaptive "conservation-withdrawal" concept of reactive depression as "passive coping" (see Schneiderman and McCabe, 1985). The foregoing constellation is such as equally to allow the speculation that some internal medicine patients are "symptomatic" because of depression, denial, and a somatic focus. For that subgroup, becoming a medical patient could be one way of seeking validation for one's distress, help in coping, and perhaps a way out via the patient role which reduces demands from others for normal performance. Rodin and Voshart (1986) considering depression in medical patients indicate that it is more common among in-patients than outpatients, and may understandably be greatest among those seriously ill. One is not to discount the possibility that among those women chronically ill "out there," even if not medically attended, the prevalence of despair is both reactive and contributory. It is a vicious circle.

Attention to neurosis, depression, denial, or manipulation of others via using the patient role as sometimes components in physical complaints, and in the phenomenon of somatizing, reflects psychologic-psychiatric investigation of these patient subpopulations. In doing that clinically, one must not ignore the more complicated psychodynamic components, i.e., the invisible highly personal meanings, conflicts, and functions derived from painful childhood family experiences which physical symptoms can represent.

It is beyond our scope here to deal with psychodynamics, but we may cite Barsky (1979) whose discussion of patients who, according to his view, "amplify" bodily sensations, is helpful. His characterization of the somatizing patient is one who is likely to be self-preoccupied, critical of physicians (after all there is a history of "failed" diagnoses and treatments), and who find gratification in suffering. This may arise from atoning for guilt, using illness to express anger, insuring being cared for by those who feel fundamentally— derived from childhood experience— unloved and uncared for, or as a masochistic self-sacrificing enterprise. Masochism can mean real pleasure (including sexual) in pain, or angrily and passively proving how bad others are by saying "look what damage you have done to me." People who want others to look bad or feel guilty about the suffering are usually complaining people who from childhood on have felt bad about themselves. Insofar as complaints or symptoms are referable to sexual organs, and do affect sexual conduct, it would be rather naive— if not plain stupid— to be so post-Freudian as to ignore the possibility of emotional conflicts about sexuality, or maternal roles and reproduction, as a psychodynamic basis for complaints. Particularly when the examining physician is a male, it would also be beyond naivete to assume that women with psychologically based complaints involving sexual reproductive organs or functions are not going to have some immediate problems, e.g., being ill at ease, not readily forthcoming, showing inappropriate emotions— typically with fear and anger— in her interaction with her physician. Keep in mind the psychoanalytic idea of transference; such a woman can bring with her to the male physician the same unconscious baggage, as attitudes and inappropriate behavior, which she learned in anguish and/or maladjustment as a child or teenager.

Schafer (1984), a psychoanalyst, offers insights applicable to some women patients as he writes of "the pursuit of failure and the idealization of unhappiness." We speak of the felt and enacted virtue in being miserable. Since misery does love company, the woman who makes a point of using illness as unhappiness also manages— intentionally even if unconsciously— to punish those around her. Their suffering lives out their love and their hate while they may be keeping their happier selves secret. As for the origins of this "entrenched" and sought after psychological suffering, it may come from trying to be like a beloved mother who was devalued by disdainful or hostile men, or a demeaning (one would now say "sexist") world around her. It can be, says Schafer, a result of being victimized by stronger others who inflict suffering and expect women to bear that. The origin of virtuous suffering and its associated complaints can be from "absorbing" the unhappiness of others into oneself, as for example when there is too little psychological differentiation (insufficient ego barriers) between oneself and others in the family. ("Let this hurt me more than it hurts you.")

This concept of "absorbing" unhappiness is central to much Greek folk healing (Blum and Blum, 1965). Healing "wise women" there (never the male healers) cure complaints ranging from headache to PMS to dyspareunia in an "evil eye" apotropaic ritual in which "the bad" is passed from the sufferer to the wise woman. Because she is a professional magician, the wise woman, rather like a lightening rod, can conduct the pain safely away from the patient, through and out of herself. Does the American psychotherapist do the same? Perhaps the challenge is for other medical health providers to develop the same insight, skill, and strength. The implication, in any event, of the idealization of unhappiness is that one group of patients with continuing complaints may be those who want to demonstrate further that they are miserable, and will fail to get well, just as they fail to celebrate joy, because that is what they have learned to do.

A further psychiatric interest in the complaining patient focuses on that diagnostic group earlier called "hysterics" and now termed "somatoform" or "somatization" disorder. Under the formal American Psychiatric Association DMS III diagnostic nomenclature this diagnosis requires medically unexplained physician symptoms beginning before and continuing beyond the age of 30, and for women the presence of 14 from a list of 37 defining symptoms. A short screening test (Othermer and DeSouza, 1985) now allows diagnosis using seven symptoms: shortness of breath, dysmenorrhea, burning sensation in sex organs, lump in throat, amnesia, vomiting, painful extremities. Symptoms such as inexplicable hyperemesis in the 9th month of pregnancy were found in a psychiatric patient comparison group who were, nevertheless, not classified as "somatizers" because they did not have a full 14 out of the DSM required 37 pre-specified complaints. Exman et al. (1985) studying such patients who express their emotional distress through the body language of symptoms notes the frequent correlated presence of depression or alexithymia (for the latter see Taylor (1984); the reference is to an emotional disorder where there is inability to match words to feelings). Observed among these patients were impoverished interpersonal relationships, little concern for how others feel, self-preoccupation, narcissistic (self-loving, egotistical, vain), fears of dependency, and a false display of dependence on physicians, i.e., "Doctor do something for me but I won't let you."

In its psychiatric diagnostic use, the "somatizing" diagnosis does, we believe, apply only to some complaining or high symptom level patients. An epidemiological study would be necessary to ascertain the size and biosocial characteristics of the population subset. By definition it excludes the pelvic pain, PMS, vaginitis, or dysmenorrhea fatigue patient who may not have been distressed before age 30 or who does not have either the screening test 7 or a full 14, as for example, functional loss of voice, blindness, paralysis, unconsciousness-fainting, amnesia, lump in throat, all of which are recognizable still as "old fashioned" dramatic "hysteria." In the meantime, we must be aware of the likelihood of misunderstanding when the obstetrician-gynecologist or health psychologist talks of somatizers (somaticizers) to psychiatrists, for the latter will have a much more specific subgroup more obviously "neurotic"— to use a term official psychiatry has now discarded—in mind.

Important for an appreciation of the emotional components which may "participate" in a presenting gynecological complaint is the finding (Byrne, 1984, cited by Eisenberg, 1984) that serious emotional distress (that classified by the investigator as psychiatric morbidity) occurred among a sample of London gynecological patients at a rate twice as great as detected in a matched community sample. It is not known to what extent this emotional distress is influential as a symptom appraisal factor motivating the medical visit, as response to illness, as co-morbidity, or as etiologically consequential.

Stone (1985) notes that reported and treated psychiatric disorder is greater among women than men. She calls attention to the interaction between normal, or abnormal hormonal affects and personality or affective (mood) disorder as such. And she reminds us that drugs used by women to treat their mood distress, (whether as OTC or other folk medication or by prescription) will in turn have effects on reproductive functions, including menstruation. One does not rule out further disruptions of mood from endocrine disturbance as a response to CNS drugs prescribed.

Dupue and Monroe (1986) offer some useful estimates of the prevalence in normal populations (unfortunately male and female differences are not broken down) of a core group of people with chronic, albeit fluctuating and intermittent, emotional and/or physical distress non specifically measured (on typical symptom inventories) and as self-characterized. These are women with irritability, anxiety, depression, or hopelessness. They are likely to be women who show high stress sensitivity— feeling vulnerable and quick to worry— they see themselves as victims, not assertive participants in life, and are, thus, aggrieved. Link and Dohrenwend (1980) use psychiatrist Jerome Frank's term for this common condition of women, "demoralization." They may feel helpless, and they are angry. Their work lives are unsatisfactory, they are sensitive, life is too often "too much." This same group appear to have a high propensity for expressing somatic disturbance, or psychosomatic complaints, from headache to digestive disorder, sleep problems, tachicardia and, we would suspect, a greater risk of pelvic pain. It may not be that this group is "under" more stress in the sense that more alien and adverse forces randomly strike them, although there is one subgroup whose expressive despair is entirely responsive to the continuing bad luck of being poor, out of work— not all of which by any means they bring on themselves— badly married and the like. Some in the negative core group may have genetic propensities, and/or suffer chronically in adulthood the learned pain of childhood, that resulting in the typical "negative affect" syndrome. Supplementing their number will be women characterizable by psychicatric depression, bipolar disorder, or sleep disorder.

What is the size of this core group, the members of which suffer chronically in their lives "out there" (and inflict some pain as well, since negative affect is hardly any joy to live with as husband, child, or friend)? Indeed such women can readily suffer lack of "social support" because they drive it away) and are more often found in the health professional's office? Dupue and Monroe, drawing on data from Link and Dohrenwend (1980), and citing Hinkle, Najman, and Thurlow propose that these chronically distressed constitute 25% of the population.

What is of essential importance for the woman's health professional to bear in mind is that women more than men suffer this broad "demoralized" condition. All studies are consistent in showing an average 10% more woman, or one-third of all adult American women, on average (lower for the wealthy, more among the poor) are so affected and afflicted. No wonder the medical practitioner's office will have a high proportion of somaticizing "over-reacting," emotionally difficult, and otherwise psychobiologically distressed patients.

Symptoms As Self-Appraisal: Two Systems In Conflict

Pennebaker demonstrates a number of variables found to predict quite successfully to varying rates of symptom reporting among normal subjects. Under experimental conditions where symptoms are mostly of autonomic CNS status, people are not very accurate about their bodily states. Women consistently report more symptoms than men and are more accurate than men in their bodily self-assessments.

That psychological laboratory finding of inaccuracy in bodily self-appraisals qua symptom reporting among the presumably physically healthy is compatible with data from physician visits. Recall that only a small proportion of self-reported illness episodes lead to the doctor's office, but even so, about half will be described as "not serious" (National Center for Health Statistics, 1978). The most common diagnosis, among general practitioners, is no diagnosis at all but for "examination" or "general symptoms" (National Center for Health Statistics, 1977). The discrepancy between women's sensitive self-evaluations versus the physician's clinical ones is further illustrated by Trussell's (1959) findings that only 22% of American rural residents' self-reported problems were found, upon presentation to a physician, to be "present."

It is data of this sort which have led to terms such as "the worried well," "the somaticizer," "the over-utilizer," or less kindly, the "crock" or "problem patient." These terms are applied more often to women because they do make more visits and do generally, in the office and out, complain of more symptoms without having any greater mortality or morbidity than men. Feminists will also contend that the derogatory terms reflect "sexism" or chauvinism among physicians most of whom are male, or as physicians, have taken on "male values" in order to successfully compete in medicine. Greek peasants, in a rural morbidity study there (Blum and Blum, 1965), show dramatic contradictions between their interpretative framework for evaluating and accounting for health problems and that of physicians. Peasants summarize the discrepancy readily, and without rancor, for there are "diseases the doctor knows" and "diseases doctors don't know."

Implied in the contrast between the self-evaluations of women, where symptoms and complaints are presented as illness, and the physician's findings of that "not present" is a conflict between interpretive frameworks, ways of sensing and defining the meaning of bodily events.

We have earlier indicated that one of the tasks before the women's health specialist, and the woman herself, fundamental to health promotion is bridging the two worlds' gap. Certainly many have experienced tension when the physician says, "I find nothing wrong" and the woman responds "but I know something is wrong." The Greek peasants may well be on to something when they speak of "diseases the doctor doesn't know," especially if that is paraphrased to say, "the woman is painfully influenced by events the doctor doesn't know." It is there, in understanding those events that lead to "unfounded" complaints, that office based health promotion is at work. That understanding is one practice which begins the expansion of mutual communication and the shared effort at change. It addresses the risk factors associated with the relatively simple business of complaint levels, for we shall see that reducing inappropriate over-use of medical facilities is fairly easy. That understanding forms the basis for the next and more difficult steps of assisting toward changes in how the woman lives and experiences her life, not simply so that "functional" symptom visits are reduced, but so that actual illness risk is itself reduced. Health promotion, here as "wellness" promotion, begins each day in the office, face to face.

Same Words, Different Meanings

When the woman's word is "pain" and the practitioner finds no physical referent, puzzlement or worse may ensue, for the patient and the healer may disagree on what is an appropriate basis in meaning for that complaint. This is a simple example of two worlds of meaning which use the same term but in different ways. A psychologically oriented care-giver may hear the patient say "pain" and, if she has been referred as without organic basis, be not puzzled; he/she may understand that a woman's anguish may be somatized or simply expressed thus in symbolic terms. (Yet a medical devil lurks here, for if the physical examination has not been thorough, physical pathology may well be present, as for example in pelvic pain mistakenly viewed as "functional.") Schwartz and Wiggins (1986), arguing for Engel's (1977) biopsychosocial approach to medicine, insist that the practitioner understand how many different worlds of meaning there are, how these meanings function as parts of life systems (family, community, medicine, etc.), and how meanings as parts of "structures" provide a kind of predictability, order, simplicity, control, and adjustment. Such theorizing (Wiggins is a philosopher) reminds us that there may be less of "concrete" or a "hard facts" agreement than the tissue-oriented surgically, technically inclined, molecularly reductionist medical scientist might prefer in dealing with the woman's world.

Yet just these complexities, nuances, abstractions become an essential focus for good science and practice. Take the findings of Brooks-Gunn (1986) on premenstrual syndrome (PMS). One hundred thirty women in a clinical sample said they had PMS. In an ordinary study, such self-diagnosis might have qualified them as subjects for the typical PMS research or treatments, which accept much variation by way of symptoms, a curiously high rate of placebo effectiveness, and frequently, clinical improvement arising from quite general life style interventions such as diet, exercise, tension-reduction and, sometimes, the charisma (or malarky?) of the "I know exactly what's wrong with you" physician. Brooks-Gunn used careful history-taking procedures to rule out those women whose symptoms were not, in fact, classically premenstrual. Only 24 women remained "with" PMS. But then, applying examination criteria as well, only 8 "true" PMS cases remained.

This work offers a cautionary tale. Since "PMS" is a medical term adopted into folk parlance, the findings tell us how much of a modern woman's language about herself is learned from physicians, or popular health readings, or the language of women speaking amongst themselves using "medical" terms. But since physicians themselves differ widely in their PMS diagnoses, i.e., it is a most unreliable classification one physician to the next, we are reminded that the unreliability of folk parlance can be but a mirror of medical practice itself when faced with psychosomatic complaints.

The moral of the story is that when women "out there" use "medical" terms for self-description, or in presenting themselves for medical care, we may not assume their system of meanings is our own. Nor is one to assume that women "out there" would agree on the meaning of medical, symptom words they use.

Cultural-Ethnic Variations

Learned styles and setting appropriate conduct studied by anthropologists doing work in cultural medicine are shown to make a difference in symptom reporting. There are cultural differences in how children are trained to interpret and speak of bodily events and allowed to express distress. Complaints about physical distress can have social, culturally approved, as well as interpersonal functions. People do use physical complaints as a way of talking about something else hidden but important in ways that vary from one culture to the next.

Zborowski (1952) showed that pain reporting was higher among Italian Catholics and Jews than among Irish Catholics and "old Americans" (WASPS). Zola (1973) in a partial replication observed that Irish, with the same disorders giving an Italian vocalized pain, would complain only of difficulties in task accomplishment. Clark (1959), in a study of Mexican Americans, illustrated how beliefs as to illness causality have functions of blame, ordering, and exoneration, a framework which reminds us that symptoms, and illness, often have interpersonal adaptation or goal achieving value as "solutions" to personal or social problems, or ways of expressing these that vary from culture to culture.

Lin et al. (1985) in a study of 3000 Asian immigrants observe that somatization per se is greater for people in transition, whether that be cultural or simply geographical. Culture teaches how one bespeaks pain; for Chinese for example, depression employs a somatic idiom. Insofar as migration represents prior catastrophic experience and is usually characterized by difficulties in adjustment, including those of language, belonging, predictability, and felt control of events, poverty, one can also understand the stress of migration. In the Lin Asian study, women who were head of household, having a large poor family, those with poor English proficiency, all had greater somatization. In general, (Blum, 1960, Barsky, 1979) somatization is more common among the less well off, those rural, and those in ethnic groups which teach one or another version of the "stiff upper lip" when one feels emotional distress. But continuing distress will likely "will out," whether as emotion, "acting out" (getting drunk, driving dangerously, a suicide attempt, etc.), or bodily complaint. If pathological processes are thereby set in motion and not controlled, whether alcoholism or hypertension or immunosuppression, it "will out" as morbidity/mortality risk.

Situational Roles, Troubles, And Complaints

O'Neill and Zeicher (1985), in a study of American working women, most of them professional/managerial, found that women who reported more work overload, uncertainty about their position, conflict in the job situation, and greater responsibility were also those who reported greater psychological distress as anxiety and depression, and physical symptomology. Stressful work related events were more often reported by the anxious-depressed-high symptom level group; also those women with more symptoms rated these more intensively. Thus, symptom intensity is associated with anxiety-depression as part of the constellation of felt work stress and troublesome work event frequency. It was also the case that women in the "I am at high work stress" group described using more of what are called "active-behavioral coping strategies" by which is meant, we suspect, doing more, more intensely, and more rapidly when under stress. That seems much like a typical Type A scurry to regain control. But, in a "no win" irony, it was also observed that those women who responded to work troubles by avoiding them, turning their backs, or otherwise doing something else, were particularly likely to be depressed, anxious and to have high physical symptom levels. It may be that the remaining two strategies (all women in the study were assessed on the basis of responses to a hypothetical case and what women said they would do, so that one is here dealing with self-descriptions again, not on-the-job independent observations), (a) information-seeking, that is, finding out before acting, and (b) accommodating to the troublesome work feature, were either best, or were the questionnaire choices more likely elected by women who, also rather calmly, described themselves on the other assessment instruments as more calm and with fewer physical complaints.

All one "really" knows from a study of this sort is that women with certain ways of seeing themselves and saying how they feel about their world do consistently differ, one style of experiencing self and work world from another, on tests, complaint levels, and when asked about work and hypothetical problems there. The ways they are said to differ are in stress response, anxiety, depression, coping styles, and coping strategies. But since some of the measures used are rather good, validated, tests, one also knows that women whose test diagnosis is that they are depressed, do seem to experience their work as more troublesome, probably do behave differently on the job than others, and certainly do have higher levels of physical complaints.

Another questionnaire study (Zappert and Weinstein, 1985) confirms the lower status and higher felt distress vulnerability of working women as compared to men, this time for graduates from a nationally high ranked business school. Beginning with the observation that women's work and life roles rally are likely to impose greater anguish— the authors cite Pitts et al. finding a higher suicide rate among female than male physicians, or women in general, and epidemiological data to the effect that poor, young, single women, whether single parents or married mothers with low paid jobs, have shown the biggest increase nationally in rates of depression. And citing Haynes and Feinleib (1980), examining Framingham study data, working women are found, more than men, to suffer more felt distress, marital dissatisfaction, anger, and fewer promotions. The recent business school women questioned by Zappert and Weinstein compared to classmate men, all graduates the same two years, had lower positions and earned less. They had more household work and worries, felt unable to control their work flow, had work related conflicts over child-bearing, and while no symptom level differences were reported, had four times more often sought mental health care.

With these data on disadvantage, role stress, and vulnerability in mind, the higher absenteeism rates reported for women are understandable. Norris (1983) reports the Bureau of Labor Statistics showing 4.3% of work hours were lost due to illness or injury by women, as opposed to 3% for men. Absenteeism is 43% higher. Women are likely to offer premenstrual syndrome as a work place clinic complaint, with one plant showing 36% of all female workers receiving sedatives from the industrial clinic. But one must keep in mind that work in itself, which many people really do not like (in spite of the Puritan ethic), may be the force leading to PMS as an acceptable complaint (Lerner, 1985). Work situations for many people are places of work powerlessness, imposed deprecation of selves, demanded mindlessness, self-blame for what others have generated and (mis)managed, and personal anger and unfulfillment. Under such conditions, body focus and the escapist "cure" of requested sedatives become substitutes, and a distorted way of expressing distress. "Opting out" does not invite cooperation, and indeed, as a "sickness," it blocks management retaliation. But, like many other symptoms and psychoactive drug use, the expression of individualized distress will not work a "cure" on the situation which engenders distress.

It is not unreasonable to conclude from the foregoing research that being a women sensitive to work situations, and to the actual disadvantages of the woman's role vis-a-vis a man at work, as stress, i.e., being stress vulnerable, is "really" also associated with feeling emotionally bad generally. At work this could be shown by either scurrying to control, or ignoring problems. This is accompanied by that self-sensitivity which expresses itself as a higher level of physical symptoms, including those referrable to menstruation, and PMS. Complaints reflect differences in experiencing self in the world, i.e., complaint levels differentiate among women, and between working women versus men.

One cannot say from such research anything about whether there are any differences in current diagnosable physical pathology between the two women's groups, or between the men and women. The best guess, thinking now of the other data about women who are depressed, anxious, "stressed," is that among some there will be chronic nonadaptive physiological differences. That would mean a heightened future "real disease" risk for these women, all else held constant.

When one adds more situational factors to the comparison of working women, in this case comparing working to non-working women, and also classifies them with reference to marital status, one finds that each situation is likely to produce differential vulnerability and differential expression of response to stress (Kandel et al., 1985, Stewart and Salt, 1981). Women under job stress tend to respond somatically, with headaches, digestive disturbance or cardiovascular symptoms including hypertension. When the pressures are at home, whether she be married or single, the woman is more likely to be depressed, nervous, or to sleep poorly. Single working women have more physical symptoms than do wives who work, whereas single women without jobs reported more depression than jobless married women. Interestingly, the women doing most— having a job, being a wife, and having children— reported less physical illness and less depression. Whether some kind of stress protection is provided by family social support stimulus variability, and multiple obligations, or whether hardier women take on more active lives, one cannot say. What does seem likely is that life situations typical for modern women do affect both the kinds and intensity of unwell responses. It is not unreasonable to expect that personality factors and resources affect the choice of life situations as well or unwell reactions to them.

A study by Carrie (1981) indicates that women with previously high levels of complaints either about menstruation (dysmenorrhea) or general health have more intense symptoms of distress later when they become pregnant. It appears that reacting adversely to reproductive system events has predictive value, or looked at another way, it a continuing situation for some women. It is paradoxical that others (Norris, 1983) report that one kind of menstrual distress, PMS, is associated with feeling exceptionally well during pregnancies. The clinical and epidemiological task that faces us here, and so often in this field, is better characterization of the subgroups so that one knows which sets of complaints in which biosocial groups of women predict to adverse later health outcomes. As we shall see in discussing obstetrical risk prediction, the field beckons.

If we take the basic data that women do report more symptoms, appear more oriented to inner states, and that event reporting is a function of change, one asks, what is there about women that is more change? Is there some sex linked predisposition that is a function simply of experiencing more change, that now independent of variables such as boredom, optimism, not being in control, depression, cultural permission for more complaint, expressiveness, higher self-care commitment among higher SEC women?

Of course there is, and it us what everyone knows about women. It is the subject matter of obstetrics and gynecology, and the condition of mammalian life. The reproductive function of women is structured for and about change: over the lifetime menarche and menopause, and during the reproductive years, menstruation with its own cycle of change over the days of the month. And, when pregnancy comes, that is certainly change, from quickening throughout delivery through the postpartum phase, all with characteristic signs and typical emotional components.

We propose that that which is universal knowledge, and for women universal experience—change as inherent in reproductive function—is a fundamental feature of their greater bodily interest and awareness. It may contribute immensely to greater symptom reporting whether or not there is underlying pathology of the sort that is a "disease that doctors know." That contribution can be conceived as independent of the other features that laboratory and epidemiological work have shown to be associated with more symptom reporting. In reality, many of these are part of the constellation which interrelates female reproductive biology with social experiences, social roles, and stress in the lives of women accompanying emotion.

Women's biological structure and role, inseparable from those social roles and personal feelings associated with reproduction-related events, can also be characterized as hardiness and hazard. The proof of hardiness is in survival rates. A higher percentage of females whether as infants surviving to one year, or as women to age 65 stay alive than do males, whether their race is white or black. That is the case for 1980 (where 84.7% of white woman survived to age 65 compared to 72.8% of white men (Vital Statistics Life Tables, 1980)) and it was the case before modern medical care in 1900. Wingard et al (1983) show that when known risk factors are controlled, the mortality risk for women remains lower than for men.

But while there is hardiness, there is also hazard in being a woman, especially if one is a woman unsupported by healthy surroundings and good obstetrical care. Consider that in 1979, U.S. maternal mortality was 9/6 per 100,000 (Who, 1983) and in 1900 60.8. In 1980 in Paraguay, it was 468.6 per 100,000. For some African countries not even able to gather statistics, World Health Organization estimates go up to 1100/100,000 (Rosenfield and Maine, 1985). Twenty-five percent of all deaths among women aged 15-49 in developing countries are maternal (compared to less than 1% in the U.S.). There is hazard in womanhood, and its control is part of civilization's advance. Civilization, including obstetrics, enhances hardiness. Health promotion is a step in that evolution.

How can a woman not be sensitive to change, ready to report its reality? How can a woman not be, in terms of probabilities, ready to attend to and to report about reproductive biological events or about sensitive bodily changes? Perhaps one should consider as analogs those complaints associated with stress vulnerability, and the statistically demonstrable greater risk of depression (remember, that in turn is linked to symptom reporting, medical visits, and disease risk). These events and concerns about them are understandable given the fundamental change and hazard which constitutes being a woman. Women know this as the wisdom of their being. As for their hardiness, that is represented in actual life span and in the discrepancy between complaints and disease findings.

Surely all women's health specialists know about their clients: they know they are undergoing greater physiological change over the days and years than are men, know the immense changes of pregnancy (or despair of infertility). Specialists work daily with the hazard and appreciate, in the office, delivery room, or from longevity statistics, the hardiness. But surely as the moon waxing and waning, there is going to be a problem in health promotion, presentation, and treatment for the big risk items if the health professional does not acknowledge and address himself or herself to the natural sensitivity of the woman, to her reproductive biology and its expressed concommitants.

The concomitants addressed in this chapter are those felt daily "out there," some of them the analogs of simply being a woman living her life. Women are reporting change, some of that real pain, disability, abnormality of the sort that doctors know, and some of it— the analogs or somaticized expressions— of the sort that professionals are not yet trained to know. We must also acknowledge that some health professionals will not want to deal with psychosocial-behavioral analogs, even if these are part of expanded definitions not simply of needed care but of a medico-legal standard of care. For these latter persons— some of them strongly technical in their orientations, many of them will not be willing to spend additional time with its economic repercussions— the solution is inclusion of psychosocial-behavioral factors in history taking and etiological comprehension, but following that, referrals of the sort we shall later discuss. If the physicians cannot do health promoting work themselves, someone else as an alter ego can do it for the physician. We are back to the two worlds that must work at becoming one if medical practice is to help the woman to reduce that illness which arises in part from the woman's life and conduct. Just as the woman's world includes others, for instance, her family or employers, so now the health professional's system is also understood to be an expanded one, including allies in behavioral health.

Summary Comment

Women commonly complain of symptoms, or being otherwise unwell. Being symptomatic is the normal state. Only a few of these episodes are brought to the attention of health professionals; most are diagnosed and treated at home. A number of factors, physical, psychosocial, cultural, and economic, influence the way bodily states are evaluated, talked about, and whether or not a care-seeking decision is made. By no means are severity of pain or disability the only factors in seeking medical care. In that sense neither are complaints nor care decisions "rational," viewed according to current standards of medical science.

The discrepancies between women's actual unwellness experience and its evaluation, and those frameworks for evaluation used by health professionals, demonstrate a contrast between two worlds of experience, values, priorities. One first-step goal of health promotion is to bring these systems into unity; the physician and nurse are to understand the influences which account for, particularly, high symptom levels "out there" where women live their daily lives. Women are to be assisted to become aware of their own characteristics and situations which may account for their almost daily varying levels of feeling well or unwell and, over time, to exert more control over those conditions that put them at risk of unwellness. Over time, too, and through the educative communication, one looks to the more accurate differentiated awareness of sensations, signs, and feeling states, which do and do not have implications— as risk, potential disease process or pathology— for physical or mental illness.

Complaints as such, when being discussed by the health professional and the patient, are to be the basis not simply for the conventional diagnostic work and assessment of treatment, and compliance, but also become a means for learning about the life of the woman— a first step in identifying what risk factors in living and in personality exist and thinking about how the woman may be assisted to awareness and her subsequent "at home" attempts at change for amelioration, and regulation.

Implied is that the physician, nurse practitioner, or licensed midwife or health psychologist are at work developing a common language and framework for looking at how bodily or emotional sensations arise to become "complaints." Those from the two worlds— the woman's real life and the professional's science and clinical practice— aim to develop a differentiated perspective, one that does not solely involve on the woman's part language referring to bodily "sickness" as an expression for changes, including distress, experienced but not, or not yet, medically pathological.

At present, the data tell us that the majority of women coming to the physician, especially general or family practitioners, can expect to be told in one way or another that "nothing is wrong." In doing that, the physician has failed to understand the problem. The act is not only one of implied rejection which can generate tension—or too many prescriptions—between doctor and patient, but it also derogates the woman's way of expressing her unwellness. This physician has missed an opportunity to find out what is happening in the patient's life, some of which may very well be ameliorable hazard, and some of which may well pose risk, if not changed, of "real" disease. To prevent disease, to promote wellness, the health professional begins where the woman is, learning about her life and sensations. Then, using that knowledge of factors which contribute to high symptom levels (including the challenge of perhaps 25% of ordinary women chronically emotionally distressed with corresponding diffuse psychosomatic symptoms) and/or to disease risk (to be presented in the next chapters), to begin a health promotion treatment plan. In this instance, since most of what has to be done is to be done by the woman, and when she is lucky by her supporting intimates, the plan must evolve cooperatively. A later section will discuss that evolution.

Based on available data, we believe that central to the fact of the propensity of women to have high levels of complaints, many more outside the medical office than in it, is the fact of their reproductive biology which daily, monthly, and over life's epochs is one of change. Women are more inner oriented, are constantly exposed to changes in function and sensation which are noticeable, alerting, often disconcerting, and are reportable. Stimulus change is what sensation is about. However hardy women are, statistically and in terms of health levels, self care, and longevity, they are also subject to and cannot but be psychobiologically aware of their hazards. These are hazards—vulnerabilities—associated with their reproductive biology and its associated, ensuing social roles and circumstances. One may posit that their hazard sensitivity has survival value not simply for themselves, but also for the species.

The subject matter of the woman's complaints is her bodily function: change, much of it the psychobiology of being reproductive. The subject matter of the obstetrician-gynecologist is exactly the same. Much that is health promotion for women will be in attention to these same matters, whether as vulnerability, sexual conduct, pregnancy, self care, or menstrual complaints. Those aspects of health promotion which are the same for women and men will be better approached in the forthcoming partnership in the treatment plan (as we shall see in a later section this may, after evaluation, call for referral). A solid doctor-patient relationship is necessary, beginning with understanding and respecting the genesis of complaints and the unavoidable self-sensing, genuinely "sensational" nature of being a woman.

4

Prevalence of Diagnosed Conditions Among Women: Behavioral Considerations

This chapter is compromised of a series of tables presenting an epidemiological array of women's diagnosed conditions, health behaviors, or service needs. While later chapters present the catalog of psychosocial-behavioral features shown through research to contribute to mortality, obstetrical diagnosed morbidity, or specific illness risk, the tabular prevalence material here will, on its face, compel a conclusion about the importance of psychosocial-behavioral components. Looking at the list of reasons for visits, services rendered, self care not taken, diagnoses made, it is evident that much of what the women's health specialist hears, sees, does, or what he or she advises as a regimen— that only sometimes to result in patient "compliance"— involves matters that are the object of health promoting work.

It would be fine to be able to say that that which is so obviously the general business of the women's specialist is recognized as such in practice. Surely the scientific data and the standards set forth by the American College of Obstetrics and Gynecologists, and the training requirements of the Council on Resident Education in Obstetrics and Gynegology persuade to that practice. But the training study data in Chapter 1 make it clear that physicians are *not* being educated to comprehend how much these human factors are their business, or to know what to do about them.

comprehend how much these human factors are their business, or to know what to do about them.

In this chapter, we also make some comparisons among, and inferences from, the statistics on diagnosis. When records from the office practitioner or his or her hospital are compared against data derived from case identifying studies of particular disorders with strong behavioral etiology and content, it becomes evident from the sometimes immense discrepencies that such disorders are highly susceptible to being overlooked in daily practice. Those data repeat or are reminiscent of the example in Chapter 1 about alcoholism.

Were there no effective treatments for such disorders in women, perhaps a missed diagnosis would not matter, unless that led to any inappropriate procedure or prescription or any otherwise avoidable risk of iatrogenic or nosocomial disease. But, happily, the darker ages are behind us and effective means for reducing risk, improving compliance, and directly intervening in the behavioral components of such disorders do exist. Thus any failure of medical awareness, interest, diagnostic acumen, energy investment, or intervention, including referrals, condemn the woman to unnecessary suffering, and usually, greater further disease risk even unto death. It also denies the health professional the satisfaction of a job well done, the patient's acknowledgement of that, and, to be practical, that continuing involvement in a necessary augmented treatment program, now as health promotion, which helps the practitioner earn a living.

Data on average office visit length are also presented for selected conditions. Time allocations are ordinarily so limited that psychosocial evaluations of etiology and risk cannot be conducted, nor is there time for health promotional interventions. When the prescription data are reviewed it allows a clear inference as to what is done instead. It is data compatible both with the high complaint levels among women and frequent finding of "no physical disorder" discussed in the previous chapter. We see that women receive more prescriptions, more tranquilizers, and on the average, prescriptions are written on about half of the occasions when there are no disease findings. As we shall see in a later chapter's discussion of negotiated diagnoses, both the woman and the physician may agree to drugs as a substitute for more appropriate but time and trouble taking interventions. As it is now, gross overprescribing suggests both parties are willing to bear the increased financial costs of such medication and the risk of adverse reactions including be said to be "acting out" the irrelevance of the inappropriate prescription. That is quite compatible with the physicians's own fundamental attitude, which is often one of uncertainty or skepticism about medication need or effects.

The health promotional effort in medical practice is, in part, one of improving the focus of attention. In the case of the pointless, costly, and often unused, adverse reaction risk prescription, it aims to improve quality of care by addressing the real situations and conduct bringing on complaints or "functional" disorders or those "general symptoms" as well as that physical pathology with psychosocial-behavioral etiology. The woman who, in her average 6 to 10 minute GP visit gets and throws away the prescription (or worse, keeps it in the medicine chest to put the family at risk), feels the care she receives is irrelevant, even if briefly reassuring. The physician who dashes off that prescription even when he is writing down (later for the Public Health Service statisticians to report to us), "observation" or "examination only" also knows what is done is irrelevant, even if a conventional impropriety. It is easy to give a prescription, the woman may expect it, wanting to be given something as proof that she feels bad, but the tacit admission by both parties of inappropriateness tells us that here is a point where the two worlds, the woman and her physician, are very close to a common starting point, however, a bad one. From irrelevance, superficiality, or uncommunicated mutual dissatisfaction with things as they are, but are not evaluated for change, the health promotional task is to find out what complaint and health related risks are really "out there" in the woman's life, and to get started on getting to work recognizing and dealing with them.

Table II
U.S. National Prevalence Data from Records

II.A   Diagnosis for short term hospital stay for women. (NCHS 1983, 1985). Ranked by order of prevalence
1. Vaginal delivery
2. Caesarean section (C-section) without co-morbidity
3. Non radical hysterectomy
4. Dilation and curettage (D & C) of uterus without malignancy

5. Abortion with D & C of uterus
6. Vaginal delivery with sterilization
Situation and regional variation: By community C-section rates vary from 5% to over 30%, with a national average about 15% (Porreco, 1985). Porreco shows no difference in outcome on mortality for a managed rate of 5.7 vs. an institutional norm of 17.6%. Implied is the interaction of physician judgemental, institutional norm and patient preference variables, all as psychosocial. Since 1984 surgical case loads for Ob-Gyn practitioners are falling. The only categories of increased surgery are caesarean and elective infertility remedial efforts. Grimes (1986) suggests that reduced overall surgery will direct greater attention to primary prevention. "In the the years ahead, social gynecology may emerge as a discipline of equal status as surgical gynecology." (p76)

II.B Office visits by women (multiple diagnoses recorded yield a sum greater than 100%, NCHS 1977)
Ranked by frequency of reason visit and time spent.
For general practitioners:
General symptoms 73%
Digestive system complaint 69%
Musculoskeletal complaints 42%
Genitourinary complaint 42%
For obstetrician-gynecologists
Family planning 62%
Pre and post operative care 42%
Symptoms referrable to genitourinary system 41%
By time spent (selected diagnoses)
Prenatal care 11 minutes
Disorders of menstruation 18 minutes
Personality-emotional disorder (4% of all diagnoses) 25-47 minutes
Note on age variation:
Disorders of menstruation peak at 70/1,100 at age bracket 25-34
Menopausal symptoms peak at 180/1,000 ages 45-54

II.C For female adolescents and youth; diagnoses for ambulatory presenting complaints referrable to the reproductive system: (NCHS, 1984, #99)

By rank:
pregnancy
contraceptive management
diseases due to viruses and chlamydiae
disorders of menstruation
other abnormal bleeding

II.D Disorders of the female reproductive system, adults (NCHS, 1977-78, #13)
By rank:
infective diseases of the uterus (except cervix)
disorders of menstruation
menopausal symptoms
chronic cystic diseases of the breast and other non-neoplastic breast disease
benign and unspecified neoplasms of the female genital organs
infective diseases of the cervix uteri and other diseases of the cervix
malignant neoplasms of the breasts
diseases of the parametrium and pelvic peritoneum
diseases of the ovary and fallopian tubes
selected diagnoses arrayed by time spent "very serious" for breast disorder, very serious modal time is 1-10 minutes
other diseases, very serious modal time 16-31 minutes

II.E Primary diagnoses in patient-physician encounters with obstetrician-gynecologists (Mendenhall, 1977)
prenatal care
medical or special examination
medical and surgical aftercare
postpartum observation
disorders in menstruation
sexually transmitted disease: infections of the uterus, vagina, vulva
delivery without complication
menopausal symptoms
uterovaginal prolapse
personal (visit) without complaint/illness
abortion with medical indications

sterility, female
uterine fibroma
other pregnancy complications
symptoms (other) referrable to the genitourinary system
other diseases of the cervix
diseases of the parametria
other diseases of the uterus
malignant neoplasms: cervix uteri
other female genital diseases
other malignant neoplasms-uterus
infective disease-cervix uteri
benign neoplasms-ovary
moniliasis
abortion - spontaneous/unspecified
cystitis
symptoms related to abdominal/lower gastrointestinal tract
observation without medical care need
pre-eclampsia/ eclampsia/ toxemia
The foregoing account for 88/1% of all patient diagnosis and 84% of physician time.

II.F   Non illness care (NCHS 1980-81) for obstetrics-gynecology office visits
Non illness care: 61.9%

II.G   Office practitioner diagnoses*, both sexes, seriousness of complaint (NCHS 1978) Selected findings
Not serious: 48.2%
Findings (selected) by rank:
  examination without finding disease
  orthopedic pain and swelling
  among the remaining top ten: benign hypertension
                                abdominal pain
                                prenatal care
                                neurosis
*Median visit length; all visits: 6-10 minutes

Possible diagnostic error in the finding of no disease, or in the "not serious" judgement.

Duff and Hollingshead (1968) report that over half of the cases in their hospital study had been misdiagnosed. Prutting (1978), comparing autopsy findings to antemortem diagnoses, found 40-50% of the latter to be wrong. Brook et al. (1976) in a review conclude, "in the last 60 years, nearly 1000 studies have been done to assess the level of quality of care delivered . . . virtually all . . . have detected basic problems. . . ." Mechanic (1976) reported that physicians who see proportionately greater numbers of patients than their (matched) colleagues are more apt to view patient complaints as trivial or inappropriate. Blum (1958) found physicians who saw very large numbers of patients daily in practice to be at greater risk for malpractice suits.

II.H New pain presented in office based care: (NCHS, 1984, #97)
By rank:
  ear ache
  chest pain
  headache
  genitourinary

II.I Urinary: office visits: (NCHS 1978, #39)
Remarks: Cystitis ranks first among diagnoses. Incontinence in the U.K. (citation by Cartwright, 1982) studies yield slightly varying rates: from .02% in women 15-64, to 3.5 - 7.1% or 8.5% having significant regular incontinence, to 45% reporting, in health surveys, some degree of urinary incontinence. The discrepancy supports the Lancet 1977 conclusion as to likely prevalence underestimation. In the U.K., only about 10% of urinary incontinent women consulted a physician. The decision for most not to bother was based on expecting no treatment efficacy (a realistic appraisal according to the Lancet editor).

II.J Sexually transmitted diseases: (See Schofield (1979) and Hatcher et al (1986) McCormack 1983, The Nations Health, January 1985 and July 1985.
As an aggregate these now are the most prevalent serious infections among (sexually active) adults and the serious infections or obstetrical risks most likely encountered in ob-gyn care. Venereal disease per se (syphilis, gonorrhea, chancroid, lymphogranuloma venerium,

granuloma inguinal) constitute a minority. Diseases capable of either non-sexual or sexual tranmission,[1] nonspecific urethritis, trichomoniasis, genital candidosis, scabies, genital warts, exoparasitic infections, molloscum contagiosum, genital herpes,[2] chlamydia trachomitis, Reiter's disease, mycoplasma hominis, Gardnerella vaginalis, mobiluneus, acquired immune deficiency, hepatitis B (AHB Ag), cytomegalo virus, mononucleosis, enteric disease, acute urethral syndrome or cystitis, cervical intraepithelial neoplasia (CIN), mucopurulent cervicitis, pelvic inflammatory disease (PID),vulvovaginitis (trichomoniasis, bacterial condidiasis) pediculosis and phthirus pubis combine to achieve STD dominant infectious prevalence. Chlamydia trachomitis is estimated to be the most prevalent female STD infection. Condylomata acumenata (genital warts) is the most common viral STD.

II.K Prescriptions: prevalence on office visits and compliance: (NCHS, 1979)

By rank, the most common disease categories generating prescriptions are:
    disorders of respiration and circulation
    central nervous system (including tranquilizers and sedatives)
    endocrine disorders (for electrolytic balance and diet related conditions)
    antineoplastics

Prescriptions for women:

Women receive more prescriptions for psychoactive drugs than do men (Verbrugge and Steiner 1985, citing Abelson et al). They receive 73% of all tranquilizers (Nation's Health, 1985). Women receive more prescriptions per capita annually and spend more on medications. When complaints are held constant, they receive more prescriptions than do men at a rate of from 1 to 18% greater prescription incidence. With complaints held constant, women are particularly likely to receive prescriptions for obesity, and during those visits when no diagnosis is rendered. Prescriptions are given to about 30% of women receiving no diagnosis, 20% getting an "examination" as diagnosis, and almost 60% when the complaints are "general." Fifteen percent receiving "observation without need for further care" get a prescription. Prescriptions are also a physician and visit characteristic, i.e., GPs and family practitioners prescribe

60% more than do specialists, solo practitioners more than group or hospital-based physicians.
Prescription compliance prevalence: Data and comment:
An overall compliance rate of 50% is commonly estimated. This an averaging of quite varying rates depending upon patient, physician, setting, etc., variables almost all of which are psychosocial, including doctor-patient interaction styles. Some work shows conformity to be as low as 20%. Even when patient motivation is presumably high, and the regimens quite simple, compliance is by no means complete. One study of oral iron prescribed to pregnant women found 69% compliance (for reference see Blum et al., 1981, Cartwright, 1984, Kirscht & Rosenstock, 1979) Lenenthal, Zimmerman and Gutmann, 1984).
Physician expectations no doubt play a role; Cartwright (1984) reviews work showing, in the U.K. (in 1964) that physician expectations were for a placebo effect in 11% of prescriptions, an uncertain therapeutic effect in 55% and only in 24% a reasonable assurance of an intended therapeutic outcome. General expectations may also be brought to bear. In the U.K. almost half of adults surveyed contended that physicians were too quick to give prescriptions; on the other hand, when patients expected a prescription from a visit they almost inevitably received one.

II.L Sexual dysfunction in women: (Jospe, Nieberding & Cohen, 1980, Watson and Banber, 1980, Knesper et al., 1985).
Percent of all patients in current care for emotional or mental disorders (men and women) with psychosexual dysfunction; Psychiatrists: 2.1%, Psychologists: 3.3%, Primary care physicians: 3.3%.
In contrast, lifetime prevalence estimates for self-perceived sexual problems to approach 100% for women. A preliminary study indicated current marital and sexual problems in 16% of married women. The majority of patients experiencing surgery, immobilization and other serious medical intervention report sexual maladjustment. Over half of women undergoing radiation therapy for cervical cancer are experiencing sexual disabilities 8 months after treatment. Sexual dysfunction, also associated with depression as well, is reported by 67% suffering cancer of reproductive organs. After chronic illness, 78% of women report decline in sexuality.

Specific illnesses associated with sexual malfunction include vaginal infection, cystitis, trauma, atrophic vaginitis, balanitis, leukoplakia, bartholin cyst, allergic responses to vaginal sprays, PID, leiomyoma, endometriosis, uterine prolapse, anal fissure and hemorrhoids, pelvic mass, ovarian cysts, ovariectomy, adrenalectomy, mastectomy, hysterectomy, as well as events such as rape, ostomy, obstetric trauma or poor episiotomy, and systemic illness such as diabetes, renal disease, etc.

One may also not know important information about sexual practices. For example, a study (Smith et al., 1985) of lesbian and bisexual women suggests that only about one-fifth were asked by their physician about their sexual preferences/practices, less than half reported these to their physician. Male physicians, not homosexual, were reported to react negatively to such disclosure. Among those not disclosing, fear of an adverse effect on their care was listed as constraining communication.

Discrepancy data:

Gynecologists and urologists seriously underestimate the prevalance of sexual dysfunction in ill women under their care, with an average estimate of 15% by specialists as compared to psychiatric, psychological evaluation (these more thorough and accepted here as better prevalence estimated (see above)).

With respect to patients in current care for sexual dysfunction, as a percent of all emotional distress being treated, one observes that the current care load for mental health professionals itself does not reflect the estimated prevalence of psychosexual dysfunction. Our inference is that reproductive or other disease related dysfunction is not brought to the attention of mental health professionals. It is also apparent from the data, that either it is not brought to the attention of, or, alternatively, recognized by primary care physicians regardless of their specialty (or general practice) status.

II.M   Alcoholism in women:

Among women age 21 to 35, 16% to 19% report conduct symptomatic of problem drinking (Wilsmick, 1984). Among women 35 to 49, the range, depending on what case finding criteria are employed, is 9% to 18%. Six percent of the 21 to 34 group are categorized as heavy drinkers. (These women were 2.6 times more likely to recall premature deliveries, 1.5 times greater miscarriage rate, three times more birth defects, and 2.5 times greater infertility prevalence than those not heavy drinkers.)

Drinking in pregnancy:

If alcohol use follows the same trends reported by Steward (1984) for diminished cigarette smoking where 42% of those pregnant do not reduce consumption, one estimates, extrapolating from Wilsneck data, a 2% regular heavy drinking rate among pregnant women. Marbury et al. (1983) in a large Boston sample asked at delivery about drinking (underreporting is to be expected), reports 0.7% recalling 14 or more drinks per week during pregnancy. Making less optimistic extrapolation from data reviewed by the Institute for Health Policy Studies (1985), one might estimate problem drinking in over 6% of pregnant women. What is astonishing is that representative population data is absent.

Discrepancy data:

In the National Collaborative Study (Women and Their Pregnancies (1972): alcoholism prevalence rate 55/100,000. NCHS (1977) survey, on office visit records, alcoholism does not appear as a primary diagnosis. NCHS DGR data, short stay hospital diagnoses (See Table II.a) for alcohol and related organic syndromes, also not segregated by sex, 3%. Peele (1984) estimates one-third of American families experiencing some problem with alcohol and 15,000,000 Americans with alcohol problems. Earlier cited, Science 229, 1985) alcoholism is the third leading cause of death implicated in 20% of general hospital admissions.

II.N Emotional disorders:

An NIMH epidemiological study (Science 1985), found over any one six-month period, 19% of the population to suffer a psychiatric disorder (80% of these do not seek mental health treatment). Examining only serious disorders, and among these depressions, the point prevalence rates are placed between 16% and 20% for the total population, higher for women. A 1985 report (the Nation's Health, April) indicates that women suffer from depression almost twice the rate of men. The more recent NIMH report on depression (Science, 1986) indicates that the likelihood of major depression is one in four for women, as opposed to one in ten for men. For persons undergoing an acute clinical episode, the suicide rate is 15%. In the U.K. Brown and Harris (1978) found 23% of working class, and 6%

of middle class women to be depressed. Women with symptoms of depression if and when electing care, usually seek general medical but not psychiatric help, and when and if diagnosed, are ordinarily treated using and usually insufficiently by means of psychoactive drugs.

Levi (1979) citing the President's Commission on Mental Health proposes a point prevalence rate of 15% of Americans in need of mental health services, with an additional 25% suffering anxiety and depression at mild or moderate levels. Eisenberg and Parron (1979) citing Rice show the range of mental disorders to constitute one of the major illness burdens in the U.S. Depending on method and criteria, population-at-large estimates can be higher, 75%, or lower, 10%, for all mental disorders.

Discrepancy:

NCHS 1978. Principle diagnoses of office visits yield a 4% prevalence for all psychiatric conditions. NIMH 1986 data suggest more optimistically that only 80% of depressions remain untreated.

Deficiencies: evaluation and diagnoses deficiencies in office practice have led to proposals for triaxial diagnostic systems which would mandate incorporating psychological states and social problems (Lipkin and Kupka, 1982). Subjective distress, or emotional disorder, is often expressed by reference to somatic symtoms as implied in Chapter III. A number of epidemiological instruments used to estimate psychiatric disorders combine questions about somatic and emotional states, with high intercorrelations between general physical symptoms and "feelings." It is not surprising, therefore, to confront, in population studies, confusion as to what may be emotional disorders, versus subjective awareness of less than perfect physical health, i.e., symptoms of organic dysfunction. Neither in etiology, nor in illness expression is that dichotomizing the rule of nature, rather it may derive from philosophical mind-body dualism. Antonovsky (1980), examining the overall disease burden is extremely critical of the single axis conceptual orientation of medicine.

II.O   Family planning service and advice requests: (NCHS, 1976 #45, 1984 #102, 103).

Seventy-nine percent of currently married fertile women used some type of family planning service during 1979–82.[3] Never married women used these services at a rate of greater than one visit per person over one year, 1982, a demand related to the fact of two-thirds of unmarried teenagers having had intercourse. Over 6 million never married women in 1982 had used infertility services at some time during their reproductive years, with fertility rates continuing to drop, with 10.6% of young wives age 20–24 unable to have a baby. By 1982 only about 53% of couples in the child bearing age (women 15–44) were able to have children. The figure includes couples where one spouse has been surgically sterilized (Nation's Health, April 1985 reporting NCHS data). Of married women earlier practicing contraception, by 1981, 41% elected sterilization, or have a sterilized husband (contrasted with 24% in 1973). There is a higher rate of infertility among black women, 21% vs. 13% for whites for all age groups.

II.P Health practices (NCHS 1979, NMMR 1982, Recent U.S.: Prevention Index '86, Prevention Research Center 1986, NCHS #119, 1986
Self-descriptive health practices:
Overweight: women more than men, 56% vs 36%
    more middle aged women
    women trying to lose weight, 46%
    women exercising to lose weight, 59%
    all adults self-estimated as within recommended weight range, 21%
Sedentary life styles and insufficient exercise:
    women more than men
    worse with aging
    fewer women than men exercise regularly, 39% vs 44%
    few women exercise strenuously, 8%
Hypertension checks and controls: more women than men have had their blood
    pressure checked within last 12 months, 79% vs 67%
    two survey discrepancy, 56% vs 86%
Regular seat belt use:
    in states with mandatory "buckle up" laws, 58%
    other states without mandatory laws, 32%
    two survey discrepancy, 56% vs 86%
Cigarettes: fewer women than men, 28% vs 33%

Problematic alcohol usage:
- have driven after drinking, 25-28%
- more men admit to driving after drinking too much, 18% vs 6%
- Men rate higher on heavy drinking by index, 13% vs 3%

Sleep: 7 to 8 hours per night, 64-66% for all adults

Meal regularity:
- missed breakfasts, 45%

Dental checkup:
- once a year or more, 74%

Brushing teeth twice a day: rare

Gynecological self-care:
- Pap smear within last 12 months, 62%
- Pap smear within last two years, 72-78%
- Least amount of pap smears done by women ages 45 and older
- breast self-examination once a year, less or never, 30%
- breast self-examination monthly or more, 32-48%
- breast self-examination by health professional within last 12 months, 68%
- least amount of breast self-examinations done by women ages 65 and older

Stress effects on health:
- more women saying that within the last year stress has adversely affected health, 49% vs 39%
- great stress felt once a week or more, 60%
- two study discrepancy, 60% vs 20%
- least amount of stress was felt by elders
- self-reported stress symptoms/effects:
  - headache, 24%
  - fatigue, 12%
  - nervousness, 26%
  - irritability, 19%
  - depression, 11%
- more women than men expressed a felt need for professional help for personal, emotional problems, 14% more women than men obtained help, 9% vs 5%

Home safety:
> smoke detector used, 59-67%
> someone in the household smokes in bed, 11%

Health care centers:
> have regular center or professional, 77%

Nutrition: minerals, sugar and fat control:
> women seek to assure adequate calcium intake, 65%
> women seek to limit fat in diet, 57%
> women seek to lower cholesterol, 42%
> women seek to assure fiber intake, 59%
> women seek to limit dietary sodium (salt), 54%
> women seek to limit sugars or sweets, 50%
> women seek to assure vitamin and mineral intake, 63%

Health professionals attention to nutrition, diet, as reported by their patients, as part of routine visits:
> Proper foods often discussed with women more than with men, 11% vs 8%
> "Sometimes" discussed with women, 18%
> Diet not part of routine visit subject matter when seeing a health care professional with women, 65%

Methodological comment:
The foregoing data derive from two health surveys, one by a Harris poll (Prevention Index) by telephone conducted in 1985 making inquiries to 1256 randomly selected adults. The other, by the Public Health Service NCHS, used household interviews, obtaining 16,780 questionnaires, that also in 1985. One is struck by the discrepancies in results. With reference to overweight (since the NCHS data show only 6% underweight) one must explain the 48% "about right" in that survey contrasted to the 21% "within the recommended weight range" on the Harris poll. For blood pressure checks within the last 12 months, there is a 30% difference between polls. For regular seat belt use, there is an uncalculated discrepancy of perhaps 13%. Breast self-examination reported monthly or more often differs by 16%, and reported great stress recently differs by 40%.

Consider these discrepancies an introduction to the problems of clinical history-taking as well as survey research on preventive care needs. How questions are phrased, the interpersonal mood established, who asks whom, and what the pressures on the person are to "fake good," and unclarified differences in definition all contribute. In survey sampling, methodology and sample size and interview training all affect outcomes.

One must be aware that answers given may not describe actual behavior. "Seeking" to control diet is not the same as doing it, "trying to lose weight" does not mean weight lost. The problems that plague the survey researcher, whilst they allow sensible caution about statistics on private habits offered for public display, may also be the problems of the inquiring health professional.

If that professional discusses health habits at all, consider the finding in the NCHH study that on only 10% of the recollected routine patient visits, proper diet is discussed; 65% of the time, women patients say their health professionals rarely or never discuss dietary matters. Insofar as the public are improving their self-care, and according to the aggregate Prevention Index they are doing so in some areas, year to year, in seat belt use up 22% over one year, smoke detector installation up 9%, stress control 10%, it would not seem to be the influence of health professionals that accounts for it.

On the other hand, index items showing declining self-care—maintaining recommended weight, doing strenuous exercise—or those items where the majority of citizens in both polls appear to be engaged in unsatisfactory self-care overall, such as weight control, exercise, breast self-examination, seat belt use, might well benefit from professional intervention. The same may be said for that minority of citizens, their numbers varying widely depending upon the health practice, who fail to be taking care of themselves.

II.Q Mortality in women: the primary causes of death for women, all ages (NCHS, 1979, Stat Abstract of the U.S. 1982-83):
By rank:
heart disease
malignant neoplasm (in order: cancer of the breast, lung[4], colon & rectum, ovary and the uterine cervix)
cerebrovascular disease
accidents
pneumonia and flu
diabetes
atherosclerosis
chronic obstructive lung disease
cirrhosis of the liver
suicide

II.R   Maternal mortality:
(Overall rate for the U.S. 8.5/100,000) Statistical Abstracts of the U.S., Kauntiz et al. 1985, Benedetti, Starzyk and Frost 1985, Russell, 1983, Ueland, 1983.
From Bureau of the Census, (aggregating those from pregnancy with abortive outcomes and direct obstetrical causes)

Equally ranked:
   Toxemia of pregnancy (eclampsia, preeclampsia)
   Hemorrhage
   Ectopic pregnancy/abortion
In the U.K., by rank:
   Abortion
   Pulmonary embolism
   Hemorrhage
   Toxemia of pregancy
For the U.S. for "non obstetrical" maternal deaths, first ranked:
   Cardiovascular
Separating abortion from direct obstetrical causes
Abortion: first ranked
   Ectopic pregnancy
Direct pregancy causes, by rank:
   Embolism
   Hypertensive disease of pregnancy (toxemia, eclampsia)
   Hemorrhage
   Obstetrical infection

Correcting for under-reporting, generalizing from Washington State less than half of all maternal deaths are identifiable as such from death certificates)
By rank:
   Hypertensive disease of pregnancy
   Embolism

Comment

Examination of the data in Table II documents the considerable extent to which women's conditions and service needs arise from and/or otherwise involve psychosocial and behavioral factors. Much that transpires in the office visit is non illness care. Much of the illness that arises has either direct antecedents in conduct and decisions— e.g., STD, intentional abortion— or have these and psychosocial features in multiple etiology or exacerbation, as in headache and abdominal pain; dietary, prenatal visits, and medication lapses in pre-eclampsia/eclampsia; hygienic measures in cystitis, cigarette smoking, lung cancer; diet in diabetes, omissions of breast self-examination, early sexuality in late emerging cervical cancer. A number of disorders can have psychosomatic components, as in menstrual disorder and genital complaints. The successful treatment in many illnesses depends on patient cooperation in regimens, whether pharmaceutical or in terms of conduct. At present, self-care preventive behavior leaves much to be desired.

Considerable variation in diagnoses dependent upon the data source and its diagnostic focus and thoroughness makes evident that serious underdiagnosis occurs in ordinary medical practice for sexual dysfunction, alcoholism and other drug abuse, and depression. These are not unique as diagnostic failures; we face a wider quality of care issue in which provision of health promotion is but an important component. One reasonably suspects inadequacies in training, and failures in history taking. The latter may be the worse when queries are pro forma, where the woman fears disapproval, or when she is busy denying to herself as well as others, significant aspects of her life style, health habits, situation, or feelings. Diagnostic underreporting may be compounded by the absence in normal practice of standard multiaxial (physical, social, personal) evaluation/diagnostic recording systems (see Lipkin and Kuptia, 1982), and the limited time which the ordinary physician spends with the typical patient, even in cases of the most serious disease. That constraint limits the diagnostic enterprise, the evaluation of psychosocial-behavioral circumstances in disease etiology or complaint, including proper understanding of the significance of pain and "general symptoms." A complementary medical failure is, as the data have shown, overprescription, particularly medications directed to the central nervous system and to diet-related conditions.

One also sees that even simple discussion of health practices such as nutrition rarely occurs as part of the medical visit.

We have examined a number of current obstetrical-gynecological textbooks. Their excellent biological scientific-technical content is, nevertheless compatible with the deficiencies, noted in Chapter 1, among women's specialty residents, and with the thrust of the data here. A good text will attend to all consequential aspects of physical illness, but it cannot be successful in the preparation of the practitioner, or as a reference volume, if it does not give due emphasis to these psychobiological, behavioral elements which contribute causally to those diseases, or make their differential diagnoses more difficult. Thus more attention is required for that widely prevalent somatization, including diffuse and multiple symptomatology. Guidance-giving attention to the serious emotional components and threatened women's role dysfunction accompanying serious gynecological disease and its disabling treatments is often absent. Practical guidance on compliance assessment and facilitation is also absent. That the major component of normal encounters will be non-illness and/or interpersonal transactions is thoroughly underestimated.

We seek here to provide a supplemental information and guidance source as remedy. Real success—not ours, but for the practice and health impact of the women's health professional—will be assured when texts, residency training, and the content of practice routinely address these matters. One must certainly agree with Romney et al., who in their 1975 text wrote, "The health care of women often does not involve disease. An education component...(exists) consisting of support and counsel concerning normal phenomena such as menarche, puberty, adolescence, sexuality, fertility control, sexual relations, pregnancy and menopause....Essential to maintenance of health in the female patient is education and information." "Psychosomatic and emotional conditions are frequent...and play a major role in such conditions as menstrual disorders, infertility, repeated abortion, lactation and chronic pelvic pain...Women need an early and ongoing education regarding their reproductive biology with methods of self assessment to prevent disease and maintain health."

There is now a large data base as to what is to be self- and health professional-assessed that constitutes risk potentially amenable to responsible self-regulation. There is also some better understanding of how the woman can be assisted to awareness and better health responsibility. We shall be addressing that risk and assistance in the coming chapters.

Summary

Statistical data on women's diagnoses show that many visits to general practitioners yield no diagnosed illness. Among these women almost half will, nevertheless, receive a prescription. Discrepancy data between known prevalence rates for disorders such as alcoholism, depression, and sexual dysfunction allow the conclusion that much disorder that is in fact present is missed by the physician. Almost half of all office visits by women are not considered serious by the physician, and even visits for very serious illnesses are ordinarily short ones. That brevity disallows inquiry into the psychosocial-behavioral factor with etiological roles in many common complaints as well as life threatening illnesses.

In 1986, the major causes of death for women were, in order: heart disease, cancers of the breast and lung, the colon, rectum, ovary and uterine cervix, cerebrovascular accident, pneumonia and flu, diabetes, atherosclerosis, chronic obstructive lung disease, cirhosis of the liver and depending on the reporting year, suicide. For maternal death in the U.S., hypertension (toxemia) of pregnancy appears first ranked. One would expect a long term health promotion impact on the majority of those.

Evaluation of emotional concomitants or of cooperation in care is limited by the current focus and brevity of the average office visit. The majority of that which transpires during the encounter with the women's health professional and the woman is acknowledged to be non-illness care, or dealing with somatization or with complaints with psychosocial-behavioral features in origin, expression, or as consequential sequalae. Nevertheless, evaluation of residents in women's health specialty training, and of excellent textbooks in the field, compels the conclusion that these areas important to disease prevention, wellness, and better quality of care are, at present, ignored. Prescribing is, on the other hand, much overdone. The proper emphasis on health promotion will increase the health professional's awareness of these data and problems and will, clinically, aim to assist the woman in a similar self-relevant awareness. Both parties will also be assuming a greater responsibility for securing those changes in the woman's conduct, and feelings, which foster disease prevention, reduced pointless medicating, wiser utilization of care, and wellness.

Footnotes

1. We do not classify cervical cancer, as some do, as an STD. We believe it is necessary to discriminate between sexual behavior as contributing to risk and precipitation, as opposed to the need to demonstrate, for the STD definition, direct transmission of pathogens. Human papilloma virus are clearly implicated but the causal proofs of the microbial model are not yet at hand. (See Singer et al., 1984.)

2. One may not know the transmission origin (sexually transmitted or otherwise) for some viral genital diseases. Grossman (1985) observes that genital herpes may arise from a dormant state after asymptomatic childhood infection under conditions of adult stress. Since 60-80% of women are seroreactive to herpes (consider that 75% of herpes B carriers never experience clinical symptoms; see also Adler and Storthlz, 1985), the stress hypothesis suggests an important psychosocial feature for disease expression.

3. Psychosocial factors are also associated with failure to seek family planning among those where pregnancy poses a risk, is unwanted, or otherwise imposes serious adverse personal or social costs, or when there is a failure to use already obtained contraceptives when pregnancy is not desired. Women having repeat abortions constitute a subgroup of special interest. Among factors identified, in small population studies, as associated with irregular contraception practices, are, in the U.K. (Cartwright, 1982) prior psychiatric disorders, and diffidence on the part of both the woman and her physician so that no discussion occurs (attributed to a general "conspiracy of silence"). Sterilization itself may present problems; in the U.K. (1982) where 19% of married women are sterilized, 21% of them have "regrets" and a further 45% reporting post sterilization menstrual problems. Are some of these "somaticized" regret?

4. It is estimated that for 1985 lung cancer will account for 18% of all female mortality, equivalent to breast cancer, and that cancer of the colon and rectum will be third ranked. The lung cancer contribution to women's deaths is up from 3% in 1950 and is attributed, by the American Cancer Society (1985) to cigarette smoking. 29% of all women smoke, as do 21% of all female and male adolescents.

5

Mortality, Diagnosed Morbidity, and Psychosocial—Behavioral Risk: Longitudinal Studies

The Work Done

There are a few studies, several quite important, of a longitudinal nature which show a relationship between overall mortality and specific behavior and/or psychosocial conditions. In the most extensive longitudinal study of natural populations, the Alameda County study (Belloc, 1973, Berkman, and Breslau, 1983), it was observed that specific health practices predicted to mortality. Those favorable to low risk were first identified as having 7-8 hours sleep, eating breakfast regularly, not eating between meals, at normal weight, not smoking cigarettes, no immoderate use of alcohol, exercise. By 1983 these factors had been condensed, with three as the most powerful predictors: cigarette smoking, physical activity, moderate alcohol use. In addition obesity and sleeping patterns remained risk predictors, all statistically independent of health status initially, of SEC, race, medical check-ups, or psychological status. However, the likelihood of maintaining good practices was related to SEC and initial health status. An important limitation for predicting mortality using the Alameda study behavior factors is that the health practices identified here do not appear to apply at all to elderly men, whereas only never having smoked cigarettes is a mortality predictor for non-institutionalized women 65 years of age and older. That finding emerges from the Massachusetts Health Care Panel Study over a five year follow-up (Branch and Jette, 1984).

Mortality in the Alameda study was found associated with social relationships. Those women with close ties to others through marriage, friends and relatives, church or other organizational memberships were, compared to isolated persons, at 3.2% less risk of death from any cause over the 20 year study period. Health practices were found to operate independently of social network presence as predictors. Psychological factors also predict mortality statistically independently of health practices. The psychological traits of uncertainty, anomie (not feeling a part of a community, being alienated), life satisfaction, being insecure socially (no resources or resiliency), being a perfectionist, and experiencing negative feelings chronically were successful predictor variables.

In Vaillant's (1979) 40 year follow up study of male Harvard students, initial mental health strongly predicted to mortality and to chronic illness, even when controlling for the effects of alcohol, tobacco, obesity, and ancestor longevity. Betz and Thomas (1979) following John Hopkins medical graduates over 30 years found that an uneven or irregular temperament (compared to slow and steady or rapid and facile; these categories were adopted from reliable ratings used by Gesell in his Yale infant studies) predicted to much higher illness rate overall and to mortality.

Thomas and Greenstreet (1973) used data on the same John Hopkins medical student population retrospectively to examine psychosocial-behavioral features related to coronary heart disease, hypertension, and tumor over a 25 year period. Students reporting becoming angry under stress were more likely to develop CHD. Those who became hypertensive were those who described themselves as not likely to become "active" under provocative, challenging conditions. These were also smokers and persons with higher initial blood pressure. On the Rorschach test one infers greater immaturity in personality at the time of original testing. The tumor group appears to deny or repress conflictual emotions and impulses.

Looking backwards over 25 years at medical students who were given the Minnesota Multiphasic Personality Inventory (MMPI), Barefoot, Dahlstrom, and Williams (1983) observed that a hostility subscale had a positive association with arteriographically documented coronary atherosclerosis (The Cook-Medley Ho score). These hostility scores "predicted subsequent mortality from all causes..." as well as CHD, i.e. the MMPI, the hostile group died earlier than the non MMPI hostile trait individuals. Shekelle et al (1983), looking backwards over 10 and 20 years in a managerial population of Western Electric employees in Chicago (N=1877), also found that the MMPI hostility scale correlated with CHD. Controlling initial health, age, blood pressure, serum cholesterol, cigarette use and alcohol intake, they further found, as with Barefoot et al. above, that trait hostility was associated with all causes of death. Low MMPI hostility scores were associated at a rate 42% less than high ones.

Keehn et al., (1974) selecting almost 30,000 army discharges, divided those discharged for psychoneurosis compared to those not. A retrospective review with much attenuation in the sample over 24 years, found considerable mortality differences in terms of higher risk of the psychoneurotics for mortality from suicide (96.6 times greater), homicide, and accidents. It was also the case that overall morbidity was slightly higher, particularly for CNS disease (vascular lesions and embolism/thrombosis) and from infectious disease, the latter attributable to tuberculosis deaths. The investigators discount, but cannot explain away, the higher general and specific CNS and infectious disease death rate. They emphasize the much higher rate for the behaviorally caused deaths.

House, Robbins, and Metzer (1982) in the 9 to 12 year Tecumseh prospective study with initial health status controlled, found that for both sexes, but for men more than women, the number of social relationships was associated with death risk. An important factor for women was church attendance. As in the Alameda study (Berkman and Syme, 1979), social ties act on risk independently of initial health measures. In a small follow-up Tecumseh sample (Julius, 1986), a group of citizens self-rated themselves for anger and its suppression. Those characterizing themselves initially as suppressing anger toward a spouse experienced double the mortality rate of others. When blood pressure was also high, mortality risk was further significantly increased. One sees here that blood pressure and anger coping, and relations with important others, act independently and interactively to affect mortality risk over a 12 year period. This parallels the earlier cited hostility findings.

Langer and Roden (1978), in an 18 month term follow up, found upon dividing nursing home elderly residents into two groups, one given additional decision making powers with respect to their lives versus one remaining passively institutionalized, that morbidity was greater in the passive group. Dramatically, those given less responsibility and having less control over their lives had double the mortality rate. (See also Berkman, 1985 and Rodin, 1986.)

In another examination of the longitudinal data for John Hopkins medical graduates, Thomas et al. (1979) observed that lack of student closeness to their parents was a factor associated positively with later cancer. Krantz and Glass (1984) are cautious about this finding, as indeed are many investigators who review proposed personality and cancer relationships. The Thomas finding is, nevertheless, compatible with the social support literature. It can also be viewed as consistent with that risk literature focusing on mental health, for the capacity for close relationships within the family is typically seen as a psychological adjustment capacity. Insofar as that is the case, then social support variables as such, particularly in populations not isolated by old age itself, are likely to show overlap with social-family adjustment measures of mental health, and with that higher general mortality predictably associated with earlier poor emotional health status. Since general mortality includes direct behaviorally caused deaths (suicide, alcohol-related accidents, etc.), any such mortality measure will be sensitive to the proportion of initially emotionally disturbed persons in the sample.

In a longitudinal retrospective study, looking back at mortality data over a 10 year span, Helsing, Szklo, and Comstock (1981) found, in a Maryland sample, that widowers more than widows were at mortality risk. And that the risk was operative for 10 years following bereavement. The study, controlling for other risk variables, cites cigarette smoking and economic status, and also observed that there was specific morbidity in association with bereavement: for men, accidents, suicide, infectious disease; for women, cirrhosis. One wonders if either alcohol use or poor eating habits as part of loneliness-depression may have been intervening factors associated with the cirrhosis death outcome. Other bereavement studies are reviewed by Goldberg and Tull (1983) beginning with Lindemann, but also Maddison and Viola, Glick et al., Maddison, Gerber, Greenblatt, Parks et al., Cox and Ford, Rees and Lutkinds, and Clayton and Darvish. There are compatible results on all follow ups; depression, insomnia, physical symptoms, menstrual disorder, physical disease, hospitalization, and mortality increase when widows or widowers are compared with controls. The only question is the duration and peak of the effect, with findings varying from six months peak to an average two years, or as in the Maryland study above, for 10 years following.

Mor, McHorney, and Sherwood (1986), using data of a prospective nature from the National Hospice Study of oncology patients and survivors, examined secondary morbidity among the recently bereaved. Physician visits, hospitalization use of antianxiety medications, and increased use of alcohol were measured among spouses and non spouses offering primary care to the dying cancer patient. Use of alcohol increased but slightly over half of the survivors made physician visits, and there was no difference— compared to population expectancy rates for similar demographic groups— in hospitalization. Health status prior to bereavement was the major predictive factor for physician visits and for the use of antianxiety medication, i.e., the least healthy also used the most antianxiety medication. When spouses were compared to non spouses— all had been primary care persons for the cancer patient— it was found that the spouses suffered considerably more secondary morbidity, defined by the criteria, than non spouses. When women were compared to men it was found that women were at greater risk, as a bereavement response, of using antianxiety medications. One cannot be sure that this is not an interaction effect influenced by physician responses to the bereaved woman. The investigators did find that the more depressed survivors had more physician visits, and they suggest that bereavement physician visits may reflect a need for psychosocial support. It is also suggested, speculatively, that women may somatize despair in the "sick role" whereas men, in this sample, more often turned to drink.

In the Western Electric Study, a 17 year follow up on about 2,000 men, it was observed that depression, reliably measured by the Minnesota Multiphasic Personality Inventory (MMPI), predicted to increased risk of cancer (Shekelle et al., 1981). This finding is compatible with the current work of Levy and her colleagues (1985) on NK (immune system killer) cells activity as a negative correlate of being "adjusted" among breast cancer patients. Women with lack of social support, including decreased communication with spouse, were in the worst prognostic category for breast cancer; indeed survival was more associated with social support and involvement (positive prognosis), listlessness (possibly correlated with either depression or passivity for adverse prognosis), rated adjustment (as noted, being "well adjusted" rather than upset, angry, and stress contributed much more to the prediction of breast cancer survival over the observation period than did disease stage at diagnosis (Levy, 1985, citing work by Funch and Mettlin, Funch and Marshall, Cohen and Cohen)).

A longitudinal retrospective study (Hibbard, 1985) in a large Oregon HMO sample utilized a household survey and medical records over seven years. Age, sex, trust, perceived control (one's action have the intended results, what happens is generally under one's personal control) were tested for association with self-perceived health and the record of physician visits for diagnosed chronic conditions. Having more social ties, being more trustful, and perceiving more control are related to better self-rated and diagnosed/visit health status. For women with less sense of control (whether confidence, resources, situation, etc.), having more social ties is associated with improved health. This finding is compatible with some of the research reviewed by Clymer et al., (1982), especially Strickland's (1978) suggesting that "internal" controllers (confidently self-directed) take more responsibility for health activities. Perhaps, they self-regulate better to avoid risk, including that from being perturbed and "stressed."

One implication of Hibbard's work is based on other findings to the effect that persons with more internal focus of control use their interpersonal/community networks more efficiently. For women, the size of the social network, when large, compensates for whatever other factors may contribute to their health risk. One thinks of older age, poverty, lack of education in association with not knowing how to cope, as well as simply having larger networds of help—available ties as resources. Broadhead (1983) reports that social supports buffer against health risk more for women than for men. Can this be related to some greater "need" for sociability, or situational depression "curable" by company? One does not know. What one does know following Cohen and Syme (1985) and Blaney (1985) is that social support is a complicated variable interacting with negative affect, interpersonal interests and skills, and coping.

In a methodologically limited but nevertheless provocative study, Grossarth-Maticek (1980, 1984) administered a psychological questionnaire to the eldest person in every 2nd household in a small

Yugoslavian town. Ten years later, diagnostic data were gathered on follow up, with 205 out of 1353 sample members diagnosed as having developed cancer. Questionnaire replies were relied upon to characterize respondents' experience and personal styles. Associations were found between the risk of cancer and presumably typical personal styles of either chronic excitement or hopelessness in response to the number of events which were designated as traumatic. Inferred as well were self-abnegation in social relationships and lack of emotional expression ("rational anti-emotive behavior"). Lack of hypochondriasis (criteria for definition not set forth) was also noted. Among these findings of stressful frequency, perhaps better characterized as subjective felt vulnerability and maladaptiveness, and of emotion suppression, the latter are compatible with the psychological distance and cancer finding of Thomas.

Blazer (1982) conducted a 30 month prospective study of the elderly in a North Carolina county. With mortality the measure, it was found that the relative risk for death, measured by a questionnaire, varied depending upon social support. Marital status and children combined to be the greatest predictor, with relative risk four times greater for unattached persons; whereas those with infrequent social interaction (visits, phone calls) or perceived lack of social support (reporting no one understanding them, no one willing to help them, etc.) experienced death at a rate about twice as great as those enjoying either more frequent personal contact or felt social support. These results are not only consistent with the Alameda and House et al. (Michigan) findings about the importance of social support, but unlike the Massachusetts work on health habits among the elderly, yield a consistently powerful predictor variable, one refined to some of the several component elements of social support as such.

Another follow-up of the elderly, reported by Kasl et al. (1980), observed what happened when people were moved from a neighborhood getting socially-economically worse to "better" subsidized housing. They were compared to people not being involuntarily relocated. Those forced to move to "better" housing suffered more nursing home and hospital admissions, more cardiac disease, and said they were in poorer health. Those who had expected the move to be trouble proved most often correct in their estimation of its adverse impact on their health.

A follow-up study after the Three Mile Island nuclear power accident was made on 709 married women (Monroe et al., 1986). Unlike other work cited in this chapter which predicts to physical illness from psychosocial variables, this begins and ends with such variables, measuring marital social support and upsetting life events to find these predict a year later to levels of depression. We include this study because of the relationship we have elsewhere discussed between depression and physical illness risk, depression as a correlate of being a medical patient, and specifically of being a gynecological patient.

Summary

The few existing prospective studies (few other than those short range convenient ones on obstetrical risk) which examine mortality per se for its association with psychosocial and behavioral risk demonstrate that mortality rates in the general population do vary with life situation, temperament and personality, events, interpersonal and emotional expressive styles, and conduct including health habits. These findings are generally compatible with those from prospective studies on that best studied and most common of chronic disease with high morality outcomes, cardiovascular disease. The features associated with mortality risk include some of the same ones which we shall see are reported for specific diseases. An early conclusion is allowed to the effect that there are general factors predictive of (and probably predisposed to) a range of morbid and fatal outcomes. One must also be aware of the arbitrary and ambiguous nature of diseases, trauma, or self-harm characterized as "causes" of death. It becomes obvious when we reflect on the labels chosen as "final causes" of death that we are but being introduced to the mostly unknown processes which initiate one person's or group's illness biologically.[1]

It is also the case, and again coronary heart disease research in relationship to personality risk variables is an example, that there is reason for caution about early acceptance of even apparently hearty findings. Aside from uncertainty about Type A personality as opposed perhaps to hostility as a refined component variable, that caution is to be applied to emotional expressive styles in relation to cancer risk. We are early on in the process of refining risk factors, how, when, and upon whom they operate.

It is important not to presume the specificity of risk factors as precursors of pathology-initiating mechanisms except where the course of physiological events, or equally evident variables such as lack of access to or appropriate use of medical care, are sufficiently known readily, replicably, to account for a fatal outcome. A cause-and-effect model has limited usefulness in the current stage of work; one is dealing with probabilities in population, and inference from those mass data to individual prognosis. The predictions upon which health promotional efforts are based are actuarial. They are slowly updated by identification of new risk factors associated with biosocial status, that is at present rather inefficient, and indeed over lifetime spans quite inexact. Knowledge of mechanisms of action pathways for perturbation within body systems will markedly improve that efficiency, as will improved methodology and systematization in risk factor identification. The usual multiple mix of classes of determinants— genetic, development, socio-environmental including pathogen exposure, life events, conduct, stress vulnerability personality, as well as neuroendocrine, immune, and circulatory system status, and also psychophysiological patterns of arousal and recovery— will play a role in influencing the course of events leading to states of wellness, particular expression of complaints, disease process, and fatal outcomes. Given this complexity, recognize that we are dealing with contextual and interacting as well as sequentially operative events moving along switching paths. Insofar as one set of those events are human choices, some made moment to moment, probability models of modern statistics are the best performers. The health professional, the public, the patient are dealing in life and in this science with uncertainty. One will not wish to overstate the promise of health through risk reduction via better awareness, self-direction and self-regulation. Nor does one ignore the potential gains.

Footnotes

1. Methodological problems

It is our hope that the clinician will become a careful, critical reader of that research which bears on disease prevention via health promotion. For that astuteness to be present, the health professional must become familiar with some of the major research problems, and typical deficiencies, in work which is done. One also hopes that the clinician as well as the established research worker will wish to begin rigorous systematic studies so as to expand our knowledge base. The following are some issues pertinent to materials presented in this chapter.

Several of the foregoing studies indicate how, in labelling traits or conditions which are assumed to be measured by a set of responses on a test, both replicability and identification may become difficult. One is returned here to some fundamental and chronic problems in psychometrics, beginning with the semantic ones associated with overlooked operationalism in concept definition. Blazer for instance examined marital status, number of living children, etc., then gave an arbitrary weight scored, and called the resulting score a measure of "roles and available attachments." Others, if not familiar with the specific questionnaire criteria, might think of a test for "roles" in other ways, as for example work, offices held, needed and respected activities. As for the Yugoslavian study, one has no idea from the published data what events were "traumatic," over what period of time they occurred, how their reporting varies over time, or what was "hypochondriasis" and how it was proven. Even with more everyday measures such as "anxiety" one finds different tests used, different concepts, as for example "state" (acute) or "trait" (chronic) anxiety, and that state anxiety is situation or stimulus aroused as opposed to that which is psychodynamically activated pre-existing conflict. As for depression, surely a consistent feature in complaint and disease risk, and as serious illness correlate, is it reactive, situational, chronic, monopolar or bipolar, with or without genetic components, or the same when measured by several of the existing often used tests? These difficulties are mentioned here not to introduce a first course on psychometrics or research design, but to warn the women's health specialist that the findings one reads are subject to much variation depending upon the focus on and care of the investigator. One major problem in risk factor identification is accurate concept identification and testing.

Control of possibly correlated, or independently acting but result affecting variables is also vital. Blazer for example wisely controlled, by measurement and then statistical manipulation, for other characteristics of his sample which were very likely to affect mortality, (age, sex, race, SEC, physical health status, self care capacity, depression, cognitive function, stressful life events, cigarette smoking). Grossarth-Maticek did not, and so we do not know how many of his Yugoslav elders who at one point in time gave answers allowing only the inference of hopelessness presumed to be a continuing reaction to events called "traumatic" were in fact already ill with cancer when selected, or were smokers or more often at risk as male, poor, or depressed.

In a later chapter on risks we include findings from the prospective specific mortality studies which have focused on cardiovascular disease. Because such longitudinal studies are similar to the Alameda study, although with a narrow focus, we take note again of that CHD work, particularly the discrepancies and changing knowledge base which bedevil the field. When the Framingham Heart Study was initiated in 1949 many CHD risk factors were unknown, cigarette smoking was not included until the 1965-67 Levine and Scotch (see Lenfant and Schweizer, 1985) 300 item questionnaire. There were limited findings on women's risk, this related to clerical work and hostile bosses

(Haynes and Feinleib, 1980). By 1972 when the Multiple Risk Factor Intervention Trial was begun, behavior was recognized as containing risk components among its high risk male cohort. By 1980 prospective studies for CHD were already showing contradiction with respect to psychosocial factors operating. The Aspirin Mycardial Infarction Study did not find Type A to be associated with (recurrent) myocardial infarction, although hostility, one component in the Type A broad assessment, was associated. Case (1985), Dembrowsky and MacDougall (1985) present similar findings; no relationship between Type A and angiograph observed coronary disease, but a significant association with hostility and unexpressed rage. Speech style also remains a component. Case et al. found in a primary male sample, no relationship between Type A and total mortality, cardiac mortality, time to death, duration of coronary unit stay, or the physiologically predictive variable of left ventricular ejection fraction. Using multivariate survivorship analysis and introducing the elsewhere so ordinarily mortality predictive demographic variables (race, education, SEC), Case et al. found these too irrelevant. It is stated that preliminary data from another prospective study (MRGIT, Shekelle is cited) also indicate no Type A association with either subsequent coronary death or non fatal MI, whether measured by structured interview or the Jenkins Activity Survey Questionnaire. In possibly relevant related work, Cromwell and Levankron (1984), varying nursing care over several dimensions of patient personality variables (whether repression of anxiety as here tested has any relationship to anger repression is not known), observed that none of the three psychological variables had impact on long term recovery, death, or further myocardial infarction incidence. They did influence length of coronary unit and hospital stay.

Such sets of findings in prospective research, usually the methodology of choice for epidemiological risk work, indicate the difficulties in securing replicability. They are consonant with the continuing process of redefinition and refinement in concepts, measurements, and outcome measures. Variations among population, as well as among measure, as discussed by Byrnes et al., 1985 on Type A measures, also emerge as sources of discrepancy. Population-dependent outcomes in turn serve to emphasize how morbidity/mortality can be clustered among groups with particular, psychosocial-behavioral characteristics, these capable of interacting with genetic, exposure, and physiological disease process variables.

Looking Backwards Is Not The Same As Looking Forward

Longitudinal studies are of two general kinds. In one, usually termed "prospective," the investigator takes a (usually) large population, specifies an idea with regard to an expected relationship between initial status (behavior, personality, etc.), tests for this, follows up, is sure that the outcome criteria are clear, and at periodic intervals tests the hypothesis for association. The other type of study is descriptive of development at a number of stages. Usually employing a larger number of measures, each based on implicit hypothesis but not ordinarily specified as to particular health outcomes, the observer watches to see what happens. Ten or twenty or even fifty years later, multiple tests of association are run to see, essentially on a catch-as-catch-can basis, what originally tested traits turn out to be associated with morbidity. The specific hypothesis testing prospective approach allows more powerful (one tail) statistical testing, but it does not generate developmental data. The retrospective, what-relates approach suffers from shotgun luck, that is, with enough initial measures some (about 5 out of 100 will be by chance) are bound to be significant. The investigators do not always tell us that trait X which did appear correlated, say, with tumor, was but one of 50 or 100 tests run. If it is but one significant finding among many non significant ones, it is essentially meaningless.

Both types of longitudinal studies suffer from defects of early reporting, i.e., students tested at age 25 are characterized as to morbidity, at say age 55. For the investigating team that is a long time to wait, but one recognizes nevertheless that the typical chronic diseases associated with psychosocial risk will not emerge as causes of death for most of the sample until even later years. Thus one cannot be sure that 30 year findings on student samples will be confirmed by outcomes that encompass most mortality, as for example survivorship to age 80. We know of no study which has contrasted its "early" 30 year findings with 50 follow up years. It is quite possible that the youthful traits of persons dying before 55 are quite different from those dying of the same disease from 56-70, or over age 71. And, as noted, it is quite possible that the statistical significance derived from tests of multiple traits and narrow outcomes (CHD, tumor, etc.).

Comment: Specificity, Uncertainty, And The Patience Mantra

The longitudinal mortality risk studies (whether prospective in fact or taking advantage retrospectively of earlier gathered data) offer demonstrations of the relationship between psychosocial-behavioral conditions and fatal morbidity, i.e., of risk condition which reduces longevity. The study variables here found to be predictors can be classed as specific food and drink ingestion habits and personal conduct, individual social relations (which can have situational, emotional, interpersonal competence, and community lack of resources components), psychological attributes whether broadly defined as mental health or temperament or by more specific traits, and stressful events and manner of emotional expression, or again, interpersonal styles. These classes of events are of the same order, with some of the same specific component predictors as will be found in long or short term morbidity, and specific disease including some gynecological illness. Such classes of events may also participate in those constellations of traits/events associated with health survey elicited complaints/symptoms.

One encounters pervasive issues here with respect to gaining knowledge. Since they are ubiquitous, and must hold our attention as we weigh the value of health promotion, including plans for clinical efforts or research, we do address them at this point.

First there is the matter of the specificity in action of risk items measured as specific in behavior. Cigarette smoking is an example. It is a predictor of several kinds of obstetrical outcomes, of CHS, several cancers and of general morbidity and mortality to which measure the foregoing illnesses strongly contribute. Considered as a specific physiological factor for illness, cigarette smoking is the focus of research on circulation and cell metabolism. For lung cancer for example, direct pathological effects are demonstrable. For low birth weight there is evidence of effects on hemoglobin levels with implied nutritional deprivation (Nilsen et al., 1984) and reduced interplacental circulation inferred from observable vasoconstriction (Mochizuke et al., 1984). Cigarette risk varies considerably depending on other maternal characteristics such as anemia (Meyer, 1978) so that both a continuum of ingested quantity and interaction with other hematological variables must be acknowledged. Furthermore, there may also be a cumulative effect operative in prepregnancy, for age of smoking onset and amount smoked prior to conception are implicated in low birth weight prediction. Yet a different order of sequence over time is invoked when one considers that cigarette smoking is also a risk factor for subsequent cannabis, PCP, and heroin use. Each of these rarer events is also an obstetrical risk factor, and all are also correlated with other maternal characteristics, many of which may seem independently to function as risk factors (age, sexual activity, non-conformity, contraceptive behavior, etc.). Smoking is also correlated with adolescent emotional status, educational level, and alcohol use, each of which may be tied directly, or indirectly—since there can be correlates here with antenatal care—with outcomes.

How specific then is cigarette smoking, not as a conduct measure but as a direct pathogen? One must not be lured into arguments of either/or kind. One may entertain the possibility that cigarette smoking is implicated across a range of actions, from independent ones on lung tissue or hemoglobin or placental circulation, to interacting ones with anemia or alcohol or cannabis, on time and quantity continua, as part of a constellation of maternal traits and situations, and separately, as a trait marker for possibly powerful other variables. For example, we know that daughter's smoking risk increases with mother's smoking, which leads to the (untested) hypothesis that for those mother-daughter pairs who smoke and where the daughter stays in a low SEC, the obstetrical risk associated with daughter's mother's height or intelligence is, to paraphrase Lillienfeld and Pasamanick (1959), a continuation of family casualty status where genetic "constitutional" and environmental factors are operative as for risk both for daughter's own at-birth morbidity and her later when-pregnant obstetrical risk.

Joffe (1969) reminds us that that which is constitutional at birth because of genetic, fetal environment, or perinatal features is affected by developmental events. Sameroff and Chandler (1975) found, for example, that persistence of neurological signs among distressed neonates is much greater among lower SEC groups. Neligan and Steiner (1983) in their fine review argue that other adverse perinatal survivors are similarly psychosocially influenced. Thus one conceives of a class of specific health pathological behaviors which lead to a range of genetic, developmental, personality, social, and medical processes wherein the specific conduct behavior takes on a differing significance depending on its context at each developmental point in a life.

The prospective mortality studies also illustrate how our measurements are in a state of continual redefinition as to best predicting components. At its most simple, one sees this in the reduction in the Alameda study, from Belloc and Breslau's first seven behavioral variables to, nine years later, five, of which three were finally selected as powerful (Camacho and Wiley, 1983). The tentative current selection of hostility as a Type A variable of greater consequentiality than the multitrait amalgam of Type A itself may prove to be another such refinement, at least for myocardial infarction.

When concepts are initially profound and set forth as theories, one must accept the scientific process to be one of both expansion and refinement. Begin for example with Claude Bernard, then to Cannon, and then to Sely's general adaption theory (1936, see also 1976), then to Wolff, then Hinkle, then to Holmes and Rahe, all refining and extending knowledge of stress events linked to physiological response and and/or illness. These are followed by better prediction from adverse events by Christensen, the work of Craig and Brown (1984) on the meaning of such events (1981), to the range of stress studies by Lazarus and his colleagues which have led us to coping strategies as stress negating responses. These are compatible with the definition of stress as an interaction event, and the work of Dohrenwend (1985) on vulnerability. That returns stress event measures to the context of personal vulnerability and resources, as we noted in Chapter 3.

Consider as part of and parallel to this the work reviewed by Drantz and Manuck (1984) on psychophysiological response pattern diversity, that in turn indebted to John Lacey. Include work done and cited by Axelrod and Reseine (1984) on multiply related interacting neurohormonal stress regulating pathways, Ader (1981) on psychoimmunology, and the new work on immune system (1985), Grossman (1985) on neuroimmunomodulation confirming that immunological responses can not only be altered by stress, but, following Ader and Cohen, conditioned, i.e., psychobiologically learned. Here too the work of Sandra Levy on high T cell activity associated with fewer involved breast cancer lymph nodes, that apparently correlated with the woman's social support and personality (repression, apathy) and also on stress and cancer, work reviewed by Sklar and Anisman (1981), which indicates the protective as well as adverse cancer course outcomes associated with noxious or "insulting" stimuli. This seems to be an important parallel set of findings; noxious stimuli at the physiological level may have diverse effects either helpful or harmful. At the psychological level, as "coping," the same range of interim effects occurs. Obviously one wants to identify the characteristics of the event-situation and of the responding person-system which mediate, account for, outcomes.

It is easy for either clinician or researcher, or indeed the interested citizen as science observer, to become discouraged by the uncertainty which characterizes current knowledge about behavioral risk and health promotion. Yet if one thinks how far one has come from Selye's brilliant concept 50 years ago to arrive at (let us dare, this one moment only, to say "sociopsychoneuroendocrine-immunology?" to use only once a German-length word, well confirming Eisenberg's (1984) worst fears about metastacizing syllables), it is all quite heartening and exciting.

Yet disappointment will be likely if one insists upon expecting the classical pathogenic model of disease causality to be demonstrable either via experimental inference or as the organizing conception for a working model of nature. Given complex interacting inner and outer processes and their environmental components to which is added, in all health behavior work, human choice, then cause and effect as sequential process may not be a workable "map." As in quantum physics and statistical theory, one works with probabilities, perhaps not simply as estimation devices but as a useful conception of how nature, when humans are choosing what next to do, works. We concur with Lachman (1984), commenting on Tyler that "at its core the principle of multiple possibilities is a thesis of limited determinism."

One does not, in considering limited probablistic versus strictly determinist models as conceptions of nature, avoid the philosophical issue of choice and freedom. Insofar as one conceives of humans exercising freedom of choice, and we do, that "free will" doctrine will be compatible with a "functional" view of adaption and behavior as information-processing, option assessing, available capabilities in readiness, and perceived best option selecting when compared against stored memories, anticipating thoughts, or innate plans and programs, whether as impulse expression or goal achievement. Because it is difficult for either the observer, or the person acting to anticipate in advance what cognitive strategy or algebra of choice will be elected, only a probability, limited-determinism statistical model, not a clinical or cause and effect one, is applicable. Thus, both research on psychosocial research prediction, and its application in health promotion, will likely acknowledge, as real, both free will and uncertainty.

The urge for specificity of cause and effect can lead to research nonreplicability if the problem of contexts is not faced. This is set forth succinctly by Christensen and Hinkle (1961) as a conclusion to their work, which showed morbidity outcomes to relate to the degree of academic training/preparation as an initial and defining characteristic in two samples of young male business managers. College graduates recently hired were compared to high school graduates doing the same jobs, of about the same age, coming from families with the same longevity, living in the same town, and earning the same salaries. The high school graduate group suffered more chronic, acute, and serious illnesses and were, although none died, judged to stand at a greater mortality risk. Some scholars have invoked competence-through-training as the explanation. But since the data analysis revealed the groups to differ in many ways, from smoking to family distress, to debts, to SEC origins, the authors/investigators were moved to write, "No matter how these data are interpreted, the interaction between these men and the world in which they live are so complex that it is a gross oversimplification to explain one to two of their categories of illness simply on the basis of the way they ate, how much they smoked, what happened to them in their childhood, or the way they reacted to their present occupations. It seems rather to be the outcome of all of these...."

The clinician or other health worker not engaged directly in research on risk complexity, may be misled into cause and effect thinking by the way in which that statistical epidemiological work which focuses on risk forecasting states its results. "Odds" or "risks" imply only that knowledge of one event leads to a better than chance prediction of another later event. We have noted how Paykel (1978) differentiates between kinds of risk: "attributed," "related," and "brought forward time." Thus when cigarette smoking is elucidated as an etiological variable in, say, CHD, it is a relative risk that the smoker is more likely to suffer a heart attack than the non-smoker, all else being equal. In that sense, and as noted in earlier discussion, cigarette smoking implicated in a sequential chain is also part of a number of interrelated chains of events where the smoking varies in the immediacy, directness, nature, and independence of effect. Yet the typical research outcome statement does not allow inference as to the nature or number of interrelated processes at work. When we are told that smoking or obesity are "causes" of disease, that is correct but understood best with the foregoing qualifications in mind. The same holds when we speak of causes of death; the certificated "cause" is an end point state, sometimes one arbitrarily selected from among several pathological processes. In Chapter 4, we saw how that reduces the accuracy of data in "causes" of maternal mortality.

But advocacy or enthusiasm, as well as an easy tendency to rely on the microbial pathogen model, may short circuit the restraint necessary in order not to oversell the data on which health promotion is based. Consider what a well known scientist in the field recently wrote, following his comment on the Surgeon General's 1979 report, and when speaking of five lifestyle factors (lack of exercise, alcohol abuse, diet, smoking, failure to use hypertensive medication) described as "causes" of 7 out of 10 diseases actually demonstrated in the aggregate to comprise the diagnosed "causes" of death for the majority of Americans. Note that here we already see several "causes" of death for each American, i.e., the combination of genetic-social-personality circumstance "causing" the lifestyle events "causing" a disease which "causes" a death. Our well intentioned writer went on to say that bringing about desired behavior change in these lifestyles would yield the result of "preventing morbidity and mortality." Now, short of the Second Coming neither of these outcomes appears likely. The Onion Principle conforms better to the historical evidence: new diseases replacing disappearing ones. Survivorship statistics can be a more useful descriptive approach to outcome evaluation. As for mortality being "preventable," well ....

At best, given the rapid expansion in risk research, the health promotion advocate asks optimistic questions. To what extent will our best efforts directed at modifying risk features significantly and favorably alter onset time longevity, complications (including emotional ones), pain, and disability? What will the evaluation of intervention efforts show by way of costs and benefits for an increase in well days? Will we find gains in well days from particular person-directed, family/community interventions?

Our emphasis here, throughout, is on systematic research: its findings, limitations, implications. Among clinicians and other caring people there can be an understandable objection to this attempt "better to improve wellness through quantification." Enkin and Chalmers (1982) also give voice to some frustration with respect to the failure to acknowledge contextual forces which confound the will. They take simultaneous aim at epidemiological research designs (the Coronary Drug Research Project) and scientific indifference to values. They comment, "The same factors that may effect a fetus adversely, such as the stresses and constraints of poverty, can also affect both a mother's motivation and her opportunity to receive adequate antenatal care. No amount of multivariate statistical pyrotechnics can take these factors properly into account... many things that really count cannot be counted" (pps. 283, 285).

Many a clinician, dealing daily with human pain and diversity, will say "amen." Yet, since much of the basis for current health promotional efforts is rational empiricism, these days such research very much a matter of counting; one must live with probability statements as best and temporary estimates. We remain advocates for risk research employing these probability and contextual maps as guides to nature and improved wellness.

One faces a further danger, if in the face of rapid change in the health behavior field, one's level of tolerance for ambiguity is breached, one may then rush to certainty about "what common sense tells you." That is easy because we all, as humans, have a lot of common-sense experience with ourselves and one another. Certainly much is to be said for that phiolsophy of knowledge promulgated by Vico (born 1668, see Berlin, 1955) to the effect that we are "given" immense knowledge about humans as compared to any other knowable realm, because observer and actor share the same systems intuitively and experientially. Thus, best bets are that what is going on in people, is happening to them from intuitions, not rationalism. Man believes he best understands that which he is, or has invented. Yes, but... Studies on memory, cognitive functioning, the irrational as such, attribution, empathy and, of great importance; inference, decisions, and information processing (see Elstien and Bordage, 1982, Eddy, 1982, Hung and McLeod, 1983 and Chalmers and Richards, 1977) warn us that conclusions we reach readily about complicated processes may well be off the mark. The work of Nisbett and Wilson (1977) or Freud, shows we may not know what is happening by way of information processing inside us, somatizing as misplaced or erroneously emphasized labelling, is the clinicians' daily proof. Thus, we must not let any sense of desperation about the present status of risk and mediating variable studies drive us to impulsive "understandings." Perhaps we should instead try the buffering relaxation therapy approach which has been shown to work to reduce maternal pre-eclampsia hypertension, using as our image or object of concentration a scientific mantra. Let us say to ourselves over and over again "provisional acceptance only, and patience."

6

Obstetrical Risk

In this chapter we consider adverse obstetrical outcomes where psychosocial-behavioral features are implicated as contributing influences. We also reflect upon the research done to date,[1] calling attention to some major trends and deficiencies.

At the outset let it be said: obstetrical risk prediction richly deserves better systemized, expanded, and methodologically more sophisticated work. The prospects for early gains in knowledge of risk are good, including the opportunity to elucidate risk derived physiological disease processes.

Caution

Let us be aware of limitations in the data to be presented here. Many of the variables presently identified as social or psychological are experimental in nature and are best considered provisional concepts "on the way" to better measurement and more exact characterization with regard to their interrelationship and their etiological role. Some "old standby" items are but gross categories which serve as shorthand markers, useful for prediction but which in themselves give little hint as to the complexity of health affecting events which are embraced by that category; socioeconomic class (SEC) is one of these, as is ethnicity. Psychological status items are too often presented in the research as if they were clear and enduring traits with strong specificity, rather than, as occurs often, being themselves situational responses better understood as particular patterns of person-environmental interaction. Anxiety (state), situational depressions, and some hypertension are examples.

Rarely considered in sufficient detail in routine studies— there are fine exceptions to be noted as in Barron and Thomson (1983)— is the role of behavioral and psychosocial variables as but elements in patterns which are ongoing and changing over time. Take the "simple" behavioral measure of alcohol use. It is correlated with other drug use (alcohol, coffee, cannabis, heroin, in terms of of both risk and moment-in-time), and depending on age of onset and style of use (supervised and learned, unsupervised and peer dictated), sexual activity, education, etc. If one looks at a constellation of drug use for individuals or groups of which drinking is a part, one will find, upon suitably classifying levels of such use, developmental association over time so that the use of tobacco-alcohol-cannabis-cocaine, for example, in turn appears to be associated with obstetrical risk. In a study of family etiology for drug abuse (Blum et al., 1969a, 1969b, 1972) mothers recollected birth and developmental histories of all their children. Those offspring with greatest drug use were recollected to have lower birth weights, more perinatal complications, more feeding problems, allergies, and learning difficulties. Furthermore, mothers from families with greater drug use were found to have more stillbirths and abortions. Yet one cannot be sure of such recollected data, which are easily biased by the mother's current knowledge of her now troublesome child. Such studies are the basis for new research, not conclusions as to perinatal problem sequelae.

Whenever a population subset, i.e., groups drawn from other than representative samples, are found to display risk factors not previously identified, and even after the necessary work of describing the pattern is done— the interrelationships among risk factors and biosocial status as through factor or cluster analysis, or covariance analysis— one cannot assume the discovery applies to all women. The cautious approach is to look for syndromes as subsets of interrelated elements in specified population groups, and where the adverse obstetrical outcome is also carefully specified. What one must suspect present is that a number of risk factors that are psychosocial and behavioral are trait markers— part of elaborate but insufficiently characterized packages, the likely group and temporal particularily of which is to be acknowledged.

Be aware that there are likely to be interaction (potentiating, synergistic) effects among items identified as variables. Nuckolls, Cassel, and Kaplan (1972) show how in the presence of one psychosocial risk factor, that greater life change events, obstetrical complications are predictable on the basis of the presence or absence of another psychosocial risk factor: membership in supporting groups, or networks. Women exposed to both these high risk elements (presence of much life change, absence of social support) have a rate of complications three times greater than those with high life change but protected by the presence of social supports. (Norbeck and Telden (1983) show similar interactions.) Lidell, (1954) showed that environmental stress can produce disorganized behavior and death in sheep and goats, but the same "psychological" stresses experienced in the presence of the animal's mother yielded no adverse results. That work in turn derived from Rene Spitz showing that babies not fondled, however, their care excellent otherwise, were at high risk of depression and death. See Field (1985) for a review of coping and separation stress, also Levine and Coe (1985).

As another interaction example, Porter (1984) has shown that reproductive failure and offspring survival rates for animals subjected to viral agents, immunosuppressants, and toxins are sensitive to even modest deficiencies in food and water available during pregancy. And Shavit et al. (1984) (see also Ader, Sklar, and Anisman, 1981) after remarking in animal studies the relationship between stress (e.g., surgery, starvation, transport), immune system suppression, and subsequent vulnerablility to neoplasia, and further noting release of opioid peptides as a stress response, then showed these peptides also implicated in immune suppression that included cytotoxic activity of natural killer (NK) cells involved in immune surveillance against neoplastic disease. Using intermittently applied (opioid stimulating) versus continous (non-opioid producing) footshock stress, the investigators find that opioid-producing, intermittent stress, but not the other, suppresses NK cells when not blocked by the opioid antagonist naltrexone, or instead, when morphine is adminstered under nonopioid generating conditions.

Such studies are illustrative of the complex and interactive nature of risk features. They may be studies at psychosocial levels where "risk synergism" is observed (Matarazzo, 1984). For example, risk of cancer of the oral cavity is greater for those smoking cigarettes and drinking alcohol than the additive risk rates for those doing either one but not both of these. Or research may focus on differential environmental exposure (as experience), immune system reponses, and pharmacological agents blocking actions. The phenomena to be addressed are complex interactions at biochemical levels, these, in turn, interacting with environmental events. For an excellent illustrative overview see Axelrod and Reisine (1984). We presume such complexity with respect to the disease processes at work to produce obstetrical complications.

Obstetrical Risk Prediction

The only area of women's health where early knowledge of multiple behavioral/psychosocial risk factors has been put to work systematically statistically for risk prediction applied to clinical practice is obstetrics risk. Antenatal care in turn has been a major practical arena for application of lifestyle advice, those health promotional interventions to assist in becoming a mother. Obstetrical risk is the field which has also generated the greatest amount of research within ob-gyn on behavioral-psychosocial factors as risk components.

The pregnancy term is particularly amenable to such predictive work because one is dealing with a clear entity, one where self-diagnosis and self-referral to medical care is early and widespread so as to achieve good sampling. Because there is concensus between doctor and patient on the diagnosis, the reason for care and the desired outcome, because there is a common interest in the role that lifestyle and self care plays in planning and having a baby, cooperation, including informed consent, for research is readily achieved. And in practice, when women are involved with self care as part of the medical and psychosocial effort, the outcome is a better one.

While recognizing the practical utility or risk prediction as practiced today, that leading to assignment to the two track high or low risk hospital care categories, one must also attend to the "third track" maternal election of midwifery home birth or an alternative birth center (ABC). That is one aspect of the "obstetrical battleground," which focuses directly on risk prediction. Here outcome criteria for risk are broadened to include not simply conventional morbidity and mortality, but also infant-child developmental features— including perinatal maternal bonding (in turn related later to child abuse) and costs and maternal/family satisfaction. Thus risk prediction is at the very heart of an issue of profound importance to consumers, physicians, third party payers, and others.

Of equal importance in these expanded outcome criteria is the inclusion of the intermediate variables of kinds of medical intervention and the settings for birth in calculations of risk. Here are found the concerns over safety, efficacy, cost, and satisfaction related to the new technology (see Chard and Richards, 1977 and Arms, 1975). Added to this debate are feelings and data about "prenatal psychology." (Verney, 1981). That is close to the explosive debate over abortion and the embryological dating of "being human" and "conscious awareness" in the fetus. Clearly the study of risk prediction whether for clinical application or health promotion touches upon powerful areas of scientific, political, social, and economic concerns.

The premise of work on obstetrical risk prediction is that medicine as an enterprise is effective and that its work is aided if one can identify components in the etiology of illness so that these may be subject to preventive or remedial intervention. In obstetrics, where etiological understanding is imperfect (for eclampsia, fetal growth retardation, low birth weight, etc.) knowledge of risk allows better preparation for effective intervention pre- and intrapartum should complications arise. These promises and possibilities have led to rapid recent expansion of research,[2] beginning from the time of Little, who in 1862 first made observations linking maternal events to infant developmental outcomes.

Baird in 1945 initiated, in Aberdeen, that epidemiological thrust which not only identified psychosocial features, poor health, and nutrition of mothers as major risk variables, but also used those findings in making an appraisal of extant obstetrical care. That critical look generated changes in clinical care which dramatically reduced perinatal mortality from placenta previa, difficult labor, pre-eclampsia, and antepartum hemorrhage. It was Baird who used clinical pathological classifications "to assist in prevention." Thus a learned policy of induction in the case of prolonged pregnancy in older primiparae, and cesarean section for intervening upon fetal distress appears greatly to have reduced mortality (see Thomson and Barron, 1983, for history), whereas obstetrical intervention appeared to be of no avail to prevent death associated with low birth weight and adverse social-environmental but unknown pathological features. Out of such findings can be generated advocacy for social medicine and improvements in public health and, when behavioral features are identified as contributory to hazard, education for health behavior. By 1986 such work in low birth rate led to legislation facilitating comprehensive (including psychosocial) prenatal care.

Ballantyne's 1902 insight and emphasis, antenatal care, has today become one of the central thrusts for preventive obstetrical work. At the same time it offers an opportunity for the development and use of risk prediction and, to date, those limited health promotional endeavors which rely on advice and regimen prescription. The combination of expanded epidemiological knowledge which has intensified prenatal care and advances in obstetrics and medicine per se, greater rates of hospital delivery for high risk cases, and associated public maternal education are all credited with the dramatic reductions in perinatal and maternal mortality and morbidity. There is also enhanced performance of survivors (Steiner and Neligan, 1983) in spite of the presence of that "continuum of reproductive casualty" identified by Lilienfield and Pasamanick (1955).

Although there can be no question as to the health advances made, the assignment of sole "cause" to obstetrics itself, including antenatal care, must be hedged with caution. Longo (1981), for example, shows that for populations as a whole, as medical attendance increased through this century, those delivering in hospital enjoyed greater maternal and infant health than others. But because these changes in health, and kind of hospital care, are themselves associated with positive changes in wealth, self care, education, and for obstetrical cases parity, age of first pregancy, nutrition, hard physical work, etc., it is difficult to assign weights to these work interdependent contributions. Excellent thorough reviews of these and related issues are to be found in Barron and Thomson (1983), Enkin and Chalmers (1982), and Chard and Richards (1977). With reference to the problem of the role birth setting per se, i.e., learning which setting is safer for whom, see the 1984 National Institute of Medicine report *Research Issues in the Assessment of Birth Settings*.

We now present a listing of psychosocial and behavioral features implicated in obstetrical complications and adverse perinatal outcomes. (See Table III.)

Table III
Psychosocial and Behavioral Features Implicated in Obstetrical Complications and Adverse Perinatal Outcomes

III.A General: outcome problems defined as "complications," "abnormal pregnancy," "difficulties."

    a. Personality and emotional factors:
       Emotional problems
       Hopelessness
       Felt inability to cope
       Anxiety
       Absence of repressive defenses and ability to deny (overlook) problems
       Upset in reponse to life changes
       Felt stress
       Presence of denial
       Psychiatric disorder (schizophrenia, depression, manic-depressive disorder now termed bipolar affective disorder)
       Puerperal emotional disorder in prior pregnancy
       Negative attititudes toward the pregacy
       Conflict about the maternal role
       Coping abilities (interacts with anxiety)
       Prior menstrual complaints
       Prior level of diffuse somatic symptoms reporting
       Social support
       Satisfaction with social support
       Uncontrolled (stressful, upsetting) life events interacting with trait anxiety
       Upsetting life events
       High level of diffuse health complaints
       Conversely, lower life change level (and high complication)
       Intensity of pregnancy complaints
       Past menstrual complaints
       Past general health complaints

b. Psychosocial biosocial status, events, conditions, milieu, related self and medical care variables:
   Age (no older age effect if delivery is in a modern tertiary care institution)
   Age at birth of first child
   Parity
   Race
   Nutrition
   Socioeconomic class level (SEC)
   Education
   Residence near hospital
   Antenatal visits
   Menstrual history
   Short birth interval
   Presence/absence of specialized high risk care
   Birth in local government hospital
   Birth in a hospital serving large ethnic minority populations
   Birth in a large hospital with large delivery service
   Hospital quality of care, including staff and facilities
   Ethnicity
   Number of children at home
   Single or married status (birth out of wedlock)
   Outside work
   High number of life event changes
   Life event changes interacting with presence/absence of social support
   Stressful life events
   Social isolation
   Socioeconomic problems
   Birth in hospital versus home (the latter risk varies with planned or unplanned birth, presence of midwife, untrained attendant)
   Receiving public assistance
   Overweight
   Inadequate weight gain
   Life stress as innoculating against difficulties
   Early menarche (relates to culture group, nutrition, state of industrialization of the society)
   Situational stress

Fatigue
High altitude exposure
Exposure to toxic substance
Among American Indians, being more tribal traditional
Among American Indians, having fewer stressful experiences (paradoxical finding). (Note the complication rate in this sample is 46%.)

c. Specific behavioral items (without regard to correlates):
High alcohol consumption
Level of cigarette smoking
Fad diets
Obesity
Dieting
Vitamin-mineral supplements
Prior induced abortions
Use of illicit drugs (cocaine, cannabis, heroin, etc.)
Excessive exercise
Sexually transmitted diseases associated with genitourinary infections in turn associated with level of sexual activity and diversity of partners
Reports of "alarming" fetal movement
Noncompliance in hypertension medication regimens

d. Complications from induced abortion:
Maternal age
Gestational age (as a function of decision change abortion)
Possible ethnicity
Possible SEC

Ref. Aubrey and Pennington 1973, Barrera & Balls 1983, Boyce 1980, Buehler et al. 1985, Butler 1969, Carrie 1981, Chalmers 1983, 1984, Chalmers, B. 1983, de Georges 1984, Edwards et al. 1979, Fagley et al. 1982, Farber et al. 1981, Field et al. 1983, Goodwin et al. 1969, Gorusch and Keys 1974, H. Ahmed 1981, Hobel et al. 1973, Hollingsworth et al. 1976, Holmes and Masuda 1974, Jones 1978, Kintz 1985, Labarba 1984, Laukaran and van den Berg 1980, Little and Hook 1979, Lotgoring 1984, Lubin et al. 1975, Lumley and Astbury 1982, Magmi 1983, Mayou 1975, McDonald 1968, Mehl and Peterson 1981, Miller et al. 1985, Molinski 1978, 1979, Naeye 1977, Nesbitt and Aubrey 1969, Norbeck and Tilden 1983, Nuckolls et al. 1971, Oakley et al. 1982, Obayama et al. 1984, Queenan and Hobbins 1983, Rayburn and McKean 1980, Reading 1983, Richards 1978, Rizzardo 1985, Sandberg et al. 1985, Sokel et al. 1977, Wrede et al. 1980

III.B Perinatal neonatal mortality (significantly associated with birth weight):
Negative maternal attitudes towards pregnancy
SEC in association with private or public hospital delivery
Sibship size
Age
Delivery planned or unplanned
Home delivery versus hospital delivery
Presence of nurse-midwife versus untrained attendant
Delivery en route to hospital
Delivery in M.D. office or clinic versus hospital
Receiving specialty care when otherwise high risk,
M.D. decisions/competence
Birth intervals
Residence near hospital, proximity to tertiary care centers
Mother's level of health and nutrition
Maternal obesity
Education
Parity
Ethnicity
Prior reproductive history
Socioeconomic class (maintained by selectivity at marriage whereby those marrying into lower SEC are in worse health, shorter, less education and less intelligent, etc.)
Cigarette smoking (note PMR may be lower in low birth weight babies born to smokers than to non smokers
Birth interval (when other factors are controlled, intervals less than 6 months operate independently))
Physician decision for nonindicated cesarean (leading to higher respiratory distress due to prematurity and PMR)
Physician's decision and mid-pelvic (Kielland's) forceps use
Prior abortion
Antenatal care

Neurotic depression in mother
Stress (fetal asphyxia)
STD infections
Season in which birth occurs (in U.S. lower mortality in fall and winter, in Norway the reverse)
Day of week of delivery (in U.K. highest mortality weekends, probably related to medical staffing and birth induction)
Hour of day, highest mortality afternoons, evening; correlates with high incidence of inductions. 3AM-6AM births lowest mortality possibly attributable to better attention/care immediately post-birth during daylight hours
Occupational activities (French data: higher mortality with long work week, standing work, few work breaks, long commute, tiring work)
Household help availability during last trimester (France)
Housing standards (France), higher mortality with crowding, absence of plumbing
Higher levels of alcohol use
More reported stress interacting with SEC
Absence of social support interacting with SEC

Ref. Bakketeig and Hoffman 1979, Bakketeig et al. 1984, Burnett et al. 1980, Goodwin et al. 1969, Kessner et al. 1973, Kleigman and Gross 1985, Laukaran and Van den Berg 1980, Leviz et al. 1971, Meyer 1974, 1976, 1977, Montgomery 1969, Morrison and Olsen 1979, Pritchard et al. 1985, Roman et al. 1978, Thomson and Barron 1983, Zackler et al. 1969, Zax, Someroff and Babigian 1977

III.C Low birth weight (LBW), (whether preterm birth normal for gestational age, or intrauterine growth retardation):
Cigarette smoking
Cigarette smoking in interaction with age
Diet
Maternal height and pre-pregnancy weight
Weight gain (low or very high)
Level of the society: technological advancement
Maternal prepregnancy nutrition
Average annual temperature (climatic)
Maternal intelligence, lower education as higher risk

Prior obstetrical history
Ethnicity, race (In U.S., LBW highest in blacks, then Latinos, lowest for whites)
Marital status, unmarried with higher risk
Hospital characteristics (care, technical adequacy)
Maternal age
Prescription drugs suppressing the immune system
Self-administered drugs of abuse
Vitamin deficiency
Physical stress including occupations, including long work week, tiring work, long commute, paid employment itself vs housewife status, standing work, work interacting with hypertension, work outside home
Psychological stress including occupation
Environmental toxin exposure
Lack of exercise
Prior induced abortions
Experience of prenatal medical care including nutritional
Participation in supplemental food programs and their availability (interacts with race and cigarette smoking)
Birth interval, parity with higher risk for multiple pregnancies
Housing quality and density, pregnancy environment as a function of atttitude
Leisure time, activity during pregnancy
Alcohol use
Attitude toward pregnancy: ambivalent or negative
Exercise
Life stress, including events triggering uterine contractions
High symptom levels (somatizing)
Anxiety
Lack of emotional support from husband
Unusual fatigue
Mother receives ultrasound feedback (+r with higher birth weights)
Alcohol use levels
Smoking by father
Experience of intensive prenatal care interacting with SEC
High density protein supplements taken (-r), nutrition supplement for cigarette smokers
Experience with anti-smoking treatment (interacts with time of prob-

lem onset, diagnosis of hypertension or infection, amount smoked)
Maternal schizophrenia
Ego defect in psychologically immature women
Mother's education less than high school
Father's education less than high school
Father low occupational level
Contraception not ordinarily practiced
Pregnancy unplanned
Infection-preventive rubella innoculation history
STD, e.g., cytomegalovirus, HSV 1 and 2, chlamydia; all practices associated in turn with STD risk
Marijuana use. Possibly marijuana in interaction with other psychoactive compounds
Quality of hospital care (hospitals rated on staff and equipment)

Ref. Berkowitz 1981, Brown 1985, Chamberlain & Garcia 1983, Cnattinguis et al. 1985, Creasy et al. 1980, Eisner et al. 1979, Enkin and Chalmers 1982, Field et al. 1985, Greve & Schroder 1977, Hebel et al. 1985, Heminki and Starfield 1978, Knorr 1979, Kuera et al. 1977, Lotgoring 1984, Meyer 1976, 1978, Oakley et al. 1982, Reading 1983, Sandbert et al. 1985, Schramm 1985, Sokel and Hobel 1984, Thomson 1983, Williams 1979, 1980, Wortis cited in Oakley et al. 1982, Wynn and Wynn 1981, Zax, Sameroff and Babigian 1977

III.D Spontaneous abortion:
Infections associated with sexually transmitted diseases in turn associated with sexual behavior
Type of contraception (pills, IUD, condoms, rhythm method)
Exposure to environmental toxins, including anethetic gases
Smoking
Alcohol use levels
Age
Cocaine use
Coital frequency associated with age
Birth order among siblings
Immaturity associated with inability to accept responsibility
Feminine role conflict in women with active career goals
Stress
Conception delay with age-related chronic anovulation and develop-

ment of uterine and/or pelvic pathology, as fibroids, endometriosis
Interaction of husband-wife: husband's antagonism
Women's father absent or perceived as inadequate, with postulated impact on psychosocial development and subsequent marital relations, including maternal dependency
Nausea reduction by anti-nausea agents
Lack of social support
Workplace environmental toxins
Prior psychosomatic reactivity
Possibly, workplace exposure to video display terminals - 20 hours a week or more
Possibly, father's workplace exposure to toxins (DBCP)

Ref. Butler and Brix 1986, Chasnoff et al. 1985, Harlap and Shiono 1980, Hemminki et al. 1983, Himmelberger et al. 1978, James 1978, Kline and Stein 1984), Kline et al. 1977, Kroger 1962, Mann 1956, 1959, McDonald 1968, Roman 1983, Smithells 1983

III.E Infections in pregnancy (including perinatal and postpartum):
Sexual behavior associated with STD
Attitude toward pregnancy and associated self-care
Person level of health and nutrition
Possible status of immune system related to stress and perceived control
Immunization behavior (rubella)
Age
SEC and marital status
SEC in association with sexual behavior
For hepatitis: acquired immune deficiency syndrome (AIDS)
Use of injectable drugs including self-injections
Ethnicity (associated with antigens)
For toxoplasmosis: food sources and environmental exposure
For chlamydia: age and marital status, sexual behavior
For chorioamnionities: SEC, nutritional status, possibly coital frequency before delivery
For puerperal sepsis: SEC, nutrition, hospital environment/management/procedures, choice of birth setting and assistants, possibly sexual intercourse prior to delivery, possibly frequency of vaginal examinations

Geographical, regional, cultural variations in infectious agent prevalence (and possible immune status). (Example: Hepatitis B surface antigen carriage is 50 times higher in Taiwan than U.S.)

Ref. Anderman and Horstmann 1984, Joklik 1985, Lammen et al. 1985, Laukaran and van den Berg 1980, Lumley and Astbury 1982, Peckinham and Marshall 1983, Pritchard et al. 1985, Pritchard, MacDonald and Gant 1985

III.F Fetal birth anomalies and malformation:
Chronic alcoholism and alcohol intake including prior obstetrical history
Absence of prenatal care
Maternal age
Paternal age
Multiparous status leading to minor gynecologic pathology
Race
Experience of prenatal care (associated with amniocentesis, fetal monitoring and induced abortion)
Ethnicity (associated with genotypes)
Sibship order (associated with parity size, nutritional vitamin deficit and associated prenatal care prescribed)
Antileptic drugs
Prescription medication interactions with age (young and old at greater risk)
Environmental
Nutrition-diet
SEC
Climate
Chronic disease exposure/experience
Diabetes
Hypertension
Obesity (see below also)
Smoking (cleft palate, neural tube) SEC
Psychological stress
Vitamin deficiency
Possibly, copper-bearing IUDs
Low SEC

Teratogenic medications:
Anti-nauseants such as meclozine, trifluoperazine or

cyclozine
Cytotoxic drugs
Stilboesterol
Folic acid antagonists
Androgens
Synthetic progestagens
Phenytoin
Oral hypoglycemic drugs
Corticosteroids
Anticoagulants (coumarins)
Tetracyline
Thalidomide
Cholesterolemics
Cytotoxins and antineoplastics
Salicylates
Rifampin (antituberculosis)
Amphetamines
Anti-acne, Retinoic Acid
Pesticide
Mercury
Industrial solvents
Industrial chemical waste site exposure/ingestion

Drugs of abuse: possibly amphetamines (cf. alcohol above)
Caffeine
OTC compounds: possibly aspirin

Infectious exposure, including STD:
Cytomegalovirus
Herpes simplex
Rubella associated with unvaccinated status
Toxoplasmosis (exposure may include contaminated water supply)
Varicella zoster
Venezualian equine encephalitis (Note: infection risk varies with immune status which appears to be partially a function of stress-related immunosuppression)

Chronic disease:
Diabetes mellitus

Epilepsy
Hypertension

Radiation exposure: industrial/medical/dump site

Ref. Alter 1984, Aro 1984, Cohen 1986, Doering 1978, Ericson et al 1979, Eriken and Chalmers 1982, Evans et al. 1979, Globus 1969, Heinonen 1977, Hemminki et al. 1983, Hingson et al. 1986, Laukaran and van den Berg 1980, Leck 1983, Miller 1986, Nayeye 1978, Sandberg et al. 1985, Smithells 1983, Tuchman-Duplessis 1975, Vouk and Sheehan 1983

III.G Sudden Infant Death Syndrome (SID):
Note: SID accounts for 40-60% postperinatal mortality, peaks 2nd, 3rd months, has many of the same predictors/correlates as perinatal mortality. Risk increases with:
Parity
Family history of SID
Younger maternal age
Lower birth weight, thus low birth weight predictors
Postnatal growth retardation, thus these predictors
Cigarette smoking in pregnancy; its correlates
Lower, absent levels of antenatal care
Heroin use in mother
SEC: eco and education lower levels
Ethnicity (blacks) in U.S.
Unmarried
Fewer prior fetal, perinatal deaths (paradoxical)

Ref. Peterson 1984

III.H Hypertension in pregnancy (pre-eclampsia): when associated with nonrenal disease with proteinuria

Antenatal care: when associated with control
Cooperation in care associated with medication use
Cooperation of family and patient blood pressure self-monitoring
Age
Ethnicity
Smoking (note smokers may have less hypertension) possibly related to thiocynate in tobacco

SEC
Diet, obesity
Health behavior related to education levels, diet and obesity
Antecedent hypertension related to stress
Occupation (e.g., a waste water or textile plant worker, husband or wife)
Stressful environment
Oral contraceptives used, primipara status
Anxiety
Maternal (inherited) pre-eclampsia, hypertension prior to pregnancy
Exercise and exertion
Exposure to cold

Ref. Chisholm 1983, Crandon 1979, Davies and Dunlop 1983, Hemminki et al. 1983, Hollingsworth 1976, Kliegman and Gross 1985, Lindbohm et al. 1984, Lindheimer 1985, Morgan et al. 1984, Redman 1982, Rofe and Goldberg 1983

III.I Induced abortion and contraceptive behavior, nonuse or unreliable in association with unwanted pregnancy:
Variables affecting contraceptive behavior include:
Legality of contraception
Sexual morals
Social pressures
Shame and guilt
Legality and availability of abortion

Personally:
Less future-oriented behavior
Conservatism as an attitude
Less problem solving ability
Less self-esteem
Frequency of coitus
Stability of sex partner relationship, unstable, conflicted relation with partner
Adequacy of future planning, number and casualness of sex partnerships
Self-rated health
Hopelessness
Prior induced abortion

Worry about pregnancy (note, this can correlate both negatively and positively)
Poor communication with partner
Less egalitarian marriage
Poor general family decision-making
Rigidity of sex related roles
Lack of female power in the relationship (absence of feminist political attitudes probably education related)
Knowledge of contraception
Unmarried status associated with lack of male responsibility for contraception
Absence of social, communication and assertiveness skills in the woman as evidenced in the relationship and generally
Embarrassment in disclosing with physician about sexual matters associated with lower SEC status
Religious/cultural background favoring contraception/abortion

For adolescent females:
Opinions favoring permissiveness
Perceived parental approval/indifference regarding sexuality and noncontraception, guilt over pregnancy
Poor communication with parents
Lack of interest in conforming to parental norms when these are for restraint regarding sex and pregnancy
Knowledge of mother's contraceptive practice
Negative relationship with mother
Drug impairment of control & judgement
Impulsivity
Wish for immediate marriage
No prior experience with "near miss"
Misinformation, no information about female reproductive functions and fertility (varies with age, race and sexual activity levels)
Whether or not first intercourse is planned
"Would not mind" becoming pregnant
Not knowing where to get or how to use contraception
Dislike of contraception requirements, sensations
Self-esteem and felt locus of control affecting openness about contraceptive use
Level of educational goals

Frequence of church attendance interacting with race
Erotophobia, as adverse feeling and inconsistent conduct

For sexually active girls:
Acceptance emotionally and self-image of oneself as favoring sexuality as opposed to guilt
Denial
Anxiety and the need to attribute activity to uncontrollable passion or male desire
Judged self-appropriateness or fit with self-concept of sexuality
Absence of motivation to delay marriage
Passivity in face of male exploitation
Absence of sexual instruction from mother
Absence of perceived ability of oneself to control events in one's life
Presence of pregnant peers
Age-related traits of impulsivity and immaturity
Exposure to non-authoritarian styles among contraceptive providers
Occupational-educational status of mother
Frequency of intercourse (increased contraception use)
Level and adequacy of communication with partner(s)
Maturity of sex-role identity in self-image

For sexual activity per se:
Age
SEC
Ethnic status
Group and individual values
Opportunities
Supervision, when parents of disapproving daughter's rebelliousness and autonomy
For married women, increasing parity
For late abortion: young and low SEC
For pain in induced abortion: prior anxiety interacting with surgical incompetence

Ref. Adler 1980, Bracken, MB 1978, Cartwright 1970, Clark et al 1984, Day et al. 1975, Durant et al. 1984, Forreit 1978, Girard 1986, Gold and Berger 1983, Harvey 1976, Herold 1979, Joe et al. 1979, Jorgensen and Sonstegard 1984, Mayou 1975, Miller 1980, Mindick et al. 1977, Morrison 1985, Nathanson and Becker 1984, Rainwater and Weinstein 1960, Rogel and Zuihlke 1982, Steinlau 1979, Tietze 1983

III.J   Maternal mortality:
For non-obstetrical causes during pregnancy:
Behavioral items associated with cardiac disease (cerebrovascular accidents correlate with older age)
Cancer
Suicide
Illegal abortion
Accidents

For obstetrical causes: for hypertension (toxemia/eclampsia):
Obesity
Age
Race
Reduced antenatal visits
Diet
Medication non-compliance
Ectopic pregnancy in non-contracepting women or those careless with menstrual dates
Caesarean section provoked by poor patient compliance
Anesthesia
Ethnicity, including ethnicity barring access to care
Birth en route to hospital
Physician error (not sending specimens for bacteriological examination, hypertonic prolonged labor and ruptured uterus with complication, coagulation disorder (DIC) and postpartum hemorrhage)
Medical or hospital setting without trained anesthesiologist
Absence in birth setting of specialist care (nurse-midwife or trained MD) (Note in the UK about 60% of maternal deaths are "avoidable" with patient behavior and non-cooperation the biggest contributing factor, and 29% staff error during labor.)
For reproductive mortality (i.e., from avoiding maternity via contraception and abortion as well as when birth is planned):
Oral contraceptive use associated with increased mortality risk in older women

Ref. Kaunitz 1985, Maternity Alliance Report 1984-85, Russell 1983, Thomson and Barron 1983

III.K Emotional disorders and psychoses of the puerperum:
Feeling unloved by partner (associated with depression)
Undesired pregnancy
Adjustment to child-care responsibility
Number of child-care related stresses
Single or separated status
History of emotional problems
Unplanned pregnancy
Breast feeding
Antenatal hostility
Anxiety with cardiovascular hyperresponsivity
Lack of social support
Stressful life events
Poor marital relations
History of interpersonal difficulties
Negative attitude toward and conflict about pregnancy
Smoking
Felt inadequacy as mother
Homosexual conflict
Family history of mental illness
Rigid personality
Social withdrawal
Less femininity
Early dysmenorrhea (possibly emotional in origin)
Failure to attend childbirth preparation classes (interacts with husband's presence and social support)
Recent stressful events
Depressive symptoms early in pregnancy, frequency & severity of prior depression
Ambivalence toward own mother, disturbed relations with both parents when a child
Self-blaming as a trait (internal attributions for negative events)
Severe PMS followed by pregnancy euphoria
Prior PMS or PMC (premenstrual mood change) history

First trimester distress:
Neurosis
Prior abortion and reactivated distress
Post induced abortion:

Neurotic or reactive depression
Preabortion adjustment
Poverty
Family ties
Poor work patterns
Contraceptive failings

Adverse reactions to induced (therapeutic, elective) abortion (Note: strong adverse reactions are rare)
Youth
Unmarried
Catholic or other religious-cultural opposition
Identification in adolescents with infant rather than as mother
Prior mental illness
Immature interpersonal relations
Unstable relation with partner
Ambivalence
Guilt-shame
Second trimester as opposed to first trimester
Surgical stress, particularly saline and prostaglandin instillation
Absence of abortion counseling

Ref. Adler 1980, Baker et al. 1971, 1961, Belsey et al. 1977, Blaney 1985, Braverman and Roux 1978, Bruckington 1981, Butts 1969, Campbell & Winokur 1985, Carnes 1983, Garvry and Tollefson 1984, Gold 1985, Greve and Schroder 1977, Hemphill 1952, Herzog 1976, Inwood 1985, Kumar, K. 1978, Kitai and Brandwin 1979, Little et al. 1982, McNeill et al. 1983, Nadelson 1978, O'Hara et al. 1983, Paykel et al. 1980, Reich and Winokur 1979, Sacks et al. 1985, Stern and Kruckman 1983, Tilden 1983

III.L   Subsequent behavior and development (neonatal, infant, child) and mother-child relationship variables attributable to pre- and perinatal events, conditions: (We note some of these as reminders that this is an important outcome criteria measure; items are, however, but illustrative).
Separation of neonate at birth from mother
Lack of staff contact/fondling of neonate
Nutrition and care provided to low birth weight infants as function of SEC

Alternative family styles
Maternal mental health
Maternal anxiety
Increased maternal emotionality during pregnancy
Emotional upset - fetal activity- infant irritability
Ultrasound feedback reducing anxiety and fetal activity
Neonatal disability
Pregnancy complications
Quality of perinatal and postpartum medical care, including analgesics and anesthetics administered (e.g., diazepam, demeral)
Bonding failures associated with failure to thrive
Child abuse associated with bonding failure
Low birth weight
Long maternal hospitalization
School performance associated with birth weight
SEC
Birth order
Sex
Birth weight
Maternal expectations and attitudes
Absence and adequacy of parents
Emotional disequilibrium during pregnancy
Interaction of life stress and social support
Husband's death during pregnancy
Maternal prenatal toxin exposure/ingestion including drug use: heroin, cocaine, alcohol, cigarettes, marijuana
Physician decisions, prescriptions: neuroleptics, dilantin, barbiturates, thalidomide, steroids (progesterone, androgens, estrogens)
Obstetrical medications: (effects may be very short term), analgesia: demerol. Epidurals, paracervical or pudendal nerve block (e.g., lidocaine, spinal anesthesia: thipental. Diazepam for eclampsia and at delivery
Environmental toxins: methyl mercury, lead, heavy solvent workplace exposure, fire retardants (polybrominated biphenyl or PBB, also PCB
Iatrogenic diasease: retrolental fibroplasia-oxygen induced
Excessive vitamin ingestion: K

For child abuse:
Maternal age
Emotional disturbance
Family dynamics
Parental history of being abused
Baby in special care unit perinatally
Perinatal difficulties (Note some features become long range predictors for eating problems, drug use, delinquency).

Ref. Ahmed 1981, Bernstein et al. 1981, Eiduson and Weisner 1978, Eskenazi 1984, Illsley 1983, Klaus and Kennel 1976, Lilienfeld and Pasamanick 1955, Lynch and Roberts 1977, Neligan and Steiner 1983, Norbeck and Tilden 1983, Sandberg et al. 1985, Shanock 1981, Silverman 1980

III.M Labor difficulty as experienced by the mother including satisfaction, pain, duration, requested medication:
Number of surgical procedures
Days in hospital
Costs
Age
SEC
Adverse life changes as stress
Attitude to medical care
Unfavorable attitude toward pregnancy
Family support
Antenatal preparation in classes
Pleasure in prior births
Presence of emotional/social support
Control over analgesia/anesthesia given
Caesarean vs non caesarean
Being left alone in labor
Insufficient information or opportunity to ask questions
Prior experience with the same birth setting
Staff rudeness/lack of consideration
Disappointment of expectations: husband not allowed in labor room
Neglect in puerperum
Sexism in birth attendants
Baby removed postpartum without explanation or cooperative decision

Inadequate medical attention and communication
Staff insensitivity/complacency (i.e., failure to comprehend patient feelings)
Anxiety during pregnancy
Coping abilities
Interaction of prior stressful experience (adverse life events) with social support availability anxiety
For pain (note childbirth pain scores can be higher than patient pain ratings for toothache, cancer, phantom limb, etc.)
Pain ratings occur depending on obstetrical complications, age, SEC
Antenatal class attendance
Anxiety, denial
Stress
Isolation
Desensitization training
See also discussion on pain variables in next subsection.

For antenatal care satisfaction:
Private versus public clinic attendance
Waiting time
Clinic atmosphere
Doctor-patient (physician warmth, interest, non authoritarian approach)
Discrepancy between patient expectations and events
Convenience of site
Organization of services as experienced
Quality of communication (being encouraged to ask questions, being given understandable information)
Examinations experienced as painful, embarrassing or frightening
Sense of choice over events

Ref. Arms 1975, Ashford 1978, Beck 1980, Blum 1964, Bottom 1980, Bradley et al. 1983, Cranden 1979, Doering and Entwisle 1975, Enkin and Chalmers 1982, Erb et al. 1983, Garcia 1982, Hartmann et al. 1979, Klein et al. (undated), Lederman et al. 1979, Lunenfeld et al. 1984, Macentyre 1977, McDonald 1968, Perez, R. 1983, Reading 1983, Rosen 1977, Sandberg 1985, Sosa et al. 1980, Sosa cited by Oakley et al. 1982, Topless 1972

III.N   Accidents during pregnancy:
         Maternal attitude toward pregnancy
         Availability of support person(s) for meeting appointments or other schedules
         Work commitments that push transportation schedules

Ref. Laukaran and van den Berg

III.O   Preterm labor threatened or realized:
         Age
         SEC
         Number of children at home
         Marital status
         Working status
         Smoking
         Fatigue
         Prior abortion history
         Reticence for communication of symtoms of infection
         Coital demands
         Unstable housing with moving stress

Ref. Bottoms 1983, Creasey 1980, 1983, Thomas and Barron 1983

III.P   Placenta previa:
         Smoking during pregnancy
         Years and level of smoking prior to pregnancy
         Prior caesarean section

Ref. Mayer 1976, 1977, Naeye 1979

III.Q   Abruptio placenta:
         Smoking
         Age
         Nutrition
         Hypertension
         Cocaine use

Ref. Chasmoff et al. 1985, Goujard 1975, Meyer 1976, 1977, Naeye 1980

III.R   Varicose veins complaints:
         Emotional distress
         Introversion (self-focus)
         Multiple diffuse symptom presentation
         Low well-being
         History of induced abortion
         Dysmenorrhea
         Oral contraceptive use
         Workplace
         Demands
         SEC
         Neglecting body hygiene and dressing
         Obesity

Ref. Wenderlein 1976

III.S   Puerperal endometritis:
         Caesarean decision
         Marital status
         Caesarean result
         Nutrition
         Neglected labor
         Obesity
         Coital demands

Ref. Rehu 1980

III.T   Nausea and vomiting (NVP)
         Smoking
         Placebo experience
         Alcohol use levels before pregnancy
         Pregnancy eating habits (foods, frequency, amount); Iron therapy & OTC
         Use of effective folk medications as cultural heritage, social network advice
         Prior NV susceptibility
         For hyperemesis gravidarium:
         Level of symptom reporting
         Expectations of maternal vomiting
         Anxiety and emotionality

Psychological dependency on parents
Attitudes toward pregnancy
Prior sexual dysfunction
Prior chronic gastrointestinal disorder (psychosomatic)

Ref. Chamberlain and Dewhurst 1982, Enkin and Chalmers 1982, Haukins 1983, Hughes et al. 1982, Little and Hook 1979, McDonald 1968

III.U   Heartburn: posture, self-medication with OTC, smoking

Ref. Enkin and Chalmers 1982

III.V   Constipation:
Prior history of constipation
OTC use
Diet
Fluid intake
Exercise
Body rhythm consciousness

Ref. Enkin and Chalmers 1982

III.W   Pseudocyesis:
Emotional distress leading to prescription of phenothiazines in turn inducing amenorrhea, breast enlargement, hyperprolactinemia, galactorrhea, possible increase in HCG

Ref. Pritchard, MacDonald and Gant 1985

III.X   Ectopic pregnancy:
STD leading to tubal infection moderately damaging mucosa
Intrauterine contraceptive devices
Induced abortion with subsequent infection
Ovulatory agent prescribed inducing fertility
Other iatrogenic causes
Douching

Ref. Pritchard, MacDonald and Gant 1985

For other work on psychosocial-behavioral biosocial factors bearing on obstetrical risk prediction see:

Akhtan and Sehgal 1980, Alberman 1977, Aubrey 1979, 1978, Aubrey and Pennington 1973, Beck et al. 1979, Beer et al. 1980, Brazie et al. 1976, Brem 1966, Broussard 1976, Burnett, Jones and Rooks 1980, Butler and Alderman 1969, Cartwright 1984, Chalmers and Richards 1977, Creacy, Gummer and Liggin 1980, Cushner 1981, Darvey 1979, Davis 1963, Doering and Entwistle 1975, Doering and Steward 1978, Donnelly et al 1957, Edwards, Barracla, Tatreau and Hakanson 1979, Eisner, Brozne, Pratt and Hector 1979, Elster 1984, Erikson 1976, Felton and Segelman 1978, Fried et al. 1984, Golbus 1980, Goodwin, Dunner and Thomas 1969, Hartmann, Nielsen and Reynolds 1979, Hemman, Sloane and Shapiro 1977, Hemminki and Starfield 1978, Hobel 1976, Hobel and Youkeles 1979, Hobel, Hyvarmer and Okada 1973, Joffe 1969, Johnstone 1981, Hemminki et al. 1983, Klein, Stein, Strabinow, Susser and Washington 1977, Knodel and Hermalin 1984, Korenbrot 1984, Lederman 1970, 1979, 1981, Lesinski 1975, Linn 1983, Little et al. 1984, Luttman and Parmalee 1978, Lotgoring 1984, Marbury et al. 1983, Matarrazo 1984, McKinley 1970, Morison and Olsen 1970, Morrison et al. 1980, Nesbitt and Aubrey 1969, Oakley 1980, Obayuwana et al. 1984, O'Brien and Smith 1981, Pearse 1979, Porter et al. 1985, Reading 1983, Richmond and Filner 1979, Riegle 1982, Ryan et al. 1980, Shapiro, Schlesinger and Nesbitt 1968, Showstack et al. 1984, Siegel et al. 1985, Sokol, Rosen, Stolkov and Chik 1977, Stembera et al. 1982, Topless 1970, Twinning 1983, Verney 1981, Weiss and Jackson 1969, Wells et al. 1968, Wideman and Singer 1984, William 1979, Williams and Chen 1982, Wilson and Schifrin 1980, Wynn and Wynn 1981, Zackler et al. 1969

Comment

Inspection of the obstetrical risk catalogue reveals a considerable range and number of items as predictors. Many appear to only correlates or tautologies, or facets of or sequences in the same phenomenon related to obstetrical outcomes. Some are met repeatedly and appear as general risk features; others are specific. It is a matter of concern that clinical risk prediction scales in use today, for example Hobel et al. (1979), or Nesbitt and Aubrey (1969), Creasey (1980) include only a very few of these useful items, as for example the rather general ones such as SEC, emotional or social problems. A very few specific behaviors (smoking, drinking) and biosocial status (parity, age) may be included in current scales.

Although the task of research on clinical risk prediction scales is not immediately the same as that for health promotion, they are very closely related. The scale is a guide to estimating individual care needs, but however clinical, the items which form a scale's basis are derived from population studies and the applications are in differentiating among populations of women in terms of expected rates of problems. Insofar as a behavioral item suggests a control possibility, e.g., cigarette smoking, it is likely the physician will seek to alter risk by advising, making the woman aware of that risk, and working with her toward behavior change. In this way research and practice using such scales (whether formally applied or as rule-of-thumb) are but an application of the logic of that same research which recommends health promotion in communities, as well as to those women presenting themselves as maternity patients.

Some among the many now claimed variables are valid, reliable, and efficient as predictors of risk in obstetrics. One would surely expect that one of the early tests of utility would be for clinical practice by their use in better systematic scales. As in Baird's work, the addition of predictor items, delineated by specific outcomes, should lead to further efforts to identify mediating organic pathways or failures in care so that medical treatments might be suggested. Advances in the differentiation of those items leading to death, pathology, dysmorphology, pain, dissatisfaction, developmental failure, unnecessary high cost, the avoidance of iatrogenic interventions, and the development of available services in the absence of which constitutes risk, ought to generate further efforts at interventions by way of health behavior and health institution change. For those with the wisdom and ideological stomach for it, there can be moves for such reform in medical care or society as would appear useful.

Sometimes the steps are more immediate than one might think. For example, Russell (1982), in the analysis of the U.K. confidential inquiries data on maternal mortality, finds among the causes of "associated" mortality treated as not an "avoidable factor" are cardiac disease, malignancy, and suicide (also intracranial hemorrhage and blood diseases). But, unless psychiatry is entirely forlorn, some suicide is preventable and, if any of the tenets of health promotion/ preventive medicine are correct, reduction in risk of cardiac disease and malignancy is also possible. Thus obstetrics, in the very business of concern for its patients likely to die from non reproductive system causes, is compelled to enter the public health arena and the effort to alter psychosocial and behavioral risk factors. The circle is joined. Research on clinical obstetrical risk prediction and for health promotion have the same populations and goals in mind. It is for that reason that one finds it easy to recommend systematic work aimed at improving clinical scales.

Certainly there are deficiencies in the current state of the art, ones shared conceptually or methodologically with the other work going on which seeks to find and understand relationships between environments, living, personality, behavior, and disease. There are also dangers. Among these foremost is failure to appreciate the risk of overreaching that false positives carry in screening programs when there is assignment error and low actual (true) disease prevalence. We have referred to Grant and Mohide (1982) for this discussion, for insofar as false high risk assignment leads to any action in fact inappropriate, there is a financial, and possible psychological and morbidity cost. Recall that women told they might have an abnormal child with spina bifida, cardiac or renal defect, etc., may begin to smoke and drink more, that labor induction for any reason including wrong diagnosis poses risk of fetal and other distress, that seeking to prolong pregnancy via bed rest and sedation is also hazardous, or that nonstress antepartum fetal heart rate monitoring poses greater risk to patients diagnosed at risk than those not known to physicians to be at risk (Grant and Mohide). One need not go on. Silverman's (1980) work on retrolental fibroplasia is indeed the parable of all that can go wrong with (some) of the best intentions.

Resistance to further work on risk scale development may, paradoxically, be understood in terms of relative disappointment with scales now in use. As Choe (1978), Hobel et al. 1973, and Sokol et al. (1977) observe, intrapartum events are only partially predicted antenatally. Van den Berg and Oeschsli (1984), reviewing the work of Newcombe and Chalmers, Fortney and Whitehorne, Papiernik-Berhauer and then Creasey, conclude with regard to the prediction of low birth weight alone (not obstetrical risk across categories) that "it is not possible to minimize the proportion of infants classified as being at high risk and at the same time to predict a large percentage of jeopardized infants." Estimating 25% as at risk, their own limited and simply scored system, which relies entirely on sociomedical history data, achieved sensitivity (true positives) of .40 and specificity (true negatives) of .75. Such prediction inefficiency readily leads to the argument that intrapartum events are better predictors of poor infant outcomes than are antepartum ones. As Butterfield (1978) put it, "you cannot say that a birth is normal until after it is over." On the other hand, as Chard and Richards (1977) remind us, it is also unwise intervention that can make a normal birth abnormal.

As it stands now, sensitivity and selectivity— for obstetrical risk assignment is a screening procedure— can be rather good for prediction accuracy, if one has populations that "fit" whatever prediction scale is selected for them, i.e., if the scale happens to contain items discriminating among that population, ones that are reliably measured. For example, looking at the already self-selected population of women interested in out-of-hospital births (OHB), that group high on SEC, self care motivation and low risk, and fortuitously choosing a prediction scale, one can be accurate four-fifths of the time or more by using a rough, practical criterion (Institute of Medicine, 1984). Findings are reported to the effect that 20% of the women accepted for OHB settings must be transferred to hospital, whereas 15% assessed as ineligible experienced no complications. Further, 98% of pregnant women labelled as low risk will have live babies post neonatal period. The IOM report acknowledges less predictive ability for neonatal morbidity, and argues for research "to perfect and extend the reliability of risk assessment methods." One can only concur, especially after one reads the sophisticated work of Molfese and her colleagues (1985) which provides a good deal less optimistic evaluation of obstetrical risk prediction than that offerered by IOM.

On Methodological Matters: Risk Prediction

Consistent with our argument that the clinician be aware of problems in research, and wherever possible, contribute to research through his or her own activities, we footnote some of the major issues which we deem to be part of improved obstetrical risk research. We deal with scale comparisons, the very serious problem of practitioner history-taking inadequacies, arbitrary scoring, statistical inefficiency and interaction, single vs. multiple observations, and limitations imposed by research environments. The footnote also examines important areas of debate as to predictive importance, namely antenatal care, the hospital role, what SEC (socio-economic class) might mean, and again the very serious matter of practitioner diagnostic unreliability and, finally, the impact, if any, of childbirth preparation.[3]

Allowable Conclusions

In spite of methodological problems, it is reasonable to conclude as follows:

(a) There is strong evidence for the role of psychosocial and behavioral variables in a variety of illnesses and care seeking processes which are of interest in obstetrics.

(b) Some of the factors identified are specifically etiological for particular outcomes. Even so, it is good to recognize that some (smoking, age of onset of sexual activity, alcoholism, SEC, prenatal care, anxiety, social supports, etc.) are also trait markers, indicators of a broader set of events linked to outcomes.

(c) Outcomes themselves, even when described as medical diagnoses, are by no means necessarily singular entities. Diagnoses in both obstetrics and gynecology share some of the same problems in measurement (reliability, criteria) that affect psychological variables. Medical diagnoses of outcome are interrelated with other consequential patient features (for example, emotions, self care capabilities, compliance), and are affected by biological status changes over time.

(d) There is insufficient work done which seeks to identify optimal classes of events to be used in predicting to optimal outcome criteria; necessarily that work is systematization as such, and leads to arrays of subsets of predictors dependent upon particular features of population, setting, measurement, and context for levels of accuracy of forecast.

(e) There is an implied emphasis on prediction so as to improve intervention, but it is here that some of the greatest uncertainty arises, for intervention studies are themselves as yet inadequate in number and, on occasion, sophistication. At what point does declining mortality attributable to cesarean delivery become rising morbidity because of caesareans, and what patient, physician, setting variables contribute to that? It is not demonstrated what antenatal care—when and for whom and how done—is most cost effective. It is only partially clear under what circumstances home births are as safe or safer than hospital births and for whom, with the present data not sufficient to provide guidance by way of education for health promotion to women about to select a birth setting.

(f) Decisions and volitional events do themselves intervene at all points (from sexual behavior through antenatal care, interaction with the physician, compliance in care, self-health help, the judgment adequacy of the hospital staff and physician, anesthetic and surgical interventions employed, etc.). One, therefore, acknowledges that the physician who utilizes any prediction scale is himself/herself influencing the content items of that scale by how well the history and examination are conducted and by his or her own sequential role— diagnosis, advice, care, operative skill, a good experience or bad for his patient. Along the way the physician himself or herself is a subset of variables upon which final outcomes depend and who must be entered into the prediction scale. The physician becomes the Heisenberg principle realized in obstetrical risk prediction.

(g) Since some portion of many outcomes is attributable to one or another psychosocial-behavioral feature, the physician's goal is to optimize and control outcomes via effective intervention effects, which in this instance means shaping the woman's behavior toward greater sensible self-awareness and self-control.

(h) Since some portion of obstetrical risk is iatrogenic, a function of the wrong, or avoidably risky medical interventions, from unnecessary damaging anesthesia through mid forceps use through unindicated surgery, outcome control also means being alert to the epidemological and clinical research data on intervention itself— as for example the "obstetrical battleground" over elected birth setting, and the "new technology" and also malpractice. Thus, health promotion must interest itself in the quality of care provided.

Summary

The use of risk factors for outcome prediction is, in the women's health arena, most extensively and systematically done in the easily studied and delineated area of obstetrical risk prediction. Scales developed to date have not, however, been as successful as one would wish, and they are generally characterized by disagreement, insufficient forecasting accuracy, and inattention to the now broad range of pregnancy outcomes affecting psychosocial-behavioral factors. One waits for a new generation of scales to remedy some of these defects. That cannot occur until obstetrical diagnosis and record-keeping demonstrate consistent reliability, and until obstetrical-medical history taking is itself improved.

Many dozens of psychosocial-behavioral items have been identified as having utility in obstetrical risk forecasting, with some of these consistently replicated, and some linked to pathological outcomes by research on demonstrated or possible physiological mechanisms of action. On the basis of such work one expects that obstetrical risk prediction can become a model for other work integrating psychosocial features into reproductive biology and, simultaneously, demonstrating the effects of improved intervention.

Fundamental problems exist with respect to evaluating and understanding the impact of some commonly accepted but nevertheless uncertainly operating risk-related procedures, as for example antenatal care and classroom preparation for birth. There are also challenges better to evaluate for risk and its perinatal clinical interventions which are the "new technology," as well as anesthesia, and increasing caesarean rates. To improve prediction and thus practice, it is important to combine epidemiological, clinical, medical, and health psychological research. One appreciates that the business of risk identification for health promotion for women's self care and in evaluating the impact of new medical interventions are all also aspects of the effort to improve quality of care as such.

Footnotes

1. We attempt in this and following chapters to be thorough with respect to identifying features identified through research as bearing on the relationship of obstetrical and gynecological conditions to psychosocial status and events. Nevertheless our citations are not complete. For one thing, we have exercised the rule that research work cited in the bibliographies of review and overview articles which we do cite need not be, except in a few instances, separately cited. For the literature prior to 1974, we have not run Medlar/Medline/Psychoinfo/BRS computer searches; thus citation for the years before 1974 will primarily be of particularly salient work.

2. In the bibliography of the National Institute of Medicine, 1984, publication on birth setting research, a doubling of citations, 1976-1981, over 1970-1975.

3. Comparing Scales

It is a welcome study that addresses methodologically the accuracy of prediction comparing antenatal with postpartum prediction. Molfese, Thomson, and Bennett (1985) examined the content, reliability, and predictive utility for discrete outcome variables of five scales. The scales are those of Zax, Sameroff, and Bagigian (1977) Littman and Parmalee (1978), Nesbitt and Aubrey (1969), including the Labor Index of Aubrey and Pennington (1973), Hobel, Hyvarinen, and Okada (1973), and Brazie, Searls, and Lubchenco (1976). Molfese found that infant outcome measures are better predicted by antepartum scores than by intrapartum ones, whereas maternal outcome is better forecast by intrapartum item. While the magnitude of difference is not great, the finding is consequential if for no other reason than encouraging further work on antepartum scale development.

Molfese et al. make several observations about scale construction. Combining the scales they analyzed, they incorporate 195 items (as we know, few of these are well delineated psychosocial and behavioral measures). The scales differ not only in content of items, but also in the criteria used to judge risk. They give as an example different cut off ages for maternal age: 15, 16, 17, 18, and 19 and 30 and 35 years. The proportion of items intrapartum versus antepartum varies, and cutoffs may not be clearly defined. Multiple items are likely intercorrelated or redundant, when they deal with aspects of a single possible, thus giving undue weight problem. Intrapartum items are more homogenous across scales than antepartum ones, and scales differ considerably in the domain and extensiveness of items included for both ante and intrapartum observation. The greater heterogeneity of antepartum items is comparable with the lack of data from systematic observation of psychosocial and behavioral risk item forecasting efficacy which assist in scale construction. That was particularly the case during the earlier period when the scales examined by Molfese were being developed. In the absence of such systematization, investigators developing scales were forced to use rather arbitrary item selection procedures.

The performance of the five scales was examined; Molfese did this by utilizing medical records for two maternity samples, a practical procedure which may suffer from the unreliability of diagnosis and inadequacy of medical records. The following findings beyond the earlier noted differential accuracy to infant versus maternal conditions for ante versus intra partum forecasting respectively, were made. As one would expect, the highest intercorrelations (agreement among scales) are between the scales whose items deal with similar categories or domains (e.g., parity, prior Rh problems, thyroid problems, etc.). Total scale intercorrelations (agreement in risk categorization) range from a low .07 to a high .65 on antepartum subscales, and .26 to .85 on intrapartum subscales. The low end of these tells us that one obstetrical risk scale in use may have essentially no agreement with another scale in its high and low risk two track assignment.

The highest accuracy for all scales, according to Molfese, was incidence of primary caesarean section, although differences for one scale predicting to maternal sample I versus II could vary from $r=0.10$ to 0.31 with a range across scales from $r=0.07$ to 0.41. The lower accuracies among these by no means inspire confidence, and are a far cry from the kind of accuracy one strives for in scale development. One is reminded of criticism of scale validity in obstetrics by Lesinsky (1975). It is surprising that in Molfese's work primary caesarean incidence would prove the overall best predictor given the considerable variation in average caesarean rates by hospital or community (about 7% to 30%) by surgeon, depending upon hospital or community situation. Generally, unreliable outcome measures must be poor tests of predictive capability. Indeed that measure becomes suspect of contamination in any case in practice where the same physician making the intrapartum assessment for the scale item also makes the cesarean decision, for both judgements may rest upon a single set of judgmental standards, that is, they arise from the same set of events and their evaluation.

The relatively poor ability of these five scales to forecast discrete outcomes speaks for the state of obstetrical science at the time of their development. When underlying relationships are understood and quantifiability measured, predictive ability can be good. Molfese was aware of difficulties and avoided contamination among same event outcome measures, i.e., did not test predictive success to both caesarean and general anesthesia, or from the need for anesthesia to caesarean, for these were aspects of the same surgical event.

Thus one does not fault either scales or obstetrics for its poor performance in risk prediction, but rather uses the demonstration of its relative deficiency as an argument for expanded research. Since one knows that one feature contributing to impaired prediction is lack of careful definition of standards for judgement, whether as a basis for rating patients as to their status on an item or as a basis for those decisions used as outcome measures (in obstetrics any intervention, from epidural to caesarean, where rates for like patients vary considerably), there is further impetus for the clarification of diagnostic entities and judgements, and intervention ones, for scientific as well as clinical reasons.

It is likely that the next generation of obstetrical risk prediction will benefit from the incorporation of systematized psychosocial-behavioral items, and after more work on the too many loose measuring devices now employed. It is not likely to be a dramatic improvement even though this area is the least attended to, and in present scales the most primitive one, until there is simultaneous progress in the understanding of the mediating pathways by which psychosocial events become pathological outcomes. The identification of new items with forecasting competence will, when employed to focus attention on possible mediating pathways, stimulate the identification of new classes of physiological events which are reproduction and environmentally responsive so as to become pathogenically active intrapartum. In other words, given any evidence from new items of biological-environmental-personality interaction, one must attend to neuroendocrine, circulatory, neuropharmacological, autoimmune or other substrate processes. One expects that research on behavioral items will also lead (as it has in cardiovascular and cancer studies in stress effects) to identification of substrate events.

4. History Taking Inadequacy

With respect to methodological problems in clinical risk scale construction, if one is now to test as one should the growing array of psychosocial predictors, the problems are the same order as those encountered in other studies in the several disciplines involved, with the added hazards that arise when item identification and patient classification derive from inadequate history taking or a failure to insist upon studies of diagnostic reliability. These are quality of care failings. Hall et al. (1980), Chng and Hall found for example that 25% of the histories taken in their antenatal care study omitted significant prior disease notations with the consequences that whereas 88% of women with significant medical histories (at risk) were referred to specialists (in the U.K. system), only 58% of women without adequate histories were so referred. Similarly, although a prior low birth weight infant was a recordable item, only 32% of the histories recorded the fact; again risk assignments differed. In the adequate history group, 90% were referred to specialists against 59% of those with inadequate histories. Similar findings are reported for retained placenta and prior perinatal mortality. It may be that the same philosophy of specialist referral is found in history taking among those physicians doing poorly at both, i.e., not that it is a matter of missed information leading to inadequate low risk assignment, simply a sloppy approach to risk assessment and to care. Yet it is this kind of unreliability which puts both the women and the risk scale research project in jeopardy. We reiterate the warning that any research which relies on extant records, on diagnoses among personnel not trained especially for inter-judge reliability, or on "routine" history taking is in trouble.

5. Arbitrary Scores

Some scales tend to rely on arbitrary arithmetic values and may incorporate elements that are never finally tested against outcome criteria. Although it is the case that Hobel et al. show only an inconsistent advantage of a stepwise regression method applied as a statistic to increase power (as opposed to arbitrary weight assignment), their work demonstrates an overall advantage for statistically derived weightings. With techniques such as multiple discriminant analysis, including interaction analysis, one may achieve refinements in description of predictor items' power. There can be confusion when medical interventions occurring in response to an intrapartum event are included, with the same algebraic sign and without independent test, in scales that also list the event itself. Thus, if the intrapartum signs include both breech presentation and forceps intervention, we may have such high intercorrelation that the latter item is essentially useless, i.e., there has been no attention to item analysis. Alternatively, without the luxury of random assignment trials (or natural laboratories providing an analogue) one does not know whether an observed morbid outcome is a consequence of the forceps intervention or of the decision-determining preceding fetal presentation (see Chalmers and Richards, 1977). The principle to which we allude, in common with Molfese's work, is that intervention-by-way-of-response must be studied independently for its own effects before incorporation into a scale.

6. Inefficiency

In the usual case when the reliability of factors used in a scale is unknown, one cannot assess resulting inefficiencies. To date the relatively low efficiencies of scales—for example, a high rate of false positives achieved by expanding a "high risk" category to include, say 50 percent of all patients—tend to be reported as general scale effects. Analysis of item or subscale analysis, either to low overall contributions, to variance, or of cutting-point strategies has been limited. One can find claims for "satisfactory" current scales based on relatively small improvements over chance expectancies, i.e., with a scale, one does only 12 percent better in categorizing than without it. The question of economy arises; is that scale worth the trouble? Wilson and Schifrin (1980) conclude that the average high risk assessment of 25% of women yields about half of observed morbidity/mortality for scales in use, and imply that cutting point efficiencies cannot be achieved by items now in use, i.e., to predict 90% of morbidity, 90% of cases would have to be assigned to the high risk category. This is a case of zero efficiency.

The question concerns not only economy, but also specificity of outcome criteria. Were one to know that general obstetrical morbidity is forecast at a rate 15 percent improved over random assignment, but that all of that 15 percent will be cases at an alternate birth center requiring transfer for hospitalization, cheers would be loud. But that specificity in forecasting is rarely seen, except in narrowly defined hypothesis-testing research. The demand then in scale research is that one link specific items and classes of items to efficiencies with respect to particular sets of hard, i.e., reliably measured, clinically consequential items. The question of triage also enters in; if a scale superbly predicts neonatal mortality from gross uncorrectable congenital anomaly, but is of little help in identifying cases for whom obstetrical intervention may make a difference, is it not time to work on the revised edition? There are other problems, typical not simply for obstetrical prediction but for other medical or behavioral prognostic work. Hobel's findings do not replicate many of the items with predictive power in Stembera's work. Molfese's five scales rely of differing item domains. Why? Different diagnostic criteria? Differing medical diagnostic instrumentation or calibration? Differing operational definitions of outcome? A sample of women different in some "fundamental" way, i.e., genetic, nutritional, or other individual or environmental traits that interact or correlate with test items, so that in one study, factors contributing to heavy meconium staining are pathological, and in the second study they are not? Implicit in the question of disparities is the need to relate prediction scale development to etiological understanding, where necessarily one deals with multidetermined morbidity and is required, for understanding, to identify etiologically processes in which pathological outcomes are facilitated or retarded by individual and environmental structures and whose phenotypic representation is the predictor trait. We emphasize with Aubrey (1980) that it is abundantly clear, when the domain is pathology, that risk studies cannot be separated from adequate diagnostic understanding.

Almost invariably, scales developed on one population suffer attenuated accuracy when applied to new, biosocially differing populations. That is the case for the Hobel scale (Baruffi, 1984). One sees it in the difference in prediction success in the two Molfese samples. Implicit is the likelihood that, for risk prediction, some of new biosocial features will affect perinatal outcomes and, further, that populations which differ biosocially will include among those differences significant health status characteristics that make individuals differentially liable to adverse effects, or which differentially have buffered them against pathogens. Our future studies must cover heterogenous populations and will probably have to be differently applied to those subgroups to be identified or homogenous with respect to risk.

7. Interactions

These common findings in the application of predictive scales remind one of the wisdom of Ader (1980) observing that a fundamental observation of psychosomatic medicine is that when populations of individuals are exposed to the same environmental pathogens, only some individuals develop disease, and "all pathological processes are subject to the influence of psychosocial interventions of one kind or another." It is this logic which allows Ader to view pathogens as "superimposed stimuli," a view which reflects Axelrod and Reisine's (1984) quotation from Claude Bernard—what they view as "one of the most cogent statements framed by a biological scientist," to the effect, "The constancy of the 'milieu interieur' is the condition of a free and independent existence." Obviously none of the pathogenic, or buffering experiences of pregnancy—or those which are risk features arising before conception— allow that sublime isolation. Indeed it is the principle of life to be "irritable," i.e., environmentally responsive, in a self-organizing way and it is the principle of interaction between organism and environment, including self-induced actions, which is fundamental to work in behavioral health. Thus, when we examine prediction error in obstetrical risk scales we are looking at a special case illustrative, in unexplained variance—often large—of the variety of features which are asssumed to be affecting pregnancy outcome. The task becomes one of finding traits which mark groups homogenous in exposure and response to environmental pathogens, and of identifying interactions which qualify and specify outcomes. This implies knowledge of the kinds of interactions which were illustrated in the introduction to this chapter.

As an example of methodology where the availability of a large number of cases allowed a search for differential perinatal mortality risk for subgroups of mothers, one calls attention to the analysis by Meyer, Tonascia, and Buck (1974) of the Ontario Perinatal Mortality Study, 1960-1961. By identifying 52 subgroups of smokers grouped for other risk features as well, and controlling for these variables when shown to affect smoking itself, it was possible to refine risk estimates. For example, the increased risk of perinatal mortality associated with light smoking among low parity, non-anemic young mothers was less than 10%, but with mothers of high parity, at public hospitals (low SEC), with previous low birthweight births, and hemoglobin less than 11 gm, when there was heavy smoking, mortality risk increased 70% to 100%.

8. Single Vs. Multiple Observations

One of the features of prediction work is improvement dependent upon sequential observation. For example, child developmental deficit emerging at 18 months is only somewhat predictable prenatally, becomes more efficient perinatally, and improves upon observation of the infant. It is not simply that proximal events are better predictors than distal ones. Examining extant scales, one sees within any one time period, e.g., "prenatal," items of varying duration and time of occurrence. Some are a record of prior life history. Some are status or event reports (i.e., low socioeconomic class, measles during pregnancy, vaginitis). Except for studies with controls for immediate status as a subsidiary variable depending on a long-acting condition, e.g., fever-influenza, or residential crowding as a function of socioeconomic class, little attention has been paid to the reformulation of these time-dependent variables by attending to periodicity, incidence, or duration, i.e., chronic or acute characteristics.

One can also examine reliability as a function of measurement method (recall vs. record vs. direct observation), and by intercorrelation devices, such as factor analysis, one can seek to identify processes as global factors of conceptual worth. For example, almost no attention is paid to onset, recentness, duration, periodicity as qualifying descriptors for those life-style variables important in disease etiology and treatment outcome, as for example nutrition, exercise, stress, smoking, illicit drug and alcohol use, cooperativeness in medical care.

The temptation of global one shot measures is the same problem which arises in psychophysiological stress research where quantitative levels are observed, but time sequence changes are not. Levine and Coe (1985) make this point about cortisol measures of adrenal response as labile depending upon environmental-organism circumstances, time of day, reproductive state and genetic variables (Levine and Coe were working on mother-infant separation stress.) Individual differences in base lines, also labile, must also be taken into account, as Campbell and Cohen (1985) remind us about immune system components in blood, for there is "enormous" inter-individual variability in "normal" levels of monocytes, macrophage, interleukin 1, interleukin 2, inducer and suppressor cytotoxic and delayed-type hypersensitivity T-cells, IgE antibodies. Insofar as one expects, and we do, obstetrical risk prediction to investigate such stress and immune levels, as in the work of Adamson et al. (1971), Lederman et al. (1978), and Schnider et al. (1979), the reminder as to insufficiency of simple index measures applies to all areas of work, at least until demonstrated otherwise.

The foregoing methodological comments are meant to call attention to the disparities in effectiveness of existing risk prediction methods and to suggest that much remains to be done in this important area. Required procedurally is more attention to variations in measurement and in definitions of factors and outcomes, to more sophisticated statistical methods, to the points in time when traits have power, and whether these are independent, sequential, process, or contextual variables. Useful conceptually is greater cross disciplinary work so the prediction efforts test items drawn from several domains, e.g., obstetrics, behavioral medicine, environmental toxicology, sociology, psychosomatics, and psychology. Important too are approaches, either initially or after factor analytic or covariance studies, which derive traits for testing from theory, i.e., from an integrated intellectual framework rather than relying entirely on ad hoc available medical history data or impressionistic clinical experience.

9. Research Environments

The reality of research environments—that one can usually only afford to do immediate, retrospective or short term prospective studies on accessible (typically clinic) small populations—means that even when statistically significant findings emerge, one has only made the first step on the road to finding risk factors of potentially general usefulness that would guide disease prevention efforts. One must learn if the finding is reproducible, efficient in terms of conceptual and operational refinement, and independent in terms of contribution to outcome explanation. One must learn if a variable's influence is limited to particular groups, i.e., is part of that particular matrix of events which the study sample in its present and historical environment, and its morbidity outcomes constitutes, or whether factor will be a useful risk predictor across a range of population subgroups. Even with this done—and one is describing either a program of studies or the slower evolution of work in a field with all of its accidental components (does it become fashionable to study, do people have the expertise necessary to study it, will ethics committees allow it, will communication among investigators be facilitating, is there time and money for the work?)—showing a relationship by no means proves that the risk factor can be altered—whether that is an environmental, personality, or behavioral item. And accomplished change by no means guarantees any early demonstration of a change in outcome prevalence. The independent variable may turn out to be a trait marker only (something else was really happening with observed covariance not related to a physiological mediating disease pathway), outcome effects will be shown to be related to prior rather than immediate influence of the variable (as when smoking before pregnancy yields a higher association with adverse outcome than smoking during pregnancy when the latter is behaviorally eliminated), or large scale social or medical changes will intervene to overwhelm any impact demonstrable from whatever it is we may succeed in altering.

Current Conflict Areas:

10. Antenatal Care

The success attributed to an intervention and used as the basis for prediction may be claimed to be only an illusion, as for example for antenatal care as argued by Enkin and Chalmers (1982). Or Silverman (1980), citing Morris et al. who, examining decline in infant mortality in the US, propose that ony a fraction of that decline could be attributed to the success of organized maternal and infant care projects. Twenty-seven percent was attributable to a change in maternal age/birth-order distribution of births. Hall et al. (1980) showed that the majority of pregnancy-related admissions to hospital for other than delivery were for conditions judged not presentable or detectable by antenatal care. Controversy abounds!

11. Hospitals

Consider hospitals themselves, and that current obstetrical battleground over home versus hospital births. A review of that literature (for example, ACOG

1978, 1979, 1980, Ashford 1978, Aubrey 1977, Brown and Isaacs 1976, Burnett et al. 1980, Cloosterman 1978, Cox et al. 1976, Darney and Rooks 1979, Declerq and Darney 1982, Dingley 1979, Estes 1978, Euland 1971, Fedrick and Yudkin, Tew and Barron, National Institute of Medicine 1984, Hazel 1975, Holmes 1929, Longo 1981, Mehl 1977, Pollinger 1977, Summary, Frontier Nursing Service 1958, Taylor 1976, Thomson and Barron citing Chalmers et al., Van Alten et al. 1976) allows no simple conclusion applicable to all maternal groups. One may say that home births are often safe, and often unsafe, that some hospitals are safer than others, as are some interventions — some of which are more justifiable than others— so that covarying, content and interaction effects, and distinct population characteristics must always be considered when evaluating outcomes as a function of intervention. More practically, given Baird's results in Aberdeen, the real fall in maternal and neonatal mortality/morbidity over this half century, the fact that hospital deliveries are by far the most prevalent and, overall, hospital attenders do better, one may safely conclude (although Tew (1979) reviewing data on stillbirths disagrees) that hospitals and their obstetricians at least have not prevented great improvements in maternal/neonatal health and, obvious in many obstetrical pathology groups, have contributed to observed improved health. How much solely and for whom must remain open questions.

12. SEC: What Is In The Basket?

One of the most compelling areas for research, and for understanding as one moves toward the application of clinical risk prediction or office-based health promotion, is as noted in Chapter 3, for the better characterization of the operational components in those items which are undifferentiated basket categories, or processes, including some diagnoses. We have referred to this in an earlier chapter, but it requires further comment. Illsley's work on SEC is exemplary in showing how "class" changes in time with respect to size and membership, but how its contribution to health involves assortive mating self-selection in marriage (or now in the US outside of marriage) for height, diet, living conditions and standards, intelligence, education, occupation, physique, and health. Buss (1985) offers comparable data on self-selection of likes as assortative narcissism (quoting Thiessen) in mating, leading to even greater class or family differences over the generations in physical attractiveness, height, mental abilities, and other socially valued traits.

When each investigator selects his own concept and measure, there can appear to be diversity of traits as contributors to outcome when there may be commonalities, as for example with depression, which may also be reflected in measures of hopelessness, low self-esteem, emotional disorder, negative affectivity (Watson and Clark, 1984), and the like. Listings of what are most likely intercorrelated events— as in findings with respect to STD— can contribute to the impression of great diversity when a more efficient statistical logic should lead to findings of clusters, discriminant weights, factors syndromes, and one hopes underlying covariance specified by population, setting, and time characteristics.

12. Diagnosis

There often appears to be the assumption of diagnostic reliability and singularity, accompanying reports of specific psychogenic etiological features. Leck (1983) warns of unreliability in diagnosis of fetal malformations in neonates, as do Vouk and Sheehan (1983) a problem which is reified, if not multiplied, in hospital or other medical records. The diagnostic problem leads to varying estimates of malformation in populations, typically from 2% to 5%. Further unreliability in rates for estimating teratological effects expands if early events (fetal loss, spontaneous abortion) and later ones (infant behavior, development aberrations) are included—arguably they should be—as outcome measures.

Thomson and Barron (1983) make it clear how difficult is the task for maternal disorder when a single diagnosis is required. That problem is illustrated by Macintyre (1977) in her discussion of the long chain of social and medical events which constitute the evolution of a diagnosed or otherwise singularly classified pregnancy outcome. One therefore is beware of misleading of specificity in some of the claims, particularly of risk factor-disease outcome studies, for one may be dealing with labile or interchangeable diagnostic entities (depending on time, criteria, interest) and constellations of etiological features. Consider for example that emotional problems appear again and again as etiological for a number of obstetrical and gynecological conditions with the implication of specific causality. But when one also considers the phenomenon of high levels of symptom reporting as such, which in turn correlates with neuroticism, being a gynecological patient (Eisenberg 1984, citing Byrne), having pain, being a repeat medical visitor, being sensitive, stressed, etc., one sees that any gynecological work up should expect to find emotional disorder appearing in the history. Or, if one takes "floating" diagnostic groups such as PMS, dysmenorrhea, pelvic pain, etc., one would not be surprised to see each carrying a similar burden of psychosocial history. This is all compounded by the fact that these conditions themselves may produce reactive emotional components and their sequelae.

As an illustration of the need to identify substrate psychobiological features as the active component accounting for outcomes in processes classified by external behavioral markers, let us look at that type of antenatal care which is childbirth training.

14. Childbirth Training

In the first place, the predictor item, antenatal care, can broadly include both medical clinic attendance and childbirth class attendance; we have not found studies which in the same population compare women doing either one and not the other. One assumes medical antenatal care, especially in the UK, is the more common and that in the UK or the US the usual self-selecting motivational, educational, and opportunity features which predispose to safe pregnancy will also be associated with the Lamaze, Read, or other "method" attendance. It is by no means demonstrated that antenatal training method attendance influences the range of outcomes which are employed as pregnancy risk measures, although we shall see that it does affect satisfaction.

Wideman and Singer (1984) and Beck, Geden, and Browder (1979) review the evaluation studies that purport to prove that "method" women request less analgesia, have fewer cesarean sections, postpartum infections, premature births, toxemia-eclampsia, postpartum hemorrhage, perinatal lacerations and perinatal mortality than comparison groups. These studies ordinarily do not sort for biosocial status preselection or for those negotiations which will enter in, as in the "natural childbirth" group, in the selection of physician and birth center to reduce the chance for anesthetic or surgical interventions as a physician elective. Further, examination shows that many of these studies rely on patient recollections of their own history—a method not known to be better than reliance on medical records and probably worse—since studies have shown that women have quite poor recollections of postpartum events and that human memory shapes itself in terms of expectations, i.e., one's "theory" of how events should have unfolded. Thus, as Wideman and Singer tell us, the one study based on chart review (here now assumed to be the better measure, but itself faulty), Lamaze women given antenatal care compared to antenatal medical care groups only experienced satisfaction and less distress but lost any advantage in length of labor or obstetrical complications. Robitaille and Kramer (1985) in a study of 1,747 primiparous women found those participating in prenatal courses were higher SEC and less often smokers so that, when these items were controlled, no birth weight differences were attributable to ante-natal courses per se. Such reductions in smoking as did occur could not be attributed to training.

Some workers have sought to identify the component processes in birth preparation class training, i.e., the most likely psychological behavioral events interacting biologically, as for example to reduce the stress response whether rated cardiovascularly or as felt anxiety. They consider preparation method gains as possibly dependent upon how much and what kind of information is given as in turn affecting discomfort (i.e., procedural and/or plus sensory information and its effect on cognitive restructuring). Respiratory training is a control elsewhere demonstrated to be able to reduce autonomic responsivity to stressors (one presumes that varying with degree of threat and ability to plan for it), relaxation training, with its passive concentration and imagery ("imaging," including conditioned imaging as generating efferent impulses, rather akin to gating theory in pain control), and coping strategies and social support. Wideman cites Sosa et al. reporting that simply the presence of a supportive layperson in a maternal preparation group leads to fewer perinatal problems, fewer cesarean sections, shorter labor, and more alert neonates. But Wideman and Singer propose that other processes may also be operating. With respect to social comparison (related to reference group and dissonance theory), they note that a number of studies show that simply being with others who share the same situation reduces anxiety and discomfort, thus class qua group may reduce anxiety later affecting delivery. Here one thinks of the range of animal studies, e.g., Liggel (1954, 1956) showing that for social animals—and primates and humans are such—the presence of fellows favorably alters a range of stress responses, providing crowding or other "behavioral sink" stressors are not built into the environmental architecture. What then are the cardiovascular and neuroendocrine mediating pathways common to these mammals whose positive effects are indicated by the trait marker of social support?

Commitment and conformity are also possible components, for much research shows once public avowals are made to important groups (e.g., peers), there can be strong motivation to experience what was undertaken. These generate self-fulfilling prophecies. Perceived self-control is another possible variable: the authors review studies showing that subjects who believe they have control over potentially noxious stimuli report decreased negative affect. Those pregnant women, for example, confidently anticipating their control capabilities during birth, later requested and received less analgesia/anesthesia during parturition. Wideman and Singer conclude that while data from work outside of childbirth does show that information, controlled respiration techniques, conditioned relaxation, visual focusing techniques, and social support are effective in reducing anxiety and discomfort, one cannot be sure these account for the (somewhat uncertain or contradictory) Lamaze or other method effects, since other processes, as noted, may also be at work.

A rather different analysis of both childbirth preparation and the psychological outcome criteria for assessment of "risk" is offered by Lumley and Ashbury (1982). Read is charged with, beginning in the late 1940's, generating expectations of fear and pain in labor "if she does not do what she is told," with these anxieties in turn claimed by Read to be associated with a range of medical risk outcomes (hemorrhage, respiratory failure in the infant, etc.). Read's information giving approach, his "intractable belief in his own theory," is said to regard women either as agreeably rational or alternatively deluded and beyond help, a view so persuasive that it has led, say Lumley and Ashbury, to the unexamined assumption in medical psychological research that anxiety must be a negative emotion with adverse medical consequences. Excluded from thought, and thereby research, they imply, are views of anxiety as adaptation to real stress facilitating coping behavior. Lumley and Ashbury then offer studies indicating that high anxiety levels are and also are not associated with obstetrical abnormalities whereas moderate levels are associated with better postnatal adjustment. (Studies on denial also show quite contradictory results.) Ashbury cites her own work indicating that knowledge (a la Read) and anxiety are unrelated, i.e., that while "method" prepared women were more knowledgeable about reproduction, they were not less anxious. Lumley and Ashbury may be over-reaching; since early psychiatry and physiology of Freud and Cannon, anxiety has been appreciated for its alerting, warning role, and its presence as an adaptation facilitating mechanism has long been recognized. Nevertheless theirs is a reminder here to question the assumption, made in "method" training and for risk categorization, that anxiety is always undesirable. Indeed one might ask if there are circumstances in which "method" training may induce denial/repression of potentially adaptive anxiety with a resulting failure on the part of the "method" committed woman to bring symptoms of consequential pathology to her physician's attention.

7

Women's Conditions Linked to Psychosocial–Behavioral Factors

In this chapter we examine the illness of women, including some suffered by women and men, for which psychosocial-behavioral risk features have been identified. We do not present or evaluate individual studies, but, rather, continue with the tabular presentation of a catalog of findings. It will be seen that a number of these discrete items repeat those already reported as relevant for obstetrical risk, complaints, general morbidity, or to mortality as such. Such reappearing items may be assumed to demonstrate experimental replicability either as risk factors for morbidity as such, or for several illnesses with parallel or underlying similar course, i.e., common pathways. When a risk factor is reported in relationship to only one disease it may be specific in etiology, it can be a marker for a subpopulation whose other experiences, characteristics, predispose to or are associated with specific disease etiology, or it can be discovery waiting to be tested for a possible role on other morbidity.

When there are only one or two studies on a disease, and reporting findings, of say, psychological etiology, the rule of caution in acceptance should be observed. Uterine myoma, for example, where only two studies are reported, must be seen as allowing much less confidence with respect to psychosocial factors in risk, than coronary heart disease where a number of studies reach consistent findings, albeit as we saw in Chapter 6 these too are under constant refinement.

The tabular approach to data presentation is intended to convey the fact that a broad range of psychosocial-behavioral items have been associated in the etiology of disease risk and to suggest thereby the range of conditions which constitute the subject matter of health promotion risk control and research. One must keep in mind that for many of the more exotic items listed, strong evidence is lacking as to their weight in relative and attributable risk, and their role in physiological mechanisms of disease process. Absent almost entirely in the literature are data on the relationship one to another and to underlying, initially statistically generated covariance of the psychobiological items. To learn how now discrete items may functionally knit together, one looks forward to systematization through future research.

By no means is it to be assumed that the listed items are to be given equal credence with reference to their etiological role. We have seen, in other chapters, how even the most replicable of factors, from stress through social support to antenatal care, Type A, alcohol or cigarette smoking, are subject to quite complex interpretation. And the quality of research, including representativeness of samples and control of other possibly influential variables, differs markedly.

Our rule of thumb, based on examination, is to have most confidence in (a) those general factors repeatedly shown to influence general morbidity and mortality (SEC, social support, stress, etc.) as a review of Tables II through V suggests, (b) those specific trait and lifestyle factors (e.g., diet, self care, depression, anxiety) repeatedly linked either to general morbidity/mortality or specific illnesses, and (c) conduct factors repeatedly shown (cigarette smoking, overeating, sexual conduct) demonstrably linked to particular diseases, especially where a mechanism of action is implicated. At present our advice to the clinician is to examine the foregoing particularly among the array, and to take note of those items about which he or she does not presently inquire in history-taking, or does not attend to when spontaneously presented by or inferrable from the conduct of the women. These items can be incorporated into a reference list to be consulted as a guide when reviewing the status of patients whose particular problems or disease course presents a puzzling etiology or course. The items are also a reminder to the women's health professional about those aspects of conduct, situation, or life styles in her world "out there" which should be addressed in, by, and with the patient as part of health promotion.

Following presentation of Tables IV and V below, our discussion will offer some cautions with respect to too quick an assumption that an illness shown etiologically associated with a risk factor can be prevented by reducing that factor, or providing a "buffering" condition. Problems in risk screening which arise when there is uncertainty as how best to characterize a risk trait are noted, as are considerations of cost for either screening or intervention. Public policy debates invariably occur as a function of dollar costs for such programs, and we allude to these. In closing this chapter we offer our view that, compared to men, women are being shortchanged by public policies and perhaps personal values, which provide less by way of research funding, screening programs, or insurance coverage for alleviating interventions for women's behavioral health related conditions.

Table IV
Diseases of Women, and Men, Associated with Psychosocial and Behavioral Risk Components

IV.A   Coronary heart disease:
Occupation
Bereavement
Social support network status (married or living with a partner versus single)
Church attendance
Network of friends
Membership in clubs, civic groups or other organizations
Frequency of contacts with others, perceived support available from others, etc.
Social mobility (income/occupation/class) within one's life span
Status incongruity
Personality type A[1] (competitive, striving, speedy, aggressive, impatient, sense of urgency, hostile, domineering as evident in voice, information processing efficiency, need for control)
Type A interacting with occupational mobility age range 45-54
Type A modified hostility and suppressed rage voice pattern of comment/control only
Smoking risk is potentiated in women taking oral contraceptives
Cigarette smoking

Smoking effects by raised lipids and lipoproteins as demonstrated.[2,3]
High cholesterol diet
Duration of anxiety, hostility and depression in response to adversely challenging events (threatening, esteem-damaging, noxious).
Non-adaptation in threat perception
Stress as a cluster of major life changes
Events experienced as severe threat in interaction with the absence of ways of dealing with the events (coping)
Stress defined as mobility including changing residences, jobs, upward class mobility among lower classes, number of promotions (particularly if out of the class of one's family of origin)
Culture changing migration, particularly when sacrificing social supports and traditional lifestyles for a fluid hard driving cultural ethos (as in the U.S.)
In one's occupation; excessive work and responsibility
For women, clerical work with nonsupportive supervisor
Other possible factors: personality traits of anxiety, irritability, depression, trait hysteria and hypochondriasis, syndrome of emotional drain, (somaticizing, fatigue, giving up, general malaise in situations giving rise to rage and frustration, and to despair and hopelessness)
Depression, over-control and constriction in imagery
Life problems perceived as intense occurring chronically
Being sedentary
Sleep disturbance
Vital exhaustion and depression
Anger under stress
Sudden emotional trauma
Work overload with low decision power
Joyless striving for women
Hostility, especially cynical hostility
Exposure (climate, housing) to cold, for CHD with arteriosclerosis

Catecholamine and cortisol stress response secretion levels CHD risk: There is only an hypothesized association between these and CHD. Under challenge secretion rates are less when personal control (sensed or real) over the situation increases. Lack of control is also associated with learned helplessness and in turn depression. Psychological arousal when both effortful and distressing increases neuroendocrine response levels characteristic of stress response to daily hassles. In general, women in the same challenging situation as men report less intense effort and secrete less catecholamines. For men, secretion levels are associated with many "success" variables, not so for women in traditional feminine roles. Women with non-traditional aspirations, (engineers, bus drivers, lawyers) respond to achievement demands with same secretion levels as men. Traditional women when challenged in traditional roles, e.g., maternal child illness care, show same secretion levels as fathers.

IV.B Angina risk:
Number of life problems, interpersonal discord, degree of marital intimacy, financial dissatisfaction
For CHD, excessive overtime work
Survival risk greater for those with fewer prior life changes
Crescendo effect in life changes during period before attack
Specific traits in Type A: time pressure, achievement/ambition motive, excess job responsibility, rapid work and movement, seek responsibility, competitive, hostile, obsessive, overcontrolling
Voice patterns suggest command/control

Also widely reported:
Cigarette smoking
Obesity
Sedentary living
Undetected-uncontrolled hypertension
Higher cholesterol as dietary function
Diabetes and its control
Recently widowed
Involuntary unemployment
MMPI scales high (negative effect)
Presence of social intimates acts as buffer when other high risk factors present

IV.C Venous thromboembolism:
For women: oral contraceptive use after age 30, and oral contraceptives combined with cigarette smoking
Illustrative citations: for CHD, angina, vascular disease studies

References: Appels 1983, Appels and Mulder 1984, Anderson 1985, Baker et al. 1984, Ball 1982, Beral and Kay 1977, Brahn et al. 1974, Case et al. 1985,

Chelune & Waring 1984, Chesney 1983, Cohen 1979, Dombrowski et al. 1983, Dombrowski and McDougall 1985, Chen 1983, Craig and Brown 1984, Eisenberg 1979, Frankenhaeusen 1983, Goldziher 1980, Hamburg, Elliot & Parron 1982, Haynes and Feinleib 1980, Hatcher et al. 1986, Herd 1984, Herd & Weiss 1983, Jain 1976, Jenkins 1976, Kannel et al. 1976, Krantz & Glass 1984, Krantz & Manuck 1984, Lanson et al. 1977, Marmot and Morris 1984, Mathews et al. 1977, Meade 1982, Morrison et al. 1979, Patel 1983, Pettite et al. 1978, Rabkin and Struening 1976, Realini & Goldheizer 1985, Rosenmann et al. 1975, Russell-Briefel et al. 1985, Salonen 1982, Sarason & Sarason 1982, Schneiderman & McCabe 1985, Smith & Forohm 1985, Surgeon General's report 1979, Webber et al. 1982, Zeichner and Dickson 1984.

IV.D Hypertension:
  High automatic reactivity to psychosocial stressors measured by circulating catecholamines and elevated cardiac output
  Active coping response challenge; greater suppressed hostility in association with high plasma renin
  Possible sodium retention influencing renal functioning as a stress response
  Greater reactivity to a variety of stimuli
  High reactivity to work stress
  Personality traits of anxiety denial-repression appear risk associated (correlates with reduced resting alpha EEG and exaggerated frontalis muscle myography response)
  Race (blacks at higher risk)
  Chronic stress, psychosocial stress
  Occupational stress
  Maternal anxiety
  Overweight
  Heavy alcohol use SEC (inverse relationships)
  Setting
  Oral contraceptive type used
  Smoking
  Dietary salt intake in those already at risk
  Medication non-compliance in those at risk
  Oral contraceptive use in women
  Chronic conflict situation exposure
  Suppressed hostility under frustration in association with anxiety
  Overt hostility and competitiveness as interacting traits

Alexthymia (inability to specify or express feelings)
Neuroticism
Among women, poorer relations with family and friends
Living in an industrial nation
High pressure jobs
High stress plus high salt diet, and potassium
Defiant assertive behavior (defensive, abasement, submissive)
Cultural instability
Living in disadvantaged neighborhood
Crowding (prison cells)
Self-medication with amphetamine-like compounds, e.g., ginseng as a "health food"
Reduced calcium intake

Ref: Anderson 1985, Baker et al. 1984, Collington et al. 1985, Craig and Brown 1984, Harlan et al. 1985, Henry & Stephen, 1977, Herd 1984, James and Kleidbaum 1976, Kok et al. 1986, Krantz, Baum & Smizer 1983, Krantz & Glass 1984, Krantz & Manuck 1984, Levi 1979, Pettiti & Klatsky 1983, Rayburn, Zuspan & Pehl 1984, Schneiderman & McCabe 1985, Schwartz 1982.

IV.E   Stroke:
       Blood pressure
       Cholesterol levels
       Diabetes
       Cigarette use, potentiated by oral contraceptives

Ref. Hatcher et al. 1986, Robbins and Blankenbaker 1982

IV.F   Rheumatic heart disease:
       Increases as unemployment rates rise

Ref. Marmot and Morris 1984

IV.G   Cancer without reference to sites or multi-sites:
       Residence
       Accidents
       Work exposure to carcinogens (both agents & worker compliance with safety measures)[4]
       Diet characteristics: lower risk with adequate

consumption of fresh vegetables, fibers, vitamin A
as beta carotene, foods rich in vitamin C, seafish, reduced dietary fat, reduced intake of salt-cured, smoked and nitrite-cured foods.
Adequate weight control
Alcohol ingestion
Cigarette smoking (for women, work stress influential on smoking)
Father's smoking in interaction with race and sex and victim smoking
Psychosocial: lack of parent-youth closeness
Suffering interpersonal loss
Felt vulnerability and repeated life trauma
Traits of repression and aggression and other deficits in the expression of emotions.[5]
MMPI trait depression
Personal experiences including loss of important relationship, sexual disturbances or unresolved tensions involving parent figures.

Ref: American Cancer Society, "Taking Control" 1985, Cohen 1979, Fox 1981, Goldberg & Tull 1983, Grossarth-Maticek et al. 1984, Kissen et al. 1969, Klerman and Izen 1977, Krantz and Glass 1984, LeShan 1966, Levy 1985, Solomon and Amkraut 1982, Sandler et al. 1985, Shekelle et al. 1981, Sklar and Anisman 1981, Young and Erhardt 1980.

IV.H   Cancer survival time or quality of life:
Psychotherapy, counseling
Social, intimate support
Absence of death wish
SEC status associated with health care use and access
Health care & access associated with risk status and factors such as isolation, age, depression, inconvenience, fear of cancer, embarrassment
Use of ineffective unorthodox treatments instead of effective ones
Clinical depression associated with altered immune function)

Goldberg & Tull 1983, Levy 1985, Moos 1984

IV.I   Skin cancer:
Primary melanoma for which in the U.S. are rising faster than for any other cancer except lung
Occupation (skin exposed)

Vacation patterns: intermittent intense exposure
Childhood blistering by sun
Incidence increased with age
White race
Lower latitude residence
Interacts with skin burning reaction and dysplactic nevi

Ref. Fitzpatrick and Sober 1985

IV.J Cancer of the bladder:
In women:
Cigarette smoking
Coffee consumption
Use of phenacetin containing medications

Ref. Piper J et al. 1986

IV.K Pneumonia-emphysema-bronchitis:
Cigarette smoking
Possibly alcohol consumption
Probably nutrition status

Ref. Robbins and Blankenbaker 1982

IV.L Gastrointestinal pathology:
Ulcers - As a marker for disease susceptibility: In animal studies, high response to stress/challenge clinically; in humans, possibly, hard driving, relentlessly active and reactive emotional stress, chronic severe stress emotionally.
Cigarette smoking

Ref. Kagen & Levi 1974, Weiss 1984, Steptoe 1984

IV.M Sexually transmitted diseases:
Number of sexual partners
Age
Duration and intensity of acquaintance with sex partner (casual or other)
Partners' sexual activity with others

Information levels
Use of prophylaxis
Self-detection of symptoms
Date of last medical examination and speed of self-referral
Adequacy of friends' information and levels of information re: treatment
Location of clinic vis-à-vis one's residence
Felt risk of exposure leading to self-care & caution
Chronic psychological capacity
Locus of control (internal or external)
SEC
Education level
Residence area
Self-esteem level
Attitudes toward society (destructive-psychopathic-anomie)
Alcoholism and alcohol hospital admission
Drug abuse and drug abuse admissions
Injuries from interpersonal violence
History of non STD infectious disease
Psychiatric disorder history
Police record including violence in relation to police
For women: abortion history
For homosexuals: number of contacts
Level of somatic complaints and hypochondriasis
Accident history
Family of origin (stability versus divorce or single parent)
Particularly important for women: SEC, ethnicity, capacity for sexual restraint during infectious periods
For women: stress may invoke latent genital herpes
Transmission via donor semen for artificial insemination
For Acquired Immune Deficiency Syndrome (AIDS): sexual practices & contraception use, sexual behavior of partners, for infants, infection from mother. (Note: transmission via blood transfusion and hyperdermic needles is also common).
Malnourishment and compromised immune states

Ref. Aral et al. 1985, Day et al. 1975, Hayes et al. 1976, Joklik, WK 1985, Leiva et al. 1985, Lundin et al. 1977, Med. brief 1985, Mayou 1975, Morton et al. 1979, Niemiec 1978.

IV.N   Postoperative recovery and adjustment: measured by depression, disruption in social life, reduced sexual function, work disruption (not physically indicated), slow recovery, and complications
Preoperative denial-repression
Hypervigilance
Failure to receive realistic preoperative prediction about what is going to happen and how one will feel
Failure of patient and MD to discuss emotions and adjustment problems postoperatively
Trait anxiety
Neuroticism
Absence of counseling
Preoperative anxiety
Perceived operation as threat, for example, to self and to spousal relationship and satisfaction
Special information-giving by nurses and relaxation instruction reduce hospital times and facilitate recovery

Ref: Cohen & Tazaras 1982, Janis 1983 a 1983 b, Johnson 1982, Mathews and Ridgeway 1984

IV.O   Infection vulnerability:
Experienced stress
Psychological ego strength
Discrepancy between goals
Motivations
Goals versus performance
Recovery rate associated with depression

Ref: Greenfield cited by Plast & Friedman 1981, Jemmott and Lock 1984, Imboden, cited by Solomon and Amkraut 1982, Meyer & Hagerty, cited by Plast & Friedman 1981

IV.P   Rheumatoid arthritis:
No "arthritic personality"
Present: significant psychological stress, e.g., emotionally charged events
High marital dysfunction
Psychological conflict
Delayed psychophysiological recovery times

Ref. Anderson et al. 1985

IV.Q Traumatic injury from traffic accident
Accident risk increases with:
Personality immaturity
Low impulse/tension control
Paranoid features
Alcohol use
Recent personal conflicts
Work-money crisis
Minor tranquilizer use
Adverse life change
Risk taking
Belligerence
Hyperactivity
Rebelliousness
Age
Seat belt use
As suicide equivalent

Ref: Tsuang et al. 1985

IV.R Diabetes:
Diet: meat eating as etiology
Sugar/carbohydrate use
Self-care failures (with self-care training and self-monitoring 50% reduction in emergency visits and decrease in coma over 2 years by 66%
Use of estrogen oral contraceptives may reduce risk
Early age pregnancy and longer breast feeding reduce risk
Physical and emotional stress increase blood glucose levels
Relaxation training produces better glucose processing
Biofeedback trained subjects can accurately estimate glucose levels, allowing better self-care via diet, exercise, medication

Ref: Cox et al. 1984, Hopper et al. 1984, King and Cobb 1958, Rabkin & Stuening 1976, Snowden & Phillips 1985, Solomon 1981, Stein & Charles cited by Ader 1981, Surwitt 1985

IV.S   Osteoporosis:
Osteoporosis is primarily a disease of older women, with an estimated 15 million cases in the U.S. As the population of elderly women increases, prevalence is expected to increase.
Age
Sex (female more than male)
Race (white women more than black)
Weight (underweight as risk)
Cigarette smoking
Failure to engage in weight bearing exercises to increase calcium absorption (assuming adequate calcium intake)
Bed rest and immobilization (in turn sometimes psycho-social as with depression)
Possibly: dietary calcium intake, care in not consuming iron at the same time calcium supplements are ingested
Possible risk items include alcohol use, possibly dietary components including vitamins A, C, magnesium and protein
In treatment: failure to comply with estrogen therapy, exercise and calcium supplements
Calcium absorption requires vitamin D (vitamin D toxicity must also be avoided)
Inadequate calcium intake in adolescence, youth as well as middle and older years
Health education information inadequacy: recommended dietary allowance (RDA) of 800 mg is too low; thus following recommended RDA is insufficient
In pregnant women, simultaneous mealtime iron and calcium intake (iron inhibits absorption)
Anorexia nervosa with amenorrhea

Ref: Brotman and Stern 1985, Fanelli 1985, Greenwood 1984, NIH Osteoporosis Concensus Report 1984, Science (dietary calcium) 1986

Table IV above is not complete. It is, however, illustrative.

We now set forth factors found etiologically associated with conditions and diseases of the female reproductive system.

Table V
Conditions and Diseases
of the Female Reproductive Tract

V.A Premenstrual syndrome (PMS)[6] (also termed Premenstrual mood changes or PMC):
Mood status: a function of personality and immediate environment including stressors and stress reaction
Onset and severity associated with life stress; severity greater for women with underlying psychological disorder
Diet: excess refined sugars, salt, dairy products
Vitamin & mineral deficiency: zinc, magnesium, B6
Prior neurotic traits
Culturally learned expectation of suffering in association with menses
Strong suggestibility, as measured by powerful placebo effect
Oral contraceptive use (inverse relationship)
Tubal litigation (possibly a trigger)
High somaticizing
Sense of helplessness
Prior chronic pain (unsubstantiated)
Depression (prior)
Use of psychotropic drugs
Social withdrawal or poor social adjustment
PMS appears primarily as a magnification of ongoing moods and exaggeration of already present monthly mood fluctuations with emphasis on negative affect and symptoms referrable to stress
Symptom intensity correlates with estrogen levels
Risk factors include history of depression, affective disorder, family history of depression, erroneous cultural beliefs about cyclicity
Undesirable life changes
Feminine role conflicts
Smoking
Prior history of menstrual, sexual or fertility differences, i.e., U.K. patterns differ from U.S.[7]
Occupational level (higher levels, less PMS risk)
Educational level
Working vs not working (less with those employed)

A correlation with physician visits for help-seeking may reflect only syndrome presence; not excluded, illness self-definition and help-seeking as independent variables
Culturally, family-generated expectations
Age (greater 20s and 30s)
Hostility
Impulsiveness
Impaired social functioning
Irritability

Ref: Backstrom and Mattson 1975, Chihal 1985, Faratian 1984, Foresti 1981, Friedman (1982), Friedman and Jaffe 1985, Goldstein et al. 1986, Golub 1976, Gruba and Rohrbaugh 1975, Haskett 1980, Hopson and Rosenfeld 1984, Hovey and Hovey 1984, Kashiwagi et al. 1976, Keye 1985, Norris 1983, O'Brien 1985, Olasov and Jackson 1986, Osofsky & Keppel 1985, Petterson 1975, Rubinow et al. 1985, Rubinow and Roy-Byrne 1984, Ruble and Broods-Gunn 1979, Shukit et al 1975, Siegel et al. 1979, Sloss and Friedrichs 1983, Steege et al 1985, Woods et al. 1982, Young and Erhardt 1980.

V.B   Amenorrhea, including galactorrhea-amenorrhea, hyperprolactinemic amenorrhea (prevalence about 0.1%):
Psychological distress
Emotional disorder
Stress adaption
Family dynamics with absent alcoholic father or violent father
Low level of knowledge re: menstruation
Negative attitude toward sexual body parts (guilt, shame)
Difficult relations with sex partner (implied sexual problems)
Adverse life events
Perfectionistic (may herald anorexia nervosa)
Life stress
Daily hassles
Exercise including that done for stress relief
Dieting and slimming
Depression
Hostility
Anxiety
Higher level of somatic symptoms: latter may be symptomatic of rather than risk factors for hyperprolactinemic amenorrhea

Emotionality associated with extreme stress
Increasing age
Nulliparity
Not breast feeding
Oral contraceptive use
Medication: dopamine, phenothyazines, butyrephenone, antihypertensives, opiates, tricyclic, antidepressants, tranquilizers, amphetamines, in turn related to psychological status of the women and physician prescribing tendencies.

Ref: Bullen et al. 1985, Ellison & Lager 1985, Fava et al. 1981, Gold 1985, Hatcher et al. 1986, Katz & Cooper 1977, Mozley 1980, Nunes et al. 1980, Oakley et al. 1982, Sakiyama and Quan 1983, Schreiber et al. 1983, Speroff 1985, Wynn & Wynn 1981, Zacur et al. 1976

V.C Dysmenorrhea: (Prevalence: 40-80% of women)
Emotional distress
Maternal dysmenorrhea
Life stress and change
Poor acceptance of female role, extreme feminism
Psychological repression as a trait neuroticism
Impulsivity
Depression
Anxiety
Self-focus (introversion)
Dependency
Self-dissatisfaction
Rejection of one's own body
Poor felt general health
Not playful — no leisure activity
Age
Parity
Possible work exposure to cold temperature
Adverse life change
Difficulty in relating to important male figures
Family encouragement, modelling, adopting a sick role for menses in adolescence
Mothers having greater menstrual distress

Ref: Bloom et al. 19787, Friederich 1979, Gold 1985, Iacone and Roberts 1983, Jordan 1982, Lawl and Davis 1981, Wengrad 1953, Whitehead et al. 1986

V.D Menorrhagia and other dysfunctional uterine bleeding:
Psychological disturbance, especially depression and sense of vulnerability
Stressful life change
Other health stress
Obesity
Work-induced masculinization
Hypertension related to stress
Adaption of sick role to express personal difficulties
Neurosis

Ref: Greenberg (1983) Klerman and Izen 1977, Romney et al. 1979, Tudiver 1983

V.E Pelvic pain, abdominal pain
Life stress defined by frequency of recent adverse life changes
Psychosexual factors including distressed sex partner relationship and other sexual dysfunction
Levels of anxiety
Competing stimuli (whether work, social involvement, exercise, etc.) determine threshold levels as do sensed threat
Field dependence as primary trait
Prior and concomitant emotional distress are antecedents
Immediately, sexual stimulation without coitus may be associated with transient pain
Women are more pain sensitive and report more chronic pain than do men
Pain onset and persistence is associated with depression & prior depression

Observations on prevalence and organic pathology:

About one-third of gynecological out-patients present with pain. Rates of organic pathology vary widely, depending on study population and investigatory criteria. UK studies show from one-third to two-thirds of gynecological pain patients are without observable pathology. Since some pelvic pain patients will be diagnosed as pelvic inflammatory disease, it is well to note diagnostic disconfirmations, i.e., upon laparascopy no positive findings and thus the inference of psychosomatic distress, of from one-third to one-half of "PID" patients. Again the data are from UK studies.

> From the general literature on pain, one finds identified with chronic pain:
> Anxiety
> Depression (often as a response to pain)
> Degree of neuroticism (depression and anxiety) influencing threshold
> Manner of pain expression as function of personal styles and culture group membership
> Acceptability of pain as opposed to another complaint or explanation of distress as a function of culture group membership
> Personality traits of introversion-extraversion
> Interpersonal manipulativeness and alienation (from others)
> Pain endurance as a trait
> "Health index" as a composite of invalidism
> Depression
> Pain preoccupation
> Pain games
> MMPI scale scores high on hypochondriasis
> Psychasthenia depression
> Hysteria
> Psychasthenia
> Schizophrenia (i.e., general neurotic, affect or bizarre trait elevation)
> Test results of field dependence and external locus of control supporting concept of trait lack of self-environment differentiation (i.e., alternatively ego strength, boundary strength)
> Somaticization and high symptom reporting levels
> Schizophrenia as pain barrier
> Prior or current psychiatric illness
> Emotional distress-damage
> Absence of coping skills
> Obsessive attention to body cues
> Lack of life styles
> Involvement and social stimulation

Interpersonal/family reward or gain for symptoms
Pain-proneness as an aspect of depressive disorders or pain and depression occurring simultaneously as a shared pathway presentation
Predictability and control
Expectations of pain
Peer behavior

Risk factors in personal histories:
Unstable family background including family pathology
Psychiatric visits
Heavy use of drugs and alcohol
OTC self-medication
Marital sex partner-instability
Poor sexual adjustment
Financial stress
Sleeping problems
Radical weight change
Prior psychosomatic illness, heightened automatic reactivity with gastrointestinal or circulatory system change, postulated pelvic congestion
Other members of the family reporting chronic pain (implies learning, social modeling)
Frequent medical visits
Own frequent surgery, prior surgical intervention for pain
Adverse life circumstances
Inability to verbalize or distinguish emotions as in alexithymea depression without response to anti-depression drugs
Pain reporting as less acute-specific (e.g., dysmenorrhea pain reports differ from specific discomfort from intrauterine device)
Observations on prevalence: The majority of non-schizophrenic psychiatric patients report (non-organic) pain
Much pain reporting in medical outpatients has emotional components; in one study 23% had pain attributable only to psychosocial features
The majority of chronic pain patients in pain clinics represent failed medical-surgical intervention for pain
Pain and depression are not only often jointly presented, but most often appear to arise simultaneously, not sequentially

One-third of American adults have experienced chronic (tissue-pathology inappropriate) pain episodes

Ref. Beard 1977, Blumer and Heilbronn 1982, Bonica and Albe-Fessard 1976, Bradley and Van der Heide 1984, Brena et al. 1981, Cohen and Lazarus 1979, Craig and Brown 1984, Crue, Kenton, Carregal and Pinsky 1981, Drossman 1982, Eisenberg 1984 citing Byrne, Hendler, Henker 1979, Jamison et al. 1976, Katon et al. 1985, LeRoy 1977, Long and Wise 1982, Melzak & Wall 1965, Merskey 1980, Ng 1981, Pearse and Beard 1984, Pierson 1984, Raener et al. 1979, Romano and Turner 1985, Romney et al. 1979, Rosen 1977, Smith and Duekson 1980, Smith, Merskey and Gross 1980, Sterbach 1976, Taylor 1949, Taylor 1984, Taylor and Duncan 1952, Terman et al 1984, Timmermans and Sternbach 1976, Wolff 1977, Wolff, Cohen and Greene 1976

V.F   Pelvic inflammatory disease (PID):
Sexual activity: multiple partners, early onset, frequency
STD: gonorrhea, chlamydia
Ethnicity (black greater)
Age 14-44, possible 30-34
Being single but formerly married
Delay in medical visit after becoming symptomatic
Medical error: non sterile procedures
Type of contraception, with condoms as low risk and IUD as high risk
Exposure to infected semen: reduced as a function of condom use, increased with IUD's

Ref: Aral 1985, Newton and Keith 1985, Pritchard et al. 1985

V.G   Menopausal adjustment and distress:
Education & social class (better adjustment)
Work status (implied involvement, stimulation as safeguarding features)
General self-perceived health
Correlates of prior, current nervousness
Depression
Headache
Traits of self-confidence and felt adjustment
Emotional distress as psychiatric morbidity

Surgical menopause as in bilateral ovariectomy, or hysterectomy which may be so defined is associated with more chronic illness, medication use, self-rated poor health

Women undergoing natural menopause report fewer menopausal complaints than the hysterectomy-overiectomy group. For hot flashes: sensitivity inferred finding, placebo effects.

Overweight vs underweight (greater fat associated with greater estrogen production)

Emotional stress

Smoking in excess

Alcohol use

Self-care for hot flashes: low caffeine and alcohol consumption, eating frequent small meals, avoiding high temperature environments

Lowered risk of atrophic vaginal tissue change among sexually active women

Ref: Ballinger 1977, Gold 1985, Greenwood 1984, LaRocca 1980, McKuldy 1985, Tulandi and Lal 1985

V.H Galactorrhea:
Paternal deprivation in childhood predicts to higher prolactin levels.

Ref. Sobrihno 1984

V.I Cancer of the breast:
Note: Breast self-examination: breast cancer. Survival rate a function of practice and frequency of breast self-examination (BSE), lag time to visit to physician. Note, 35% of U.S. sample say they refuse to visit MD for breast examination even though breast CA is 2nd leading cause of death for U.S. women. 84% of all malignancies are first found by the women herself. BSE is associated with smaller tumors at diagnosis and fewer involved lymph nodes — in turn correlated with mortality risk. BSE associated with age and education, personal confidence in being able to do BSE, confidence that BSE works. Only 25% of U.S. women practice BSE, in spite of mass education efforts: Absence of BSE. The more a woman depends on her physician (believes MD controls her health), the less likely is BSE. U.S. poll data suggests many women think any lump means

CA, and that any breast CA is fatal: delay in medical visit. Denial and repression appear to operate to inhibit BSE and MD visits. Among those judged competent in BSE are more likely than those incompetent when doing BSE to discover their own cancers. U.S. women overestimate actual prevalence of breast CA: fear may retard visits. Those not practicing BSE say (50%) it would make them worry unnecessarily. Most women do not share such fears with their husbands and lack that social support. Possible relationship to belief in one's own susceptibility, and being socially/familially involved with other people ("support networks").

Anger suppression found in some studies of etiology as are other deficits in emotional expression
Migration among ethnic groups
Heavier alcohol consumption and greater prior abortion history
Obesity in women over 40
Delayed childbirth and failure to nurse newborn
Cigarette smoking - a dose response relationship
Dietary fat intake
Fibrocystic disease of the breast only in association with other factors among which behavior-related factors are being nulliparous or having the first child after age 35

Ref: Alagna & Reddy 1984, Assaf. et al. 1985, Barlar 1984, Cates 1982, Derogitise et al. 1979: see discussion: Temoshok 1982, Fisher et al. 1969, Foster et al. 1978, Gambrell 1984, Greer & Morris 1975, Huguley & Brown 1981, King et al. 1985, Kilata 1985, Krishmer 1980, Labrum 1980, Love, Gelman and Silen 1982, Melamed 1983, Reddy 1984, Schecter et al. 1985, Sklar & Anisman 1981, Young & Erhardt 1980, Williams, de la Fuente & Rosenbaum 1976.

V.J Cancer of the cervix of the uterus:
Multiplicity of sex partners. Early age on onset of being sexually active. 75% of herpes related cases had occurred within 15 years after first coitus. Onset time is becoming briefer - with an increase in women in the 24-35 age group
Gonoccocal infection (perhaps as multiple STD or sexuality correlate)
Exposure to herpes simplex virus II and HPV 5, 6, 10, 16, 18 as STD
Use or non use of condom or diaphram as contraception
Genital warts via STD

Number of sexual partners of husbands'(married women with husbands having 15 or more partners outside of marriage have nearly 8 times greater risk)
Cancer of the penis or urethra in male sex partners
Poor sex hygiene (prophylaxis)
Smoking
Lower risk in women making regular visits for Pap smears
SEC and delay in visits
Failure to secure Pap smears in high risk groups
Mortality risk associated, in young age group, with speed of lab procedures for Pap smear analysis and recall the function of expenditure limiting of public policy
Failure to respond to recall after Pap screening: age and SEC are correlates
When CA present, survival rate a function of visit frequency. These in turn associated with ethnicity and SEC
Some studies show prior to CA onset there is a loss of parent, other bereavement, or history of parental rejection
Personality trait and experience studies (be cautious in accepting)
Extreme suppression of emotion as trait a risk factor, as is social isolation (in turn related to superficial and interpersonal relations)
More disturbed family backgrounds
Increased risk with separation and divorce
Very high risk for prostitutes in prison (promiscuity history plus isolation/deprivation)
Trait helplessness/hopelessness, hopeless prone personality
Adolescent school difficulty
Low risk in rural women, nuns, Jewish women (possibly related to sexual behavior)
Race: survival rate factor
SEC: family income and educational levels, survival rate factor
Age at time of diagnosis: survival rate factor

Also implicated:
Smoking
Alcohol beverage consumption
Age of onset of smoking
Diet with cruciferous vegetables and fat

Ref: Bergren & Sjostee 1984, Buckley et al. 1981, Clarke et al. 1982, Clarke et al. 1985, Franceschi et al. 1983, Furgyik & Asted 1980, Graham 1979, Klerman & Izen 1977, Labrum 1980, Levy 1985, Lyon et al. 1983, Marshall et al. 1983, Martin & Hull 1984, Mayberry 1985, Reid et al. 1984, Sadeghi et al. 1984, Sansom et al 1975, Schmale & Iker 1965, 1966, Siebold & Roper 1979, Singer et al. 1984, Sklar & Anisman 1981, Smith et al. 1980, Stellman et al. 1980, Steinhorn et al. 1986, Syrjanen 1984, Tranethan et al. 1983, Wright et al. 1984.

V.K   Endometrial cancer:
- Risk increases with obesity
- Chronic anovulation
- Infertility
- Use of exogenous estrogens
- Extreme stress (death of spouse) can lead to immunosuppression and increased risk
- Hypertension
- Oral contraceptive use (reduces risk)
- Premenopausal smoking

Ref: Andersen 1984, Hatcher et al. 1986, Kolata 1985, Labrum, 1980, Levy 1985, Smith et al. 1984

V.L   Ovarian cancer:
- Reproductive history of no children
- Not married
- Oral contraceptives (reduce risk)
- Use of talc for feminine hygiene
- Residence in industrial nation (excepting Japan)
- Migration from low incidence to an industrial nation
- High animal fat consumption
- Coffee use
- Heavy alcohol consumption

Ref: Demopoulis et al. 1979, Gwinn, Metal 1986, Hatcher et al. 1986, Weiss et al. 1977

V.M   Uterine myoma:
- Psychosomatic/emotional personality variable

Chronic anovulation
Frustration over childlessness

Ref: Ilm & Pokhilko 1983, Fellman et al. 1983

V.N Gynecological surgery: adverse postoperative responses (Adverse psychological outcomes are more common for sexual-reproductive organs than others, for example cholecystectomy, at a rate of 30 to 80% among women of reproductive age.)
Pre-operative lack of confidence in own femininity
Absence of social support
Lack of coping skills, resources
Anxiety denial or extreme anxiety
Poor quality of care interpersonally, medically, post-op
Prior psychiatric illness, personality distress
Consequential marital problems
Finding that operation was unnecessary upon tissue audit
Absence of counseling, support group
Pre-existing depression

Ref: Youngs and Wise 1980, Goldberg & Tull 1983, Gittin and Pasnau 1983

V.O Vaginal discharge/pruritus, vulvovaginitis:
Particularly in young women: crab lice
Venereal warts
Trichomonas, Gardinella or Candida as STD
Diet-urinary sugars as chain of events
Oral-genital sex
Trichomonas exposure from bathing/swimming
Stress and increased non infectious discharge as complaint
Oral contraceptive use
Antibiotics
Trauma/stress
Dieting
Chemical sensitization to sexual lubricants and diaphragm gels
Lost tampon
Emotion liability

Ref: Peirson 1984, Dodson and Friederich 1978, Friederich 1985

V.P   Vaginal lesions:
       Digitally inserted tampon use

Ref: Berkeley et al. 1985

V.Q   Chronic vaginal infection:
       Candida albicans patients report more unsatisfying marriages prior to infection, more sexual problems prior
       Separation or divorce can lead to recovery when medical treatment has failed
       Coital activity in contraception barrier vs. convenience methods
       Yeast infections following antibiotic medications self or inappropriately medically given or for avoidable cystitis

Ref: Kinch & Steinberg 1975

V.R   Vaginismus:
       Psychological variables responsive to behavioral treatments

Ref: Reamy 1982

V.S   Attendance at gynecological screening: public clinics
       Poor information levels
       Incorrect expectations
       Prior gynecological examinations - or current expectations - felt unpleasant
       Lower intelligence levels

Ref: Hesselius et al. 1975, Wenderlein 1978

V.T   Infertility (Estimate rates for prevalence for primary psychosocial determinants vary from 5% to nearly 50%, with 20% in the U.S.)
       Stress
       Emotional distress
       Psychological defenses
       Depression
       Smoking
       Alcohol use
       Subsets of personality and marital problems
       Low coital activity

STD outcome
Homosexual preferences affecting sexual conduct
Low capacity for orgasm affecting sexual conduct
Residential geography (a global variable)
Ignorance of reproductive cycle (example: 40% of college women believed ovulation took place during menstruation), and exposure to education to fertility data in fertility clinics
STD resulting tubal obstruction or other pathology: from 20% to 40% of all infertility may be so caused

Ref: Band & Wilcox 1985, Belsey 1984, Drake and Redway 1978, Elleberg and Koren 1982, Freiderich 1979, Hare 1983, Hatcher et al 1986, Herrenkohl 1979, Humphrey 1984, Lalos et al. 1985, Lux et al 1983, Mosley 1976, 1980, Olsen 1983, Sorenson 1980, Sverre-Pederson 1984

V.U Cystitis/urinary tract infection, retention disorder and distress
For bacteria: marital status
Age
Emotional stress
Use of vaginal diaphram
Other contraception
Non sterile vibrators leading to vaginitis[8], then cystic disease via colon infection
Anal intercourse prior to vaginal without washing penis or dildo, iatrogenic from bruising via urethral dilation[9]
For those with cystitis, exacervation, recurring: male and female hygiene measures before and after intercourse
Diet[10] (tea, coffee, alcohol, excess carbohydrate)
Exposure to chlorinated water in swimming, allergies[11] to sprays and douches, tight jeans[12]
Nylon pantyhose reducing air circulation[13]
Recent intercourse
Use of diaphram
Tampon use
Soft drinks ingestion associated with increased urinary pH

Ref: Foxman and Frerichs 1985, Henry & Stephens 1977, Almy 1982, Kilmartin 1980, Kunin & McCormick, Shapiro 1985, Struab, Ripley & Wolf 1949 (a) 1949 (b)

V.V   Fibrocystic disease of the breast:
Diet: caffeinated drinks, chocolate
Low parity, late age 1st birth, all factors contibuting and the sterile menstrual cycle (contraception & family planning, Western society, etc.
No oral contraception
Late menopause

Ref: Boyle et al. 1984, Johansson 1984, Parazzini et al. 1984, Rannevik et al. 1984, Vecchia 1984

V.W   Arthritis of pregnancy (prevalence 2-5%)

Gonococcal infection as STD
Age (youth), other STD contributors

Ref: Zbella 1984

V.X   Toxic shock syndrome (TSS):
Use of superabsorbant fiber tampons
Use, manner of use (time retained) of barrier contraceptives
Failure to change tampon every eight hours
Failure to rotate tampons with sanitary napkins, i.e., at night
Unclean hands, use of hands rather than inserter mechanisms for tampons
Prior STD related infections: herpes, all STD behavior factors

Ref: Hatcher et al., 1986

V.Y   Hydatidiform mole:
Geographical area of residence
Maternal age
Induced abortion history

Ref. Hayashi and Bracken, 1984

V.Z   Cervical inflammation:
STD, including chlamydia tracomatis as major contributor, thus all factors predictive of STD
Oral contraceptive use

Ref: Paavonen, 1986

Comment and Caution

A considerable range and diversity of psychosocial-behavioral variables have been identified as etiological in the specific diseases or pain experienced by women, and for their contraceptive and sexual activities, these in turn also associated with reproductive and disease risk. The literature cited varies greatly in terms of theoretical orientation, samples, methods, definitions, experimental sophistication, and subsequent reproducibility and utility. Yet it is obvious that the evidence is overwhelming as to the operation of such variables for women's contraception, reproduction, complaint syndromes, disease, and pain.

The general demonstration, and in some cases the specification (as a weight in attributable risk) of the operation of psychosocial-behavioral features as risk components has generated health promotion as an enterprise. It is, however, an enterprise based on limited knowledge as well as appealing assumptions. It also must be attentive to such efficacy data as exist. The health professional and the women with whom a health promotional enterprise is jointly undertaken, must be realistic. That realism requires, essentially, that current identification of a factor as a disease risk not itself be taken as evidence that reduction in the risk factor will prolong life, reduce morbidity, or enhance wellness. One must be specific about changes shown to work, and those not so shown. One must also be realistic about the relativity of such gains, that is, whether the effort is worth the trouble.

Kaplan (1984) offers a critical overview of claims with respect to the relationship between behavior and health. The assumptions of health promotion are set forth as (a) particular behaviors increase some chronic disease risk (b) that changes in these behaviors reduce probability of illness onset (c) that behaviors can (easily) be changed and (d) the effort is cost effective. Kaplan argues that what is missing in work to date is a definition of health which combines quality of life (wellness) with morbidity/mortality measures, and care in logic such that risk factors measured are not simply (non causal) parts of the constellation but include outcome and statements with reference to risk which tell us, using adequate statistics, what predictive role the risk factor plays. He cites, by way of illustration, the 1970 Pooling Project which combined results from six prospective studies for heart disease: over a ten year period only 10% of men with two or more risk factors developed heart disease. Obviously 90% did not, whereas 58% of those who did develop heart disease had one or no identified risk factors.

The relationship of cholesterol to heart disease was presumably solidly established, the debate laid to rest, by the report of the Lipid Research project (1984) (Kolata, 1984) results: lower incidence of CHD occurred in cholestyramine-treated initally high cholesterol men. With a decline of 8.5% in total cholesterol, there occurred 24% fewer heart disease deaths compared to controls. However, prior work had presumed to have established that dietary cholesterol had only small effects on serum cholesterol within the normal range and Stallones (1983) had shown, in seven studies reviewed, that those developing CHD did not consume more calories, fat, or cholesterol than others. The cautious conclusion, in 1986, may be that dietary change is but a small mortality risk reducer when unaccompanied by cholestyramine treatment. That is not because, statistically, cholesterol change does not reduce CHD mortality, to the contrary, but because, at least summing four studies, as CHD declined, mortality from other causes increased. And in the Lipid Research program trials as well, although CHD mortality did decline, total mortality between treated and untreated was not significantly different. Nor is the debate over. There remains no irrefutable evidence that dietary lowering of cholesterol reduces risk (Kolata, 1985).

For health promotion the point is that inducing dietary change may not always or much reduce mortality risk. Indeed Hirsch and Leibel (discussed by Kolata, 1985) suggest that, given biochemically normal cells in fat people, it may be healthier to stay obese than to make their cells abnormal metabolically. Further, inducing change is difficult. This is well illustrated in weight reduction programs which, for the short run, do rather well, but where long term loss is difficult to maintain. Similarly for anti-smoking interventions: success rates run about 20% to 30%, good indeed for morbidity and mortality expectancies for those who stop, but keeping us mindful that the many smokers are not easily capable of smoking self-control. The same is true for cardiac patient and exercise; those maintaining it are at a lower risk of CHD mortality but there are many drop outs. By no means does this argue against health promotion programs, for to reduce risk for a minority is worthwhile, but there are people whom current programs do not reach, or if reached, are not changed in their conduct. Lund and Kegals (1984) argue that the recent desirable shifts observed in popular health-related conduct may be entirely unrelated to education or intervention efforts. Implied is that claims of health promoters and practitioners of behavioral medicine as to efficacy are unwarrented, that they are riding a bandwagon otherwise powered.

There is historical precedent for caution with respect to efficacy of specific intervention, as opposed to appreciation of social, economic, or immune status of substrate as determining feature changes. Berkman and Breslau (1983) reviewing public health changes over the last 150 years (citing Evans, Drause, Linenthal, Rosen, and others) point to the general benefits of events occurring before the recent discovery of pharmacotherapeutic and immunizing agents, as for example in Western countries better nutrition, cleaner water supplies, fewer flies following abandonment of horse powered vehicles, better factory working conditions. Cholera, tuberculosis, diphtheria are examples of diseases whose prevalence was reduced prior to the introduction of chemotherapies. Hemminki and Paklulainen are cited showing that in Sweden of 13 infectious diseases with declining mortality rates over time only for three is there evidence of reduction accelerated by medicine's introduction.

Syme (1984) on methodological grounds, is also cautious with respect to the degree of impact of currently identified risk factors. While presenting a clear picture of the contribution of such variables, his review of the literature yields the illustration that for CHD, for example, even though men with the 3 major risk factors have odds 6 times greater for CHD, nevertheless, over 10 years only 14% of these developed CHD whereas of those with one risk factor only 5% did so. Conversely, of all those developing CHD, only 17% had 3 risk factors and 58% two or more. The limitations imposed on forecasting accuracy are all the more important when CHD is the illustrative case, since it is clearly defined as an outcome and disease entity, and has been the subject of more prospective work employing behavior-related risk factors as variables than any other clinical syndrome.

Given such cautions, it is consistent that Cohen and Syme (1985) in reviewing the social support data, for which there is the evidence of its role as a powerful variable, proposes that the data are best interpreted as indicating only that there is a minimal level (threshold) of social contact required for health maintentance. Furthermore, and very importantly, for all of the consistency of the risk data itself, there are as yet, they argue, no data justifying the generation of social support as a mode for health promotion.

Here we disagree, and in the direction of much greater optimism. There is much in the health behavior literature showing that for those already ill, or recovering from illness and its severe treatments, or engaged in poor health practices, one or another form of the added, guided "human touch" can make a great difference. Suffice it here to remind ourselves that "support groups," classes, home visits, family dynamics, treatments, illness adjusted persons as "expert" patients, work stress counseling groups, or indeed peer groups of almost any kind joined together in setting norms and goals and in mutual assistance make major differences in lives. And community or organizational interventions seeking to educate and mobilize awareness and to set better health norms also have positive effects (Frederikson et al. (1985)). Consider these examples of social psychological "marketing."

Studies of one of the more powerful CHD risk factors, Type A and Type B personality, are probably the most satisfying and elegant of any work on cardiovascular response patterns, and constitute a range of theoretically and empirically interrelated studies; from stressors, personality-environment interactions, to autonomic and cardiovasular functioning. As Grantz and Glass (1984) note, "unlike any other individual-difference variable studies in connection with illness, Type A behavior meets most of the ... criteria ... to establish a cause-effect relationship ... Among these ... association with clinical CHD: consistency persistence and reproducibiity of finding, the fact that Type A (demonstrable) precedes CHS and ... the link is plausible in the light of biomedical knowledge of how CHD develops."

Nevertheless here too are difficulties. In terms of development of screening tests for behavioral change, where one goal is avoidance of false positives and subsequent costs for unnecessary interventions, the varying criteria for Type A classification pose a problem, for prevalence may be from 15% to 70% (Krantz and Glass, 1984, Chesney 1981, 1985) depending on the method and group. Dembroski and MacDougall (1985) deplore the trend toward even greater inclusiveness in Type A categorization. For example, in one set of studies 75% came to be labelled Type A. Where disease prevalence is low, and where a screening device operates inefficiently, such categorization of high risk means false positives increasing to unacceptable, i.e., entirely useless levels. (See Grant and Mohide, 1982.) Chapter 5 reviews the work of

Case (1985), Dembroski and MacDougall (1985), Ruddell et al. (1983), and others, finding no relationship between global Type A and any measure of myocardial incidence risk. If it is hostility as is now suspected, which is the operative effector component of Type A, and not the global array of personal traits, Type A diagnostic screening over-reaches, and may indeed also overlook risk. The utility problem is also there, for in the Western Collaborative Study of men (Rosenman et al., 1975), while Type A had odds twice as great for CHD over 8-1/2 years, these were the same odds as for other factors, cholesterol, cigarettes, etc., all contributing clearly in a small way to outcome. Type A appears to contribute about as much to prediction as other factors, so that perhaps 5% of men who are Type A will experience CHD (our surmise: we have not found the numbers). We cannot find data telling us the odds for Type B, without other risk. Nor are any data on women available.

Of great importance to the women's specialist and his/her patients is the recognition that almost all of the CHD studies are on men, and most other prospective studies based on measurements in youth, are also men. There are happy exceptions, but the fact is women too often are disregarded as a population for research. Indeed, the field of ob/gyn by no means recieves its fair share of Federal or philanthropic funding. Women, measured by the focus of and investment in health research, are short changed. Here indeed is a "risk" factor at work.

Thinking About Costs

Kaplan, reviewing cost and benefits for intervention, uses a quality of life index (Kaplan and Bush, 1982), work also performed by Bush and his colleagues (1973, 1979, 1981) in a number of studies. Programs vary immensely in costs. Analysis of 57 OSHA programs suggests a cost of $170,000 to $3,000,000 to prevent a single death. Hypertension detection and treatment is another story; to produce one more year of life costs between $10,000 and $23,000 through screening and primary prevention programs. And for neonates PKU screening and dietary treatment yields a well life year for $7,500. It is estimated that behavioral interventions for hypertension simply to induce compliance with medication (exluding demonstrated benefits from relaxation treatements) appears relatively inexpensive. Costs features and the well year concept cannot be ignored as aspects of health promotion.

One must also be willing to incur costs, as for example for health research intended to benefit women, or for screening programs. Consider two instances in the U.K. There, where health care is government provided, and thus would be expected to be rational on the basis of public health need, there is no breast cancer screening service, even though it is estimated (Roberts, 1985) that 3,000 lives a year could be saved. Indeed one recent U.K. ob-gyn textbook argues against GPs encouraging their patients to do breast self examinations on the grounds that the resulting demands for clinical and mammography screening would impose undue work/cost loads on the National Health Service. The second instance involves cytological (Pap smear) screening for cervical cancer. An age group newly at risk are young women, with onset time for neoplasms, following HPV or other STD exposure (see Table V.J) no longer the 15 year lapse time, but within one year. But funds in the U.K. have been cut back for laboratories, and as of 1985, some smears were "backlogged," not examined for six months. A preventable cancer death becomes terminal, and in the U.K. the number of cases, and the number of young women as cases (27% under age 35) (Med Briefing, 1985) is increasing as the underfunded laboratory load increases. In the U.K. 10% of cancer of the cervix patients die; the forecast under these conditions is for an increase in mortality. Cost conscious administrators, some themselves epidemiologists, argue that it may cost several hundred thousand dollars (pounds) to save a life, simply because mass screening is costly and finds few positives.

Cervical cancer prevalence would be reduced if its inductive behavior were changed; if women had fewer sexual partners, delayed onset of intercourse to an older - less anatomically vulnerable age (that at least is the hypothesis), and screened self and partner for an history or presence of genital warts, herpes, gonorrhea, etc. But, as Brandt (1985) argues, such restraint does not occur, and so is not the "ideal" self disciplined substitute for public health/medical STD disease screening, treating, and reporting measures. But in the U.S., until AIDS, very few Federal funds were allocated for public health work on STD. These issues lead one to ask what is a life worth, who determines that, who pays for it? The woman's health professional cannot help but be concerned with these matters of public health economics and policy values. As risk factors are better identified with respect to their weight in attributable risk, and the cost of prevention- screening programs are worked out as Kaplan and Bush have done such issues will be even more in the forefront of health promotional debate.

Summary comment

A variety of psychosocial and behavioral factors have been identified, the presence of which increases the odds that a woman will suffer diagnosable physical illness, or a syndrome of bodily dysfunction, or other pain. There are other aspects of living which are identified as buffers or safeguarding features. Among illnesses and conditions reported as more likely to occur when particular psychosocial behavioral risk features are present are, as examples, cardiovascular disease, diabetes, some gastrointestinal pathology, sexually transmitted diseases (STD), postoperative recovery and adjustment, infection vulnerability, premenstrual syndrome, amenorrhea, dysmenorrhea, monorrhagia and other dysfunctional uterine bleeding, pelvic/abdominal pain, pelvic inflammatory disease, cancer of the breast, cancer of the cervix, skin endometrium or ovaries, vaginal discharge/pruritis/vulvovaginitis, chronic vaginal infection, infertility, and female cystitis.

Some risk features appear to play broad roles predisposing to a variety of illnesses; others are quite specific. They range from characterizations of biosocial status such as socioeconomic class through personality traits to items of conduct such as smoking to particulars of choice, as in type of contraception. There are methodological problems which affect replicability and which highlight important issues in identifying the course of illness and intervention events. The search for and examination of risk factors not only suggests areas for changes in social circumstances or conduct which offer hope for self-directed health improvement, but also may point the way to careful examination of, and quality of care improving changes in medical care for reproductive system and disorder.

Identification of risk factors does not allow the automatic assumption that their alteration will improve health; our knowledge must become specific about the etiological, disease process. There is a need for very much greater research on intervention, innovation, and evaluation. Insofar as women at risk can be identified, there are strong arguments for self- and public health screening programs. In the case of expensive programs counter arguements based on economic cost are offered. These may well determine public policy. For the clinician with responsibilities for individual patients, their self care and screening may and must be pursued; nevertheless the health care professional, as long as he or she is an advocate for women's health and for models of rational care, will not be divorced from public health and related economic policy issues.

Health promotion takes place, then, not only in the office where it is directly attentive to the patient's health status and her risks in her world, out there, where she lives, but also to the world of women generally "out there" and how sensible prevention, screening, and treatment is most wisely, and compassionately provided. As it stands now, women's health is shortchanged by low research priorities evidenced by available funds. Insurance programs are also inadequate for behavioral health care, as the Institute of Medicine, in its report on low birth weight prevention (1985) emphasizes. These constitute women's health risks themselves, ones policy derived. A woman's health will also be shortchanged if her health professional does not act for risk assessment, as for example cognizant of the data in Tables IV and V, as part of evaluation, and diagnosis and then when appropriate, for health promotion.

Footnotes

1. CHD risk associated with Type A: Type A prevalence increases with education level and occupation. When SEC and work are controlled, prevalence for women is the same as in men. For women, as American masculine work roles and stresses are adopted, it is expected that CHD risk will increase.

A methodological problem exists because of a tendency to overclassify Type A. Chesney (1985) and Dembroski and McDougall (1985) have observed that is in some studies, for example the Multiple Risk Factor Intervention Trial, the majority of persons are so classified. Such overclassification through attention bias is elsewhere found, as for example in teratogen studies where, for antiemetics following thalidomide, biased reporting of limb reduction deformities occurred to skew, even while underreporting both the kinds of defects and the alleged anti-nauseant source (Weber, 1983).

2. Note, interactions occur suggesting that, in general, psychosocial behavioral features are most likely to operate synergistically to potentiate risk in people where already present is dietary induced hyperlipemia (Ball, 1982).

3. Failures to replicate these studies require the cautious conclusion that psychosocial variables are not yet proven to be linked with cancer risk. Animal studies do demonstrate that stress can facilitate tumor growth, that predictable stress may protect against that. Social isolation is associated with enhanced tumor cell growth. Sklar and Anisman (1981) conclude "stress does not cause cancer but influences the course of neoplastic disease." Response to diagnosis and or treatment may be related to the future course of disease.

4. Levy (1985) lists as occupational agents linked to cancer: aromatic amines, arsenic, asbestos, benzine, bichloromethyl ether, cadmium, chromium, ionizing radiations, isopropyl oil, mustard base, nickel, polycyclic hydrocarbons in soot, tar, oil; ultraviolet light, vinyl chloride. For a more complete discussion of the potential effects, carcinogenic and other, of about 400 toxic substances likely to be encountered occupationally, see Proctor and Hughes (1978).

5. Premenstrual affective syndrome (PAS) is sometimes described separately, for example Friedman et al. (1982), Kashiwagi et al. (1978) as part of an effort to describe more unitary subentities in a postulated PMS catch-all category. Freeman (1985) supports that effort, but, using the reasonable criterion of marked change and severity in symptom intensity pre and post menstrual days (one can also say self-sensitivity), it is observed that emotional symptoms predominate and that only 5% had only "physical" complaints. Were a random sample to be taken, it is not known what proportion of now PMS diagnosed women would be PAS, that is, without any physical complaint. What is shown (Haskett et al. are cited) is that the "true" PMS patient has fewer complaints on general symtoms measures over the month; on the other hand, a good deal of research emphasizes that initially higher levels of distress complaints are one of the characteristics of those with PMS diagnosed. For our purposes we believe the conceptual and statistical psychophysiological work has not been done to demonstrate the efficiency of the PAS diagnosis. Here we make no distinction. It is estimated 5-10% of all women require PMS-related treatment.

6. PMS has been successfully used as a legal defense in two homicide cases in the U.S., beginning with axe killer Lizzie Bordon. This illustrates cultural expectations, as evidenced in jurors. Rabin (1985), reviewing Hafner and Boker on violence among the psychiatrically ill (a high PMS risk group) observes that (in homicide generally) women more than men kill family members or other intimate persons much more frequently than men when suiciding. They term this "extended suicide." A Texas study (Peterson et al.,1985) showed interpersonal conflict a common precipitating factor, along with alcohol and other drugs, in women self-inflicted gunshot wounds. In this sample psychiatric disorder (other than impulsive violence) was not a common characteristic. Chilah reports suicide more common in the luteal phase. Suggested is the possibility that a rare but consequential outcome for the depressed or impulsive high PMS risk women in conflict situations is suicide or murder as a sequential crescendo of risk to which the clinician must be attentive.

7. Most pain research has addressed itself to more prevalent chronic pain complaints. Since chronic pain presentation, in the absence of tissue pathology appropriate to the fact of level of pain reported, has major psychosocial components which are similar regardless of the reference site for pain, one would assume that functional pain referred to reproductive organs would share antecedents and correlates in common. The limited work done on pelvic and abdominal functional pain supports that assumption, but does not assist us in saying how it is likely that these reproductive sites have been selected other than by invoking rather general notions such as "learning" and, more psychodynamically, to assume that is where historically trauma and felt hurt reside, or where pain complaint yields a currently desired psychological result (sex avoidance, sympathy, etc.).

It is an arbitrary decision here to examine pain as a specific syndrome with psychosocial antecedents as opposed to considering it under general morbidity, for one may well consider chronic pain, even though normally referred to a site (or region), as having much in common with high levels of symptoms presented. Both represent psychosomatizing as a response to prior and current person-environmental interactions.

8. These factors, identified by Kilmartin in a self-help lay women's guide, not, to our knowledge, epidimiologically validated. They appear sensible enough to warrant inclusion here.

9. Ibid.

10. Ibid.

11. Ibid.

12. Ibid.

13. Ibid.

SECTION III

Case Examples

8

The Experiences of Six Women

Anecdotal clinical experience is useful in medicine only as it may lead to the discovery of a principle of pathophysiology or serve to illustrate repetitive and reproducible observations. Recognition of patterns of symptoms or of associations among a number of related variables often heralds the elucidation of cause-effect relationships necessary for clinical validation. In obstetrics and gynecology, symptom patterns and associations are important clues that often lead the clinician to assessments relating repetitive cyclic or periodic events to physiological adaptations. These may include weekend cycles, menstrual cycles, or pregnancy. The following clinical case reports serve to illustrate the importance of considering clinical symptoms and findings in the broader context of the patient's living environment, her emotional maturity and experience, and the incentives and disincentives for the control of symptoms and for achieving wellness.

One Woman's Fiery Vulvo-Vaginitis

Mrs. A.C., a 36 year old para 3013[1] woman, is a successful travel agent. She presented in the medical center by referral for severe, unremitting, intractable monilial vulvo-vaginitis that recurred about every two or three months over a period of 3 years since the weaning of her youngest child. Her husband, a realtor, had a bilateral vasectomy at that time. The patient's reproductive history was eventful for regular menses after age 14, mild dysmenorrhea during the college years (her B.A. from a prominent Eastern University was in English), and conceptions without delay at ages 23, 24, 26, and 27 years; the third pregnancy miscarried at 9 weeks and required a D&C for control of bleeding. The children, now age 13, 11, and 9, weighed between 7 lbs 6 oz, and 8 lbs 4 oz, at birth, all vaginally, and are healthy and well adjusted. Child care is aided, at this time, by a live-in housekeeper. The diagnosis of vaginal moniliasis was by repeated recognition of abundant mycelia and spores in wet-mount preparations of leucorrhea and by sporadic cultures for monilia. Therapy locally and systemically had been intensive and prolonged with the major commercial antifungal agents and with gentian violet, all used as recommended (and longer) but without permanent relief. She also used intermittantly vinegar or boric acid douches and had introduced plain yogurt into the vagina in personal efforts to rid herself of the problem. Marital friction was but one consequence of her repetitious dyspareunia-producing vulvo-vaginitis episodes. The patient had undergone cervical conization for severe cervictis and had a hemorrhoidectomy, both 3 or 4 years prior to the current consultation.

The patient had correlated the peak occurrence of her episodes of vaginitis with stressful events in her life. Spring and summer months were worst when the travel business peaked, when busy children's activities were maximal, and when her husband's business hours were most irregular and demanding. Upon further inquiry, the patient could recall that many of her infection episodes occurred just after menses which were characterized by 8 or 9 days of bleeding. These periods started and ended with a couple of days of spotting and were heavier than usual; cramping was notably, and pleasantly, reduced on those occasions.

Comment: The clues of stress-related, periodic episodes of monilial vulvo-vaginitis and symptoms of anovulation were the secret to understanding this woman's situation. After assuring that a fasting plasma glucose was normal and treating the current infection with an anti-fungal preparations, she was advised of the environmental basis of monilial overgrowth and the role of a stressful lifestyle in producing anovulation. The presence in the vagina of blood for 8 or 9 days monthly promotes a basic pH in which yeast thrive and invade the epithelium. This circumstance was demonstrated and the concept reinforced over a four month interval during which basal body temperatures (BBT) were recorded and postmenstrual pH was measured. The patient was instructed to douche once postmenstrually with a commercially produced buffer preparation. She reported a year later that she had remained free of recurrence of the problem. Another therapeutic approach to utilize, if it became necessary, could have been the addition, during anovulatory cycles diagnosed by BBT, an oral progestin for promoting a normal menstruation.

A Girl's Painful Sexual Maturation

M.C. is a 21 year old woman who has grown successfully into young motherhood after experiencing a stormy adolescence characterized by sexual promiscuity and recurrent pelvic inflammatory disease. M.C. is the second child among three female siblings who grew up in the modest home of their parents in a Midwestern city. Her first coital experience was at age 13 years following a junior high school dance. During her freshman and sophomore years of high school she developed casual sexual relationships with six different high school boys (history reconstructed from her diary). In these encounters, numbering a total of eleven, M.C. used no contraception although four of the boys used condoms. She was generally aware, from biology class, that having sex midway between menses could result in pregnancy. She believed that she wouldn't get pregnant, however, and didn't ask her partners to withdraw before ejaculation within her. During the summer after her sophomore year, she had her first episode of acute gonococcal salpingitis. Treatment was with probenecid and penicillin. Her special friend during junior year was on the football team. They had sex about weekly using foam sporadically or condoms, or sometimes nothing for contraception. Her academic work suffered in part because of an evening job at a movie theater. She contracted gonococcal salpingitis again that spring and was treated with spectinomycin. Her symptoms of pelvic and upper abdominal pain did not clear up as rapidly as previously. Repeated therapy with ampicillin was temporarily beneficial but she experienced dysparenuia and several episodes of gardnerella vaginitis. Empiric therapy for chlamydia trachomatis with tetracycline produced some relief of symptoms. Thereafter, she had an ectopic pregnancy diagnosed at eight weeks gestation, for which a laparotomy and salpingectomy was done. Her reproductive health has been further complicated by abnormal Pap smears and cervical biopsies containing severe dysplasia. Cryocautery successfully treated this lesion. After high school graduation, M.C. moved to

California and worked as a salesperson in a plant nursery. She found a young man with whom she developed a supportive relationship and conceived. Her pregnancy was uncomplicated and she is using oral contraception at the present time.

Comment: M.C. is an example of a large segment of young women whose health history, sexuality, hygiene, and risk-taking behavior contain a significant number of unhappy and painful experiences. This group is characterized by an active coital history starting at a young age, many sexual partners, and irregular use of contraception. Of particular interest is the belief among this group of young women that their health is controlled by chance and/or the power of others, such as boyfriends, parents, or health care professionals, other than by themselves. The higher frequency of acute salpingitis and its sequelae such as ectopic pregnancy or infertility reflect, at least in part, personal attitudes and behaviors that prejudice them for repeated sexually-transmitted infections. Preventative care may be discouraging for such individuals unless specific education and support is offered with the goal of self-determination in regard to health choices.

Cyclic Symptoms as a Manifestation of Metabolic Endocrinopathy

M.B. was a 32 year old P2002 teacher of Italian heritage seeking help for symptoms of cyclic depression, weight loss, nausea, lightheadedness and weakness. During the 2 to 3 days prior to menses, she usually lost about 10 lbs. and was bedridden from headache, nausea, and weakness. She became anorexic but craved salt during these days of the cycle and regained her weight by mid cycle when she felt well enough to function at home. She had resigned her junior high school teaching position in mathematics a year earlier due to "burn out." Indeed, she had lost about 10 lbs, down to 110 lbs body weight over the prior 2 to 3 years. Her history was otherwise unremarkable except for some skin allergies, successfully controlled with OTC antipruritics, and she had constipation. Her menses seemed to be shorter, only 3 days instead of her usual 6 day flow, but these occurred regularly. She uses a diaphragm for contraception but had noted a decrease in libido.

On physical examination, the patient (height 5'6") appeared thin and unanimated. Her blood pressure was 98/50 and the pulse 88; postural change (standing) increased the rate to 110 and decreased the pressure to 90/40. The skin of the elbows, knees, nipples, and lips was mildly hyperpigmented and buccal mucosa had spots of prominent pigment; ancillary and pubic hair were sparse and the skin was dry and of sallow color. The thyroid gland and the breasts were palpably normal, the latter without galactorrhea. The abdominal and pelvic exams were normal and the patient's muscle strength and deep tendon reflexes were judged to be normal, though barely so.

Laboratory assessments indicated a hematocrit of 35% with normal differential, but a thyroid stimulating hormone (TSH) concentration of 14.4 U/ml indicated excess secretion and a 1:40 titer of thyroid anti-microsomal antibodies was found. An 8 am cortisol serum value was 2.5 mg/100 ml and this level increased only to 3.0 following an IM injection of 25 units of cortrosyn (synthetic ACTH). Gonadotrophins, prolactin, serum electrolytes and blood sugar values were normal.

Treatments with dexamethasone 0.5 mg BID and levothyroxine sodium (Synthroid) 0.1 mg QD produced a dramatic effect for this patient. Her cyclic symptoms abated over a 2 to 3 month interval and her menses and libido resumed their normal pattern. She gained about 10 lbs and within 12 months began a part-time business. The endocrine consultant reported that the etiology was primary thyroidism and adrenal insufficiency. An etiology for the combined endocrine gland disease was not evident.

Comment: Patients with endocrinopathies have a component, perhaps mild, of mentation difficulty, either disorders of thinking or emotion control. The relationship may be either primary or secondary and may be pronounced by the menstrual biorhythm. The gynecologist is the primary physician for many younger women for whom an internal review of systems is important as part of health maintenance. If adult family members accompany the patient to the office, a moment of inquiry about the family members' perceptions of function may be helpful. Frequently, a spouse will have identified mood swings, etc., that the patient is oblivious to or is denying, perhaps. Even more important is the need for a menstrual diary for a prospective documentation over a couple of cycles of symptoms, eating patterns, and body weight. Sometimes basal body temperature (BBT) information, in addition, helps one consider gonadal hormone factors as occurs with sporadic anovulation, progesterone allergy, etc. Occasionally, one finds to the patient's surprise that the periodicity of symptoms is unrelated to the menstrual cycle. Other circumstances in the environment must then be considered.

Just a "Touch" of Pregnancy

A 16 year old girl had amenorrhea for 8.5 months following a positive "home" pregnancy test. Morning sickness and breast tenderness and enlargements were followed by quickening at 17 weeks "gestation." Monthly abdominal examinations indicated "normal progress" and the patient gained 11.8 kg above her "pre-pregnancy" weight. On admission at 38 weeks, she had darkened areola and a milky discharge was readily expressed from both nipples. The abdomen was enlarged to the size of a near-term pregnancy but neither the uterus nor a fetus was palpable, and no fetal heart sounds were heard. Pelvic examination revealed a well estrogenized vaginal mucosa and a small, soft cervix. A tense, rigid, distended abdominal wall prevented palpation of the uterus or adnexa. A presumptive diagnosis of pseudocyesis was confirmed by sonography which demonstrated a uterus of normal size and a 3x4 cm. adnexal mass. A radiography of the abdomen revealed an abundance of gas but no fetal parts, ruling out an abdominal pregnancy. The patient was described as very anxious and quite suspicious about being hospitalized before the onset of labor.

Following hospital admission for endocrine and psychiatric evaluation, base-line levels of the greatest pulses of leutinizing hormone and prolactin were elevated up to five-fold. Other hormones (FSH,TSH, GH, and insulin) were in normal ranges and the estrogen and progesterone levels were consistent with luteal phase. The psychiatric diagnosis was mild depression.

On the second day of hospitalization, the patient was informed about her false pregnancy, which she related had been initiated by a first coitus with her boyfriend. Thereafter she had stopped attending high school but continued living with her parents. Within 30 minutes of receiving the information that the pregnancy was false, her distended abdomen completely disappeared after passage of large amounts of flatus. Further endocrine testing (infusions of L-dopa and of arginine) was carried out but the baseline values of prolactin and LH obtained shortly after informing the patient of her situation were much lower than those of the prior day but were still elevated; L-dopa reduced both, and arginine increased PRL levels as expected. The patient had a menses two weeks later and the ovarian mass disappeared. A year later, she delivered a normal term male infant without incident.

Comment: The hormone levels observed in this case cannot be explained by the fluctuations of the menstrual cycle and the interpretations of the data would be more secure if elevated PRL and LH values had been found prior to hospitalization. Nevertheless, the role of catecholamines in the modulation of mood and behavior, as well as hypothalamic function, is well recognized. Pseudocyesis has been cited as a paradigm for psychophysiological interaction (Aldrich, 1972). Brown and Barfglow (1971) have formulated the hypothesis that the presence of endogenous depression has a crucial significance in the genesis of pseudocyesis. The fantasy of pregnancy appears to function as a defense against depression. Since preliminary data suggest that mental depression is associated with a decrease in CNS catacholamine activity, a postulation of a reduced dopaminergic mechanism would account for the hypersecretion of both LH and PRL. Further, the role of anxiety in producing elevated levels of LH and PRL is suggested by the prompt fall in the serum concentrations after revealing the diagnosis to this patient.

This case illustrates the significance of important life-experiences to physiological functions. The circumstances surrounding initial sexual experiences, whether guilt-provoking, forced, or loving, are important for the evoked responses. If contraception is known but not utilized in passionate moments of "first love," the expectation of pregnancy is usually great and an inexperienced person, such as a teenager, is subject to fulfilling the expectation. First coital experiences may, particularly if unexpected, represent emotional or even physical trauma, as anxiety and haste can inhibit or limit foreplay and reduce the time necessary for adequate sexual lubrication secretions. All of these and a variety of additional factors may induce a state of cathacholamine hypersecretion that affects hypothalamic gonadal functions and produces headaches, poor concentration, insomnia, and other evidences of inner tension.

Self-Induced" High Risk Pregnancy

L.S. is a 23 year old primagravida with Type 2 diabetes mellitus first diagnosed at age 11. Over the ensuing 12 years, she has had two episodes of ketoacidosis, one mild and one with blood sugars over 1200 mg%. The patient works as a waitress and lives in a small furnished apartment with her boyfriend of two years duration; he works the night shift at a 24 hour service station.

L.S. came for prenatal care at 11 weeks gestation when she developed a severe monilial vulvo-vaginitis. She reported that recent urinary sugar levels in fractional specimens had been 3- 4+ and that her last fasting plasma glucose 8 weeks before had been 276 mg%. Her pre-pregnancy weight was 180 lbs.

Initial fasting glucose was 196 mg% and the hemoglobin A1C was 12.6%. The patient was advised about the importance of accurately controlling blood sugar during pregnancy and she agreed to self-monitor her levels twice daily with a glucometer. She seemed to understand the principle of adjusting insulin dosage with 2/3 of the dose in the a.m. and 1/3 after the evening meal, according to the meter readings, and the objective of maintaining a fasting level of about 100 mg%. Over the next 24 weeks the patient was successful in improving control, with values ranging from 115 to 160 mg%. A weight gain of 40 lbs was associated with development of a large fetus and hydramnios determined sonographically. The patient missed several prenatal visits without apparent concern for the welfare of her pregnancy; no family, only a girlfriend occasionally, came with her.

At 37 weeks gestation, the patient became hypertensive (BP 168/110) and was admitted to the hospital for bed rest. Urinary excretion of albumin was 4 gms/24 hours. Apresoline therapy reduced the BP to 140/96 but the non-stress test was non-reactive and an oxytocin challenge test was positive. Induction of labor over 48 hours led to the vaginal delivery during epidural anesthesia of a 3610 gm infant girl with Apgar scores of 6 and 8. The infant developed hypoglycemia and hyperbilirubinemia. These were treated without complications. The immediate puerperium was unremarkable; however, the patient failed to return for postpartum visits and was pregnant four months thereafter, when she sought an abortion.

Comments: Patients, especially young individuals with chronic illnesses, often have difficulty complying with regimens designed to promote good health. Attitudes of rebellion may be directed towards family, friends, and health care providers, but these are destructive primarily to the patients themselves. Inadequate discipline for dietary and insulin control of diabetes is often coupled with absenteeism and blaming of circumstances (such as inconveniences with appointments and transportation, or family conflicts including finances and permanent living quarters). Denial of an effect of dietary indulgences on the pregnancy and a state of chronic depression are common determinants of the development of high-risk characteristics that necessitate expensive, invasive, and anxiety-provoking interventions which usually aggravate the marginal socio-economic balance. A pattern of prolonged irresponsibility for self-caring is often present and the frustration provoked in professionals by repeated failures may lead to impatience and the absence of constructive, supportive relationships.

Prematurity—A Legacy of Socio–Economic Deprivation

K.A. is a 19 year old, P0120, black woman who entered the hospital with premature ruptured membranes at 32 weeks gestation. She had worked as a chip-assembler during the week and had moved along with her mother into a new apartment during the weekend immediately prior to the rupture. Despite the earlier instructions and admonitions by her physicians to rest on weekends, particularly when she noted increasing uterine cramps, she failed to do so in this pregnancy, just as in her last. Her previous pregnancies, two therapeutic abortions at ages 15 and 18, and the 26 week pregnancy that ended with severe pre-eclampsia and intrauterine growth retardation had been with different boyfriends; all had refused to use condoms and K.A. hadn't been able to remember to take her oral contraceptive pills regularly. Her firstborn died in the neonatal period.

Labor began after four days of observation in the hospital. Fetal tachycardia to 180 bpm was followed by chills and fever to 102F. Antibiotic therapy was begun for the predominant organism found in the initial cervix culture. Vaginal delivery was accomplished without further evidence of fetal distress. Apgar scores were 3 and 7 and the cord pH was 7.23. Fetal weight was 1600 gms and the infant grew in the intensive care unit until 2700 grams. He was discharged to his mother's care, which was to be guided by the grandmother with whom the family lived. The patient had elected an IUD for contraception, believing that oral contraceptives cause cancer.

Comment: This young woman had experienced a number of unhappy reproductive events that had stressed her body and her family before she reached adulthood. Adolescent pregnancy can be the consequence of inadequate information or misinformation about contraception, but is also often associated with powerful attitudinal and emotional features which negate contraception.

Conclusion

The above examples of commonly-occurring clinical situations highlight the need for recognizing their psychophysiological components, whether of primary or secondary consequence. Each example is associated in some manner with *reproductive change* relating to the menstrual cycle, initiation of sexual activity, change in sexual partners, or pregnancy. These physiological events of reproduction are usually understood and given meaning in relation to the circumstances in which they are experienced. The mature, well-informed individual living in a supportive environment is less likely to experience disease or distress than is the young (and therefore inexperienced), socio-economically deprived person having similar experiences. The astute clinican will always seek to determine the environmental contexts in which patients observe and report the onset and progression of their symptoms.

Footnotes

1. "Para" refers to parous, or birth history. The numbers denote, respectively, the number of full term births, of premature births, of abortions, and of living children. The woman in this case then has had three full term births, no premature births, one abortion, and has three children living.

SECTION IV

Office Based Health Promotion Activities

9

From Poor Compliance to Good Cooperation

Recall from Table II in Chapter 4, the widespread prevalence of patient non-compliance in following recommended regimens. There is an abundance of literature identifying psychosocial features that are shown to be determinants of that behavior. The rate of non-cooperativeness is a function of the research worker's care in counting; generally the more strict the observation of what the patient does compared to what the physician recommended, the greater the observed non-adherence (Sacket and Haynes, 1976).

"Compliance" connotes a passive role where "obedience" is expected. That in itself may generate oppositional "non-compliance" among patients whose only remaining ability to resist or be self-determining is regressively, by doing "no," to feel matters are still to be under personal control (Janis and Rodin, 1982). We therefore prefer to use the term "non-cooperation" to call attention to the cooperative rather than imposed, authoritative aspects of the business of self care as recommended medically.

Regarding Instructions

A number of studies consider how well patients understand what they read or are told (see a review of Blum, 1981). Non-adherence is shown to result from patient misunderstanding of directions. In one investigation not once was a prescription label uniformly interpreted by all patients. Even when instructions were written out, more than one-third did not know the medication name, and one-fourth did not know what its use was. The average patient did not recall instruction as to when to take the medication, or under what circumstances to change dosage. Sometimes leaflet instructions are not understandable to the average patient. Using the Fleish formula for intelligibility (related to reader education level) it is observed that for working class people, hospital direction leaflets are usually beyond their comprehension even when patients read and signed a form, as in a consent form stipulating "I understand." Follow-up reveals that essentials of risk information are missed.

A national survey (Morris, 1984) found that only 60% of patients recently receiving a new prescription said the doctor had provided directions for use. Suchman (1965) reports that 37% of patients drawn from a community sample having had a series of doctor visits claimed they were not told what to expect from their illness. As time passes after exposure to information, the number remembering it falls off. Ley reports that 35% to 50% of what general practioners tell their patients cannot be recalled after a matter of minutes. Content is differentially remembered; instructions and advice are more frequently forgotten than illness explanations.

Kirsch and Rosenstock (1982), indicate that cooperation may not be associated with health knowledge defined broadly but with information specific about the regimen itself. Even so, the more that is required by way of cooperation in changing behavior, maintaining changes, or in doing many things, the less adherence. Understandably, the more a regimen interferes with normal activities, the more difficult it is, and the less is adherence. Improvements, nevertheless, can be obtained with long term, habit changing health education for self care. Nelson (1984), in work designed to improve self care among healthy elderly persons, employed classes, skill training, role playing, and making commitments through contracts. A self-help book was also employed. Improvements were obtained in knowledge, confidence, and attempts to improve fitness, nutrition, and weight control. While changes lasted over the study year, they diminished over time, and ultimately there was no difference between the intensive group and controls with respect to final health levels or care utilization. Note, however, the groups began in good health.

Wise Anticipation and Informational Pre-Treatment

The effects of the medication or regimen are to have considerable consequence for patient's conduct. Adverse side effects, for example, are an element in the Becker and Maiman (1975, 1977) adherence model stating that therapeutic effects as a function of adherence cannot be divorced from undesirable simultaneous pharmacological consequences. It is important that these latter possibilities be anticipated and discussed fully with the patient in advance—contrary to much current practice—so that drugs unsafe for some patients may be discontinued. That is also part of "informed consent." But beyond these reasons, one anticipates (here more research is necessary) on the basis of the research on pre-surgical "innoculation" with information about "what to expect" that greater patient control and less sudden later anxiety will be felt, with subsequent better adherence. If unpleasantness occurs it is thereby understood, i.e., it has been pre-treated. Felt "side effects" appear to have major implications for adherence. Examples are seen among patients already being treated medically for illnesses which have strong psychosocial components in risk. Crowley et al. (1985) for example, noting the 90% treatment drop out rate among naltrexone treated opium addicts (at 8 months), finds that there is a long term dysphoria imposed by naltrexone. While there are many reasons for non-compliance in this generally non conforming group for whom opium euphoria was a factor in their original use, the effect— whether "side" or "main"— is indistinguishable. When naltrexone blocking of opium-binding changes mood in a fashion felt as depression, this may also be a non-compliance stimulus just as is the depressive side effect in the thiazide diuretic treatment of hypertensive patients (Okada, 1985). Obviously informational pre-treatment can occur only when the physician is well informed as to potential side effects, and is not reluctant to discuss these as part of the process of obtaining informed consent in pharmacotherapeutics.

That physician communication can upset the patient is obvious, as for example in giving bad news, proposing regimens that disruptively require the patient to give up important activities, or simply frightening when uncertainty cannot be resolved. Haan (1982) cites Beeson showing that a likely peak upset phase in pregnancy will be that occurring if and when women undergoing amniocentesis are told that further prenatal diagnostic procedures are in order because there is a risk of abnormality. High anxiety in turn is readily associated with maladaptive conduct (Enkin and Chalmers, 1982). In some cases, when the women were told of the risk of an abnormal child, they increased their smoking and drinking. Again one sees that communication and its consequences, its interactional nature, are the central concern, not communication clarity by itself.

Should the physician resort to exhortation as a form of persuasion to compliance, as for example to prevent smoking that can have a negative effect? Lumly and Astbury (1982) cite work to the effect that half of women smoking in pregnancy are worried about it but cannot stop. The Institute of Health Policy (1985), reviewing prenatal class outcomes, confirm an even more pessimistic appraisal. In any event, Lumly and Astbury (1982) find that 10% increase their smoking presumably because of increased guilt and anxiety. Lumly and Astbury conclude that exhortations do not help, that there "will be no perfect child and can be no perfect mother whose life is uncontaminated by sex, cigarettes, alcohol or anxiety. Exhortations...fail to take into account the real lives and responsibilities of women."

These remarks are consistent with Surgeon General Koop (1985) admonishing physicians who fail to comprehend that medications use occurs in the context of daily lives and demands, where adherence requests must conform to these realities. Enkin and Chalmers (1982) remind us that "safe" remedies such as bed rest and sedation are associated with increased obstetrical risk (citing Mathews), whereas we are all aware that many medications are recommended without controlled trials demonstrating efficacy. To the extent that adherence failures reflect a response to noxious side effects not expected because not warned, non-adherence is to be appreciated as one form of iatrogenic illness prevention. It is a form of responsible self care.

Creating the Right Atmosphere

DiMatteo and DiNicola (1982) emphasize the importance of generating an atmosphere for communication which promotes a sense of cooperative or joint endeavor. They cite work showing, for example, an experiment in which the doctor took the time to co-author the medical record with the patient, i.e., where entries were made in consultation with the patient that positively affected understanding and involvement. Communication of fact by itself is by no means a sufficient device to assure understanding or desired reponse, for response varies with the style, relationship, and personal and emotional situation in which information is given. Thus, simply writing something down, or handing out a pamphlet by no means assures any of the outcomes sought. (It may assure the physician, but that, presumably, is not the treatment goal.) Rapport is a key element, and as DiMatteo and DiNicola point out, that depends upon establishing trust, being sensitive and friendly, and the physician being able through "self-disclosure" to share with the patient his or her own uncertainty. Such frankness also makes the physician a model for the patient, as one who can accept uncertainty and make decisions based on estimation, not certainty.

The physician or nurse can also "co-author" participation in procedures and thereby expect a better outcome. Enkin and Chalmers cite work by Campbell and Reading showing that women given the opportunity to share the ultrasound visualization of their baby early in pregnancy not only have more positive attitudes toward the pregnancy than controls (itself a variable affecting obstetrical outcomes) but are also more likely to reduce their smoking and drinking. (See also Sandberg et al., 1985.)

It is important that the physician or other health provider learn from the patient what beliefs she has about her condition, its cause, and what actions in living or in cooperation in medical care she already believes are going to affect outcome. Whatever the patient does will be based on and compatible with her already existing beliefs about, for example, whether medicine is worth taking, whether doctors really know what is wrong, whether "it will go away by itself," or whether her family can afford the medicine or advised further procedures.

Leventhal, Zimmerman, and Gutman (1984) cite a dental study comparing expectations of dentists and patients prior to the visit. The more discrepancies, the less the adherence and the less improvement in gum inflammations. Time must be taken to see what are the discrepant expectations between the woman's beliefs (her world) and the medical one. It requires patience and dialogue to work toward a concensus. Without doctor-patient concensus on methods and goals, one has little hope for compatible adherence outcomes.

What goes on between physician and patient does affect emotions and patient motivation. That in turn influences adherence.

Leventhal et al. (1984) show low mutual information exchange, active disagreements and criticism, and low perceived physician friendliness associated with low adherence. Adherence outcomes improve when an initial opportunity is given to the patient to tell her story followed by physician feedback response and instructions. The physician whom the woman experiences as a person who listens, takes time, explains, can be reached by phone, is respected and credible, cares for the woman as a person, is the one whom the patient wants to see again, and whose recommendations are more often followed.

Only in delineated areas is the physician able to persuade the patient to do something new or suspect. To be persuasive—here Di Matteo reviews communication studies—the doctor must be seen by the patient as an expert: likeable, confident, and trustworthy. As for routine adherence achievement, one recognizes that it is more readily come by when instructions and regimens are simple, not competing with habits, when there is regular follow-up, prompting and reminders by telephone or card, when the patient has explicitly agreed, as with a handshake or other commitment, when she herself makes a weekly or daily record as an adherence diary, and when she is told to do something nice for herself as a reward for applying adequate enough self-control.

Note that we say "adequate enough," not "perfect." The professional must not be impatient or irritated over failures, but rather express encouragement for any movement in the right direction. This is a fundamental principle in all "behavior modification." If on follow-up, adherence to simple regimens is missing, one must sit down with the woman to find out what she thinks about and to learn if, considering the admitted difficulties, one can jointly negotiate even partial solutions. Negotiation is also a principle in behavioral treatments which moves toward the goal of shared commitments.

Incompatible Outcomes

The nature of the interpersonal transaction with the physician also influences adherence as outcome. For example, when patients who are disappointed with an exchange, they are less cooperative (Janis and Rodin, 1982, citing others). We have not found investigations which link disappointment or understanding in turn related to adherence, to the amount of time spent with a patient. Nevertheless, given the short times typically spent with patients during office visits, one wonders what can be communicated. Consider, for example, from Table II, Chapter 4, that for "very serious breast disease" a modal one to ten minutes (NCHS #63, 1977-78) was spent with women, with one-third seen from 11 to 15 minutes, or for very serious genital tract disorders, a modal 16-30 minutes was spent. About half of all women were seen for 15 minutes or less. For prenatal care, an average of 11 minutes (NCHS # 45, 1977) is spent and for disorders of menstruation, 18 minutes. These spans include examination time. In the NCHS ambulatory care study, GPs spent 13 minutes, and internists spent 18 minutes during the average patient visit.

An American College of Obstetricians and Gynecologists study (1985) where specialists received questionnaires from patients indicated the 44% of this sample (with inevitable but unknown sampling bias) wanted more adequate information and education from their physicians.

The onus for failing to enjoy an informationally complete exchange in the doctor-patient encounter by no means falls entirely upon the physician. Malpractice and quality of care studies by Blum (1958, 1960) describe the malpractice prone patient: the woman who puts herself entirely in the hands of her physician, and passively surrenders her judgment in exchange for offering adulation to the physician. Such a patient may deny any need to worry, or be responsible for her own care, even for forthcoming major procedures requiring active pre or post operative roles. Such passive, unrealistic patients are satisfied with whatever the physician tells them, whatever little time he or she gives them, until something goes wrong, or is seen by the patient to have gone wrong. Complaints about care which eventuate in malpractice litigation are common results.

The work of Green, Weinberger, and Mamlin, reviewed by Clymer (1984), demonstrates how little the passive patient wants. This study of mostly low SEC black women revealed that almost none expected from the physician any details about their medical problem. Most would not ask questions, and almost none expected to learn about their medications effects. Low SEC, and disadvantaged ethnic status contribute to learned "passivity" as a function of resource poverty, inhibiting status inequalities, and "copelessness."

Patients claim that being given self care advice by the physician is rare even after serious illness. Butt's review (1977) indicates that a majority of hospital just-released patients claimed that they were given no self care advice at all. But we have already noted that information by itself would have guaranted little by way of recollection or self care. When Butt gave his patients a take-home tape recording of a pre-release what-to-do instructional meeting, 90% did say that was helpful. However, being pleased is not the same as adhering. Hladik and White (1976) showed that patients who said they read materials given to them upon release from the hospital said they were helpful; nevertheless, they could not answer questions about when and how to take their medication. Garcia (1982) cites Oakley to the effect that only 17% of UK mothers receiving antenatal care said they had learned anything about their pregnancy or baby from physicians and nurses there. One must wonder what is going wrong?

Time Dose-Effect Relationships

The preceding findings suggest that too short a visit simply cannot allow for the assessment and life planning collaboration which is necessary for the preventive approach. They also indicate that the time for a visit is not enough when information exchange is not assured. We know, of course, that information giving, or advice is itself not enough to ordinarily produce behavior change. But consider that time "over time," i.e., frequency of visits, is also an important feature when the treatment goal with the patient involves some aspect of living and feeling. We take our data from Howard et al. (1986) reviewing 114 studies of psychotherapy outcomes. Almost all of these investigations show a positive outcome relates to the amount of time, measured by the number of visits (here the 50 minute hour is assumed). Specifically found, psychotherapy is effective; further among diagnostic groups, depressive patients begin responding at the lowest dosages, with anxiety patients a close second; thus by 13 sessions 50% of all of these had improved. This is very important since we recall that depression is a very common disorder associated with gynecological illnesses and their treatments, and with women's emotional state "out there" in their world. The data further show that by 26 sessions 75% of all psychotherapy patients have improved.

One does not know whether such findings apply to the woman with reproductive-system-associated emotional complaints, or for health psychological interventions aimed at disease-preventing behavior change. Until that evidence is in, it would be our surmise that visit frequency is a consequential variable. For positive emotional change many relatively long visits are required. Because of that, it is our proposal that for treatments of longstanding life style and emotional aspects of women's illness, and lives, there be referral to specialists prepared to offer these time-demanding expert interventions.

Women's Sexual Problems: A Special Case of the Incomplete Medical Visit

When specific information is considered, particularly that regarding sexual functioning where the physician's own awkward reluctance plays a role (Chamberlain and Dewhurst, 1984), serious patient versus physician reporting discrepancies arise. Coronary patients report, for example, in 66% of cases studied, they receive no advice as to sexual activities; but 94% of their physicians' claim advice was given (Geere and Hesse, 1982, citing others). Cartwright (1984) citing Bone in a UK family planning survey found that single women were not asked about their sexual activity or needs. Cartwright finds in the UK the same reluctance as in the US; women were embarrassed about asking for contraceptive advice, and practitioners were reluctant to offer it unasked. Dodd and Parsons (1984) citing work by Burnap and Golden emphasize the difference between the health professional asking about sexual problems, or waiting to be told. Twice as many problems are reported in response to specific query as are spontaneously presented. Anderson and Hacker (1983), citing surveys of gynecological patients needs, report that 70% of patients receive no information on sexual adjustment before, during, or after their radiation therapy, whereas 80% of the women wanted such information but would not ask for it themselves.

Consider that 90% of women with disease at sexual body organ sites have sexual difficulties (Andersen and Jochimsen, 1985, Goldberg and Tull, 1983, Derogates and Kourlesis, 1981) with subsequent recovery dysfunction varying with the illness site and kind of intervention (O'Hoy and Tang, 1985). In post-hysterectomy patients that dysfunction ranges from 6% to 33% and/or post-radiation therapy patients 29% to 79%. When left untreated, sexual difficulties had not "cured themselves" over a two year follow-up period (Andersen and Jochinsen (1985) citing Maguire et al. and Morris et al.). It is unlikely that counseling would ever be considered unless there is adequate communication between doctor and patient, i.e., the physician inquires and learns about a behavioral condition related to reproductive illness.

The foregoing studies indicate problems for quality of care well beyond simple "compliance." They are indicative of failure among health care providers to see to it that treatment is extended to those emotional and behavioral domains necessary for a return to optimal well-being, i.e., to as full a recovery of function and wellness as is possible. That assumes here the likelihood of success of treatment for much sexual dysfunction (Kaplan, 1983) if it is applied. The larger implication is that the definition of treatment goals, one compatible with treatments available, is to be expanded to include quality of life, i.e., felt wellness as part of recovery.

Becker and Maiman (1975) in their belief model identify as cooperation determining variables in the patient: health concern, willingness, intent to comply (note: patients may attend a visit with a pre-formed intent not to return or take medication), general health, self-help activity, estimate of vulnerability to harm or role performance detriment from the illness, prior experience with symptoms or disease, estimates of regimen's safety and efficacy, and confidence in the physician. Related factors in the model are age (less adherence in young or old), costs, SEC status, side effects, complexity of regimen, feedback in the doctor-patient interaction, satisfaction with the physician, and family support for or opposition to the care recommended.

Patient emotions and personality play a role in cooperation. E. Blum (1958) compared cooperative and non-cooperative patients, and found the uncooperative to be generally more irresponsible, immature, and impulsive on a test developed to predict future cooperation ratings. Such a test is a "model" for trait variables judged to be most influential. Other psychological disabilities tend to be associated with non-adherence, including high anxiety, being socially isolated, or being in an unstable family situation. Denial or repression may also be such a factor, but since these emtional states are also normal means of coping with extreme fear, or serious illness, especially in the early stages (Cohen and Lazarus, 1982) this should be considered a common situational reponse with implications for future regimen cooperation failures only when initial denial continues chronically to disallow recognition of what is needed for proper self care.

Kirsch and Rosenstock (1982) also offer a care adherence data based "model" (really just a list). It proposes a greater likelihood for cooperation in prevention programs, requiring changes in behavior over time when the patients are female, educated, and in higher income brackets, where the woman believes there is real threat to health from the illness (or failure to change life style), believes in the efficacy of recommended action, when she is confident, self-directed, and where she enjoys social support and primary group (family, friends) stability. A prevention program cooperation list should also include hypertension based on data from studies on greater patient involvement. Diversity and frequency of encouragement and information are also factors, for the more varied and greater the contact of health education or assisting (e.g., home visitors) outreach programs, when planned using available knowledge of media, marketing (Frederiksen et al. 1984), and social pschology, the better the likely result. The Farquhar (1984) community health education programs are examples. Finally, of great importance is the education of the physician. Kirsch and Rosenstock (1979) describe Innui's work at John Hopkins where the physician was the immediate educational target. Hypertensive patients assigned to the care of physicians newly educated about factors affecting patient compliance, and exposed to data about patient beliefs derived from that clinic's survey of its own hypertensive patients, were found to have more knowledge about their illness, their treatment program, and to be more cooperative in it, and to emerge with better blood pressure control.

Communications and Assuring Support

A mother's satisfaction with pediatric care is a strong adherence determinant (Becker and Maiman, 1975). Satisfaction is in turn dependent upon the physician's attitude as perceived by the patient. When the physician is experienced as reassuring and positive, adherence is greater. The variables most predictive of dissatisfaction were disappointment, frustration, and anger over expecting but not receiving an explanation of the cause and nature of the illness. Here in this study of mothers and children, length of the visit was not consequential. How serious the physician considers a disease is not related to patient adherence. However, seriousness in the patient's eyes, or as sensed by a mother for her child, is a consequential matter. One infers that the health care provider dare not presume he or she and the woman share the same appraisal of illness seriousness. When there is discrepancy, it is the woman's appraisal which affects cooperation.

The physician's own expectations for the efficacy of a medication may well be communicated by tone of voice or by gesture, and influence patient response. Should the instance be one of those many where the prescription is, in any event, not indicated, or where physician enthusiasm does not accompany the "throw of the die" hoping for a placebo effect, or where important outcomes are nevertheless "iffy," the woman may well respond to that communicated doubt by becoming indifferent to her adherence. This phenomenon is one of the effective but unintended communication of real health care provider expectancies. In effect the nihilistic expectation means absence of support via encouragement. Not created is the needed two person group of doctor and patient working together. Instead there is the subliminal establishment of the indifferent group norm of "who cares?" or "who dares hope?" which results in non-adherence.

Important work on the role of support to produce cooperation comes from the work of Morisky et al. (1985), who examined adherence to long term hypertensive self-administered medication regimens. The investigators found that among poor rural blacks the best blood pressure control occurred in experimental groups receiving supportive home visits from a nurse or pharmacist. (In one group a family member daily measured blood pressure; this specific test involvement/monitoring surprisingly did not make a difference.) Another study found better control among patient groups enjoying a nurse-run support group, and also when family members were seen by the patient to be supportive of the regimen and its goals. Further studies cited by Morisky also show the incremental value of family support. In the Morisky et al. study, where home visitors involved family members in caring about the home management of blood pressure for a family member, where a control group received no such supportive program, there was much less success in low blood pressure achievement in the control group over a three year follow up period. A further blood pressure study by Williams et al. (1985), working with hypertensive women drawn from a household survey— primarily poor rural black residents—industrially employed—in the high risk "stroke belt" of North Carolina, found that those who continued treatment enjoyed more social support. Support here was defined (somewhat misleadingly) only in terms of work; as job pressure and job/home conflict, and spouse and friends approval of the woman's work role. There was also a questionnaire measure of perceived access to supportive resources in the event of various life problems. (For those unemployed, only a "feeling pushed" query was made.) Controlling for age, education, access to care, and income, it was found that, especially for women— and this is consistent with other findings— the sense of social support was associated with greater likelihood of continuing anti-hypertensive treatment. It may of course be that those who feel supported, or are socially competent are also the cooperators in care.

Kirsch and Rosenstock (1982) cite work by McKenney utilizing a monthly meeting with a pharmacist for hypertensive patients. Meetings included discussion and information. Adherence and blood pressure control improved during the period, but diminished after the program ended. Citing Finney, the researchers report that modification of how care was given, by better monitoring and more sensitivity to patients' needs, led to much better treatment results among hypertensive patients. Another effort utilized home visits. That too worked, as did a method employing personalized follow-ups to remind and assist. In one study (Fink is cited), a family management worker was employed in a pediatric clinic. Compared to controls, patients receiving that extra attention did significantly better in medication adherence, keeping appointments, and following other recommendations.

The Contrary Case: The Professional as Saboteur

The health professional may unnecessarily doubt and hold suspect the patient's good sense to manage that part of her life which needs managing and is directly related to bodily events. There are extremely competent health aware women whose life styles deviate from the probably conservative values of the traditional care-giver. One thinks of a woman devoted to yoga or meditation, one who occasionally uses mild marijuana recreationally, or the woman sensibly devoted to self care books with liberal ideologies such as *The New Our Bodies, Ourselves*. Some wisely skeptical, self-educating women refer to their home copy of *The Physician's Desk Reference* after every prescription received. They will call in to inquire testily about unwarned possible side effects. Some women will be judged eccentric for their health food preferences which run to vegetarianism, yogurt, and rosehips tea. It is important that the care provider's stereotypes not indict conduct that is different, but not health damaging.

Insofar as the goal in a regimen for consequential conditions as in pregnancy or for disease control recovery, one must distinguish— by the discussion which allows exchange, evaluation, judgement— the bases and effects of unusual personal choices. This is part of the ordinary exchange which addresses health risks and change. The professional sabotages the growth of further patient self-competence if disapproval is directed at that which is safely irrelevant, indeed even quite useful for the woman's much needed sense of being in caring self-control. Even with regard to the use of home medical advisor books there is evidence of needless— is it jealous or demeaning?— physician distrust.

Sometimes physicians have even refused permission for patient contact with researchers. In a study (Boring et al., 1984) of breast, endometrial, and ovarian cancer patients reached through physicians' permission, half thought that permission was irrelevant, and only 2% would have preferred not to be contacted. But 6% of physicians contacted for permission to see their patients refused it. This is being paternalistic, exercising authority without asking the woman what she wants.

For some physicians it is gratifying to have a grateful, dependent, passive woman as patient who does not think for herself, and adores or renders homage to her possibly vain and authoritarian, probably immature, and certainly self-defeating physician. As the California Medical Association malpractice and quality of care studies showed (Blum, 1958, 1962), such physicians are inviting explosive disruptions in the doctor-patient relationship. They run the risk of poorer quality of care in practice because they tend not to encourage consultation or patient shared responsibility accompanied by genuinely informed consent. If a bad result does occur, the dance between the two of them— unrealistic patient and unrealistic physician— turns into a run, each to a lawyer's office because there may well be a malpractice suit. The risk is by no means uncommon, Nelson (1984), citing Linn and Lwies, observed that a majority of physicians in one study opposed increased self-reliance by patients in their own care.

It may be difficult to distinguish between the attitude of the practitioner related to his or her own habit or enjoyment of dominance, and the tradition of medical institutions as such with their emphasis on "efficiency" through directing and "processing" patients. Yet the nursing home study by Langer and Rodin (1976) showed that greater responsibility in nursing homes given the elderly, led to less mortality, morbidity, and unhappiness. Rodin (1986), in a review, makes the important point that perhaps particularly among the elderly, restrictions on their felt choice and control can be detrimental, whether for handling stress, the experience of symptoms, physiologically, and in self health care. Some of course do not want control; thus the treatment style and milieu which offers control options to the patient is probably best. Rodin points out that offering options and the sense of self-determination runs counter to the typical approach of health care and social service institutions. In this sense, the institutional traditions of medicine can be "bad for" patients.

We do not know where the line is drawn between sabotaging health promotion, risking reduced cooperation in regimen adherence, putting the patient at risk of that encouraged passivity associated with poorer health, and making the personal injury malpractice lawyer's practice richly profitable. The latter comes via associated poor quality of care and malpractice outcomes, or medically unsubstantiated but nevertheless costly and painful avoidable disappointments in the relationship between two unrealistic, uncommunicative, irresponsible people— the malpractice suit prone patient and her malpractice suit prone physician.

Not related to malpractice now, but simply adherence success, are other personality traits of the physician. Miller (1985) cites work showing that health professionals who are either aggressive or self-abasing do not do as well as those who are courteous and respectful, who are aware of what they are doing and how they are being received (insightful), and are sympathetic (natural or emphathetic).

Genetic Counseling: When Is It Not? A Case in Point

Pregnancy deterrence, future total contraception, in response to counseling among genetically high risk parents is a special and intense case demonstrating how physician role, information flow, patient emotion, patient coping are all related to parental decision making outcome. We rely in this discussion on the review by and work of Haan (1982). For any bad news or threatening possiblity, the moment of communication of diagnosis is stressful for both physician and patient. One physician defense against the anguish felt about being a bearer of bad news is the erection of psychological defenses. The first defense is not to inform. That may be based on snap assessments of patient intelligence. As a factor in deciding to withhold information, that judgement criteria is possibly wrong. Some work suggests that, at least for advice retention, intelligence level (within the normal range and assuming communication is geared to levels of verbal understanding) is irrelevant. Further, it is found (Kirsch and Rosenstock, 1982) that physicians generally underestimate knowledge levels of patients. Such implied derogation, perhaps self-elevation at the cost of others, is incompatible with the goal of a doctor-patient partnership in generating responsible patient lifestyle control.

Physicians telling bad news are observed to use euphamism and indirection, to intellectualize, to be detached. Patients in response employ distortion and illogic, blame themselves, become very upset and depressed. "Chains of mutually transacting defensive responses (then) occur." Physicians are then likely to try to dampen, deny their own and the patients distress, rather than to acknowledge and deal with it. Yet Haan cites research with mothers of deformed babies suggesting that anguish is necessary. It must be felt and worked through. Those mothers who are calm, the repressors or stiff-upper-lipper, later coped more poorly. The same findings have been made for post-operative maladjustment.

A U.K. study (Carter et al.) is cited indicating that genetic counseling where half of those deterred from further child bearing were low risk, whereas almost one-third of the high risk parents went ahead to have babies. Haan ascribes such failure rates to one-shot exchanges, not counseling as it should be. Haan takes this failure rate to be so unacceptable as to be a malpractice equivalent. For ourselves, we believe malpractice definitions will be expanded by the courts to embrace consequential communication failure beyond informed consent.

Another study (Sibinga and Friedman), this of parental understanding of their child's phenylketonuria, indicated that even after careful information giving, half did not comprehend the genetic basis for the disability. A follow up showed that when both parents did come to a good understanding, i.e., in this instance were not so upset as to distort or repress, the child had better functioning. A Scottish and Irish study (McCrae and others) of parents with cystic fibrosis offspring observed that the majority complained of insufficient "instruction," an average one-third felt guilty for disease transmission, and four-fifths of the mothers were depressed. The inference of absent genetic counseling is allowable. A study of a range of genetic risk parents (Reynolds et al.) shows 44% not deterred from pregnancy (not all at high risk, however). In the N of 98 were five subsequent divorces interpreted as related to risk knowledge and subsequent emotional distress. Haan argues that these investigators' conclusion that the "understanding" was "adequate" on statistical grounds is not acceptable, given both undeterred child bearing and the divorce response. Like many sensitive clinicians she looks at consequences in lives, not statistical significance levels, to judge outcomes. Gath is cited for work on Down's syndrome couples where 90% reported grief two years postpartum and 30% experienced severe marital disruptions, compared to none among non-Down's controls. The work of Allan, Townly, and Phelan reported that the emotional impact of the bad news of child cystic fibrosis on mothers was such that "almost every mother stated she had heard nothing (more) after the doctor told of the nature of the illness." Leonard, Chase, and Childs' work is reported on follow up of genetic counseling among parents of cystic fibrosis children in a sample roughly representative of the national average. Forty-four percent had important memory failures for information received, 34% attributed to the diagnosis adverse effects on their sex lives, whereas none of the variance with respect to their subsequent deterred or not deterred pregnancies was attributable to information retained. Blumberg and Golbus, also cited by Haan, report that as a response to positive risk diagnosis from amniocentesis and subsequent abortion, depressive reactions occurred in up to 92% of mothers and 82% of fathers. Only one study examined genetic counseling conducted short term as genuine counseling, not just information giving. This (Antley and Harlage) found counseled Down's syndrome parents to be less anxious and depressed than uncounseled parents, to be unchanged with respect to hostility, but also 26% of the counseling cases were more upset. That outcome is attributed to insufficient time given to counseling.

Powerlessness Is Bad News

Haan is critical of methodological flaws, but allows empirical realities as demonstrated in these studies. Her own thrust of argument is that people will decide for themselves what to do and can defeat preventive efforts which are felt to be imposed by the physician. Powerlessness is not a feeling patients will nourish or want to tolerate. When the "prescription" is the traditional medical role played out, where the patient's capacity or need to be self-directing is not nourished, one may get covert combat, not compliance. That is stressful for both physician and patient and is counter-productive for both. It is an "emotionally and morally untenable position" when the physician tries, even in good faith, to assume unilateral responsibility. Haan argues that the health professional must recognize that patients need to maintain as much sense of control over options as is possible and to avoid feeling helpless so as to have a positively adaptive response to the always alien and intrusive nature of illness. Here is the emerging participating model of partnership and responsibility as far as possible.

We have encountered the concept of patient felt self-control before as central to both institutional and individual patient care stategies. Consider work on arthritis, a disease far more common among women then men, and of course, age-related. A Stanford program, based on the effort to demonstrate self-confidence, called by Bandura "self efficacy," relies on a self-help course, in which the major process appears to be an enhanced sense of coping capacities, i.e., some control over their illness. Women taking the course, compared to controls, experience less reported pain, or pain concerns, make fewer physician visits, are more active physically, and can reduce medication use. (See McLeod, 1986.)

Moose (1984) in his important book on coping with physical illness, writes, "By emphasizing the active role of the individual in the etiology and management of illness, behavioral medicine has taken a valuable step beyond the classical psychosomatic perspective" (p5). Illness adaptation then, as coping by the individual, is an active process. It is this activity which the health provider must encourage and guide. Here the medium is the message, i.e., the goal for active disease prevention and illness coping must be reflected in the events of the encounter, the transaction between the physician or other health provider, and the woman. Whatever powerlessness she feels initially, whatever passivity may be her bad habit or her iatrogenically learned response, becomes an immediate focus of the change effort. Indeed "non compliance" may be one way that the patient who feels powerless shows her health provider that powerlessness can be a contagious condition. When she does not comply, the frustrated health care provider also senses what it is to feel powerless. As with other contagious conditions, the now two "infected" parties would not wish to continue in an untreated state.

Summary

Non-compliance of patients with recommendations made by the physician is common. Many of the same general features associated with illness risk are found to affect compliance as well. Thus the health professional's efforts to improve that situation can employ techniques, and importantly, a general perspective, which have been shown useful in assisting women in compliance and for other self-directing health relevant change. The evidence, as well as social developments in society and leitmotifs in current psychobiological medicine, all point to the importance of fostering increased patient self-direction through special ways of communicating and relating. This can include sharing uncertainty, responsibility, involving persons close to the patient, and helping the woman feel "in charge" of herself.

One way to characterize the kind of change necessary in the physician or other health professional so that he or she is in a better position to work with the patient is to abandon the term "compliance" itself. It implies in the professional, command and authority, and in the patient, obedience and passivity. None of these is useful when the goal is that the patient do for herself, and do so on the basis of understanding why it should be so, how it is to be done, and because she wants to do it. The term "cooperation" symbolizes the change needed. There are a number of ways in which improved cooperation for adherence to mutually agreed upon regimens and lifestyles may be brought about. All imply that the professional himself or herself wants this to occur, is willing to communicate extensively as to reasons and goals, listens to learn of obstacles, resistance and consequential emotional aspects, and reaches out to bring in others to monitor and support the women in her change efforts. One does not hold out impossible goals, and does reward with approval all steps in the right direction. Building the woman's confidence, as well as understanding, is vital. So, too, is realizing that major changes in conduct must be fitted into an existing life, not ordinarily as revolution but as modifying steps which occur in the context of family and work. Whenever possible, one arranges for specific training, practice, and devices to augment the woman's self-monitoring awareness of what she is doing daily with respect to needed health care.

10

More on Getting Cooperation: Securing Long Term Change in Health Behaviors

Much work has been done in behavioral medicine to bring about long term changes in women's behavior to reduce disease risk, for example, obesity, being sedentary, smoking, and alcohol and drug for abuse. It is unwise to make too great a distinction between principles for health promotion for lifelong self-regulation of habits, and shorter term new actions, as in regimens for serious illness. Control of diabetes or hypertension illustrates how a medication program may also be a lifelong habit change: for diabetes, for example, medications and diet, and for hypertension, diet, exercise, medication and perhaps relaxation therapies such as biofeedback for pre-eclampsia, or other stress management. In all cases the basis for initiating change begins with the determination through evaluation that a risk or debilitating condition exists which requires intervention by the health professional aimed at assisting the woman to alter her lifestyles, habits, and situational responses.

Treatment beginnings are much the same. What was said in Chapter 9 about the elements of gaining cooperation apply to any effort requiring patient participation, from pregnancy antenatal care attendance or genital herpes medication and transmission prophylaxis to diabetes management. What has been learned from the earlier "compliance" research applies just as well to the physician's initial role in longer term changes. What has been learned more recently as principles from life, habit, and reaction change programs applies to the office encounter as it focuses on facilitating cooperation of any kind.

One ordinarily distinguishes between those activities which involve only the health professional and the woman, and those which are better managed through the involvement of supporting or expert others as well. One cannot always predict what will be needed. A self-damaging patient in acute care—for example, the immediate postoperative counter phobic Type A woman executive who will not accept bedrest—will require behavioral health consultation. On the other hand, remarkable shifts may sometimes be made simply upon advice. Probably the most widely cited of the latter is work by Russell et al. (1979). Patients were told to stop smoking by their regular physician, with one group getting an anti-smoking leaflet and told they would be followed up. A questionnaire one year later indicated that 19% of the leaflet-warning group had quit, as had the advice only group. Some in the control groups had reduced smoking too. It is unknown if any patients lied on the questionnaire, or if changes—e.g., the controls—were part of a general downward social trend in that population sector.

Wilson, in a report presented in the *Nation's Health* (Jan. 1986, p.11), indicates that physicians whose advice includes a prescription for nicotine gum, instruction on use, and "some behavior modification techniques," will yield a smoking cessation rate of 15%. That figure is close enough to the Russell et al. finding to confirm the responsiveness of some patients to medical advice regarding smoking cessation, but to leave in doubt the process at work—whether gum is much of a help.

Some lessons learned from behavioral therapies have already been set forth in our discussion of general elements for securing cooperation. Examples are co-authoring the medical record to enhance patient self-awareness of what she is doing and what it signifies for health, the use of frequent reminders and contacts, securing patient agreement to engage in or avoid an activity that, bound by a stated formal commitment, rewards progress even in small degrees. The physician rewards the patient at the next visit by encouraging the woman to reward herself frequently for improvement, with a movie or new sweater or whatever else is appropriate and pleasing. Bringing in others (for example, "support" groups), although by no means any recent discovery, is typically part of behavior treatments, or indeed, many other forms of psychotherapy. Thus one sees, for patients on change regimens, home visitors, or family or "significant other" programs to involve intimates in assessment and support. Feedback is a central concept, for it is necessary for people to see how and what they are doing in order to shape their conduct. Whether that is blood pressure monitoring at home, calculating daily calories consumed, writing a daily diary recording recommended medicine usage, exercise, rest or what-have-you, or the conversational exchange with the health professional where progress, problems, impressions, or test results are communicated, all of it assists in self-appraisal and self-correction.

These sensible, practical, easy to apply, indeed simple minded methods do, in part, work, whether in behavioral treatments or within the context of enhancing routine efforts at office adherence. Their use assumes either an initial motivation to participate on the part of the patient or if that is absent, the capacity of the professional, upon assessing with the patient what it is she wants, suffers, realizes, or expects, to identify some aspect of current interest or conduct which points in the right direction, and to begin there. "Negotiation" and "contracting" are words currently employed to describe the process whereby both parties—the professional and the patient—work their way by discussion to decide what they can agree to, if only as a short term goal or even provisional effort, and handshake on it, or sometimes write it down. The terms imply the urge for a declaration of initial interests and positions, e.g., the physician really believes the woman is at risk of serious ill health because of some bad habits, whereas she does not believe she can entirely give up, say, chocolates, or a promiscuous lover constantly reinfecting her. The gin, on the other hand, is not so essential, she says, and a nicotine chewing gum will do as a substitute while she agrees to give up two packs of cigarettes a day. "Negotiation" implies the understanding that most people can move on an upward course from where they are to some place close by, and that it is likely both unrealistic and frightening to aim for the moon until one is sure one can make it to the next block.

We repeat that such popular and useful programs and procedures work only in part, varying from person to person, generally following a sine wave course of getting better and then falling back. Most single modality, single target programs are too narrow to embrace the complexity of emotion, interpersonal interaction, uncontrolled situational stresses and temptations, psychodynamic conflicts and needs, and other influences in which the effort to secure cooperation in and personal commitment to adherence is embedded.

Janis and Mann (1983), in a series of studies, set out some other findings pertinent to the "simple" approach. Their conclusion is that adherence to difficult self-regulating practices (this experimental work emphasizes obesity control) can better be understood by thinking of a woman's state of "vigilance." That is defined as her simultaneous awareness (perception, weighing) of (a) the negative features both of adhering (cost side effects, trouble) and of not adhering, (b) optimism about the regimen as the better choice (weigh costs/benefits, believing in efficacy), and (c) not being rushed and becoming too anxious or emotional. It is implied that patients need time to weigh therapeutic recommendations. Janis finds there will be defensive avoidance, such as non-adherence or escape. Communications likely to improve adherence actions are those that enhance patient self-esteem through approval and acceptance leading to trust and reliance; those that make clear that the actions required are not overwhelming and that some failures are to be expected (and will be accepted without harsh criticism) where adherence is praised; and where the professional secures verbal agreement (or in the case of support groups such as for obesity control, public declarations) to undertake the recommended regimen. Approval is to be given only when it is sincere. It is important for the patient to be put in charge of her own conduct when the aim of therapy is the development of self-approval when the patient is engaging in desired, disciplined self-help.

In another study on weight loss, positive feedback (i.e., praise) from the counselor yielded more weight loss than when there was counselor criticism or disdain. Providing approval is limited to that self-help which is, or is moving toward ("shaping" as it is called through reinforcement) the desired goal. One does not reward the failures, and thus must not be sympathetic about patient statements reflecting lack of motivation to change health behavior. The research also shows that adherence is greater when there is professional-patient discussion about what causes worry or what is hoped for, but not at such a level of depth that one probes for and receives intimate revelations. (These findings apply to obesity, hypertension, smoking programs; not to sexual dysfunction associated with cancer treatment.) The principle is that the physician or counselor who is not trained to be, or taking time to be a psychotherapist as such, should avoid probing about psychodynamics. As a corollary a friendly businesslike relationship, one not encouraging dependency, gets the best results. An additional technique, useful in surgical or obstetrical preparation, or for chronic anxiety or pain management, is "positive self-talk," i.e., teaching the patient to practice telling herself she is in control of pain. Or, as an extension, encouraging her to use the "imaging" technique of blocking conditioned fears by "imaging" self-control— putting positive pictures in the mind, or a singular concentrating "mantra." Relaxation and yoga methods of concentration are similar.

Melamed (1984) examines programs aimed at securing self-help changes as recommended for the treatment of diabetes. Children shown films of other children injecting insulin became more skilled and reliable. Students working closely with adult diabetics to help them identify everyday habit change needs when shopping, snacking, eating out, etc., appeared to be facilitators for important gains. When children were rated over time for foot care, diet, and urine testing, and given reward points for cooperation, adherence to diet was much improved. Parents trained to offer approval also achieved good results in their children. Such results are not obtainable in conflicted, disorganized families. Using a clinical treatment case, Melamed tells of biofeedback relaxation relieving felt stress and lowering insulin needs in patients. However, in one case a severely hypoglycemic reaction occurred because the patient, the non-observant physician and the biofeedback expert all failed to lower the self-medicated insulin dose accordingly. Both patient and physician require feedback!

Melamed discusses the work of Craighead, Brownell, and Stunkard on weight control programs. Their approach, carefully considered in a thorough review of behavioral programs for self-control development by Leventhal, Zimmermann, and Gutmann (1984), examines the components (and sometimes, contexts) for real life conduct with respect to the activity requiring self-regulation. For example, with obesity programs, Stunkard et al., attend to the woman's monitoring food intake, her always eating in the same (controlled) situation, eating slowly and in small portions, enjoying and not gulping food, etc. One seeks to make the entire sequence of behaviors matters of awareness and self-control, sometimes assisted by token rewards from others or oneself. Consonant with this, Schwartz (1983) has emphasized the importance of awareness-feedback mechanisms for any successful self-regulation (as do Leventhal et al.). Indeed, Schwartz refers to the self-correcting, regulating brain as a "health care system" (1982). The hope for such self-regulatory models is that all relevant conduct by the woman becomes part of self-care as a process where each component is identified and recognized as consequential, requiring self-monitoring and self-control. This is in contrast to the mechanistic and specific obedience "model" for "compliance" which has, generally, so little success except for the most simple, short term, and salient self-care activities.

Behavioral approaches reported considerable initial success, typically in the range of 60% to 90% for smoking, eating, and similar behaviors, but as Hunt (1974) has shown for smoking, heroin, and alcohol withdrawal programs, one year later 75% of those persons previously successful were backsliders. This may not be as hopeless as the statistic suggests. Longer term studies of alcohol treatments (Blum and Blum, 1967) suggest that aging (maturing) is itself a positive factor in compulsive consumption reduction and, further, that a sawtooth progression on-and-off, i.e., backsliding and back on the wagon, can nevertheless reduce overall average consumption, where episodes of either controlled, social drinking or abstinence become longer and more frequent.

Melamed cites recent Stunkard et al. research to demonstrate a long term gain from behavioral methods, superior to pharmacotherapy for obesity. One study of 120 obese women set up four groups. One received behavioral therapy (self-monitoring, stimulus control, slowing eating, nutrition education, management of exercise, i.e., a typical multiple component behavior oriented approach). A second group received that and an appetite suppressant (fenfluramine), the third received only medication, and a fourth control group was untreated. After six months all three treatment groups were markedly less obese than controls, with both medication groups superior to behavior therapy alone. However by the end of a follow-up year, this was reversed; those on medication regained an average of 10.7 kg compared to 1.9 kg for the behavior but no drug treatment group. And of course, the no medication group suffered no side effects and experienced no medication costs. The study also proved replicable. Melamed is, nevertheless, realistic about potential goals as she notes the ordinary 50% drop-out rate from programs. She contends this may be a function of a physiological "set point" for hypothalamically fixed body weight (as in thermostatic) regulation. (But where was the "set point" when a woman, at 120 pounds until she was 35, broke loose to become a 200 pound 40 year old?) Set point theory is popular these days, but one does well not to equate compulsions or other psychologically intricate phenomena with hypothalamic thermostats.

Breast self-examination is another area to which Melamed attends, observing as a result of training, not simply the desired outcome of BSE (smaller tumor size and higher subsequent survival rates), but women's trainability as such. Giving out advice or a pamphlet is not the answer (compliance is low) (Assal et al., 1985), but training with a physical model, being helped by an instructor, doing it in a group, practicing at home with the husband's supportive presence, does lead to high proficiency and continued (over 6 months) BSE. She cites Hall showing that, with training, correct detections on the silicone model improved to the point where there was a 7% false positive rate, the same as in mass screening.

Kinds of Social Supports

Melamed describes the need for specificity in identifying the kinds of social support which are most clearly related to adherence. She distinguishes between quantity and quality, and in the latter, between emotional support and instrumental helping. Citing Kaplan et al., it is patient-perceived support from spouse, friends, and physician which is associated with improved hypertensive patient motivation, awareness of risk, actual BP control and maintenance of that control, and also reduced depression.

Particularly helpful for long term and difficult self-help are "buddy systems" such as Alcoholics Anonymous. Treating people in pairs (see Jamis, 1983) using group sessions, having buddies telephone each other often about their health behaviors, with discussion between them about their problems and temptations, and emphasis (training initiated originally by the physician or counselor) on how important the health behavior is, are all useful devices. Follow-up using these procedures showed reduction in cigarette smoking maintained over 10 years. In an analogous experiment with overweight women, those who as buddies talked daily to each other, lost more weight than women having less frequent contacts. It is also found helpful if the buddies assigned are rather like each other in background and attitude, but are not told of these similarities.

The Illusion of Control and Spontaneous Change

Even when short term success can be shown, there are difficulties of several sorts in promoting cooperation with recommended self-help regimens. For one thing, people who believe that a behavior is potentially under their control may relax and do nothing about it. Leventhal et al. (1984) point to teenage smoking where two-thirds of teenagers know smoking is potentially harmful, but two-thirds of these claim no harm in casual smoking since, they contend, "casual" smokers can easily stop if they want to. The dependency producing features, one's own addiction and related withdrawal diffculties from nicotine are denied.

Acceptance of theoretical risk and conviction about a personal risk are separate beliefs. Weinstein (1984) shows accurate knowledge of behavioral threats to health (from health statistics) in a person who believes her habits are under her self-control leads to overly optimistic appraisals about her own risk status. Whereas other people not using seat belts, enjoying high cholesterol diets, consuming a lot of alcohol, not exercising, or not brushing their teeth are rightly judged to be at greater health risk, in a student sample people who had those same bad habits rated themselves at less risk than hypothetical "other" people. Coming between what they are really doing daily and what might happen statistically (as "relative risk") is the notion that "I can stop if I want to" or "I will stop if I get in trouble." Perhaps such rationalizations are linked not simply to denial and comfort, but to some sense of invulnerability— the happy immutual delusion, "Lady luck loves me." Overconfidence too soon is a negative feature requiring doses of reality. It is a lesson most parents try to teach their children, yet it remains a primary public health lesson yet to be learned by many.

Leventhal et al., reviewing the obesity literature, find that the reasons people do change health behavior are more likely associated with how they feel (citing Knapp) than knowledge-based, intellectually valid estimates of future dangers. Women begin actual slimming in order to be socially approved, that, is to look good or to avoid "feeling tired," not because of health dangers. Cardiac patients who feel well respond less well to care recommendations (citing Gutmann et al.) than do those who are symptomatic. It is easy to deny one's illness and nurture the illusion that one is entirely well again.

Changing the self-image, for example, to accept oneself as ill but still a valuable, self-valuing person, can be part of the treatment.

Giving confidence that one can lose weight, for example, by short term success in giving up ice cream for a week and rewarding that, is also part of the road to a new view of the self.

Programs directed at the self-concept, not behavior per se, through training for assertiveness and social skills or self-management (as in time and stress management), do work to produce health changes (Leventhal, citing Wilson). Workers' stress reduction groups which aim at asserting power, being angry at demeaning work situations, and rejecting self-blame and building pride, reduce physical symptoms and depression, anxiety and alcohol intake (Lerner, 1985). Indeed the capacity to learn prideful resolve seems fundamental to most health behavior changes that do occur, and it is independent of treatments. In one experimental anti-smoking study (Leventhal, 1984), the controls did better than the treated experimental group, including not resuming the tobacco habit. One speculates either that the control group felt they were in a competition, or knew and responded to the investigator's intent (see Risenbery, 1984). Groups angered by feeling left out can competitively organize themselves and feel better for doing so.

The phenomenon of spontaneous, or at least not experimentally or treatment induced, health behavior change is widespread. Indeed it appears to be the major circumstance for behavioral health change. It can, however, be an unstable or even unwise behavior change. Consider the positive first. Two-thirds of those Americans who have by now quit smoking have done so on their own (Rosenthal, citing Schacter). That represents over thirty million people. On the other hand, among those who are still smokers yet say they want to quit, only one-third have been willing to attend any anti-smoking program. Consider smoking in pregnancy (Institute for Health Policy, 1985). About 25 to 30 percent of pregnant women smoke; among these about one-fourth quit because they are pregnant. But it doesn't last; some resume smoking while they are still pregnant, while most of the others resume after birth. Those who do quit are those who smoked less in the first place, are better educated, and are more often primiparae. The smokers are poorer and have fewer social supports. Indeed they may smoke more, or resume it, because of the "stress" of being pregnant. It is the old MARLIC principle applied now to spontaneous change; those with the most resources and the fewest problems change most easily. Psychotherapy evaluations produce similar findings: the healthier get more treatment and do better.

But change is not always for the wiser, for one can be misled, or mislead oneself. Consider dietary habits (Hall, 1985). People are buying more foods labeled "fresh" or otherwise "natural" or healthy, like salads, which they want to believe are healthy—although the salads most purchased today in restaurants are likely to be "chefs" heavy with ham, cheeses, and rich dressing. What is changing most in the American diet is convenience and "upscale" sophistication ("ethnic frozen food"), whereas a two and one-half year follow up shows that the nutrition and health conscious food purchasing group has actually grown smaller. While half of the U.S. population say they are trying to lose weight (at any one polling moment), overall calorie consumption per capita, refined sugar and corn sweetener, cheese, and vegetable fat consumption have increased with a probable overall national uptake in lipids. (A Department of Agriculture estimate is 6% per capita uptake in availability over 10 years; this may not be the same as consumption or as reflected in circulating blood levels). Apparently for the sake of this same "dieting," nutritious food such as prunes have declined in sales by 60%, although generally, happily, fruit and vegetable consumption is up about 8% (but to yet inadequate nutrition levels for complex carbohydrates). Hall attributes some of this paradox to public misconception and confusion; one poll showed primary public dietary concern to be about vitamins, minerals, and food additives, not major health risk factors such as fats, or, with respect to cancer, fibers and fats. Hall concludes "people are eating...what they always have, [but] marketers know that they have to emphasize the healthful aspects of their products." Something advertised as "natural"—which three-fourths of purchasers say is a label that influences their buying decisions, may be a product chock full of chemical additives (one "all natural" coffee cake contains monoglycerides, diglycerides, lecithin, xanthan and, no doubt, great quantities of refined sugars). Self-change, the food data show, can be guided by advertiser imposed and consumer self-selected illusion in the service of convenience, status, pleasure, and continuing bad habits.

Such data tell us that a good deal more than treatment by programs of behavioral manipulation of the sort used in behavioral medicine is at work, although "manipulation" by illusion is by no means excluded. Consider for instance Holroyd et al. (1984), who used electromyograph display biofeedback training, a technique known for good results in tension headache. But Holroyd provided bogus feedback on the screen with respect to the degree of frontalis muscle control occurring. The patients whose false feedback showed them to be gaining muscle control were those who reported less headache. One can surmise this is a matter of belief in self-control, an illusion here, but it worked on the headache. Alternatively, patients given the "evidence" and wanting to please the therapist denied their headache. We suspect it was the illusion at work— another placebo effect.

One by no means derides the placebo effect, or the importance of research on its central psychophysiological mechanisms. The phenomenon itself, which is simply a label for a process not understood, appears to play a major role in many forms of health intervention. For example, common treatments for PMS employ progesterone for good effects proclaimed by both patients and physician (Norris, 1983). In fact, in blind, controlled trials, progesterone does no better than inert materials (O'Brien, 1985). PMS women are described as particularly susceptible to placebo effects at a rate of about 50%, a phenomenon which should direct research to their sensitivity and the valence of their immediate experiences leading to pain or reports of relief.

The placebo effect shows itself as an energizing, self-organizing, potentially powerful psychophysiological response (recall Eisenberg's (1984) examples of powerful and paradoxical psychopharmacological outcomes). It can also emerge as mobilization of conduct for cognitive or social functions. As we define the effect, it is directed by expectations shared by a person in a position of relative deference or felt need working with a person perceived as more powerful and knowledgeable. The response is triggered by an immediate and direct action which is seen to be independently compelling, i.e., an external force for change which the patient directly experiences as felt change. Whether one calls that suggestibility, social support, encouragement, or magic, hardly changes the elements. In Holroyd's work it is a deception leading to greater felt self-control or mastery. It is initially illusion, but the good outcomes are real.

Taylor (1983) has described women's adaptation to breast cancer. There were three major components in this psychological process. There was a search for meaning in the experience: 95% had to explain the event, most often using a theory of stress in relationship to their marriages. Attempts to gain a sense of mastery were a second component. Two-thirds said they believed they themselves could do things to keep the cancer from recurring, for example by meditation, changing their lives, or changing their diet to include more fruits and vegetables. Many reduced medications such as routine estrogen or birth control pills, and some became more informed about the disease itself. For those receiving chemotherapy, mastery of side effects were, for 50%, practiced by imaging (making an image in the mind of something good, protective, painless, or beautiful to counteract nausea or other painful sensation), self-hypnosis, meditation, or the distraction of doing something. Self-enhancement was the third component. Surprisingly, more women said they were better adjusted or wiser after the illness than before, in spite of their disfigurement and fear. Almost all of them saw themselves as better off than others with whom they chose to compare themselves, for example, an older woman saying how much easier it was for her to adjust to radical mastectomy than for a younger woman.

Taylor views these data as demonstrating not simply the healing potential women have within themselves for psychological adjustment, but how that process focuses on one's experience in such a way as to employ illusion positively. Denial, repression, or at least selective use of fact is not such a bad thing. Since denial is a naturally occurring major psychological defense mechanism, that makes sense.

Continuing Contact and Other Essentials

Lenfant and Schweizer (1985), when reviewing the successes of the Multiple Risk Factor Intervention Trial (MRFIT) to reduce CHD, measured subjects' maintaining cigarette smoking reduction over time (they cite also Hughs, 1981). They attribute that success to "continued uninterrupted contact with patients after intervention." Since success in such behavior change depends on initial continuity of participation in program groups, then one responsibility for the health professional is to create circumstances which facilitate continuing contact. This includes an "open door" for those women relapsing. To help generate contact opportunities, one must know what is going on in the woman's life "out there" to facilitate or hinder the repeat visits that are typically part of programs for treatment. Convenient weekend or evening hours, programs held in low income neighborhoods or in institutions on buslines, subsidies or insurance programs to pay for what cannot routinely be afforded, persuading the husband not to sabotage care—indeed bringing him in to join the group, encouraging the woman to ask friends to babysit, or providing a nursery in the clinic are all examples of the professional and his or her institution going that extra mile to facilitate contact.

Martin and Prue (1985) found they got better results in a hospital-based behavioral medicine (cigarettes, stress management etc.) program by reducing self-monitoring from daily to weekly (a paradoxical effect). For patients living many miles away, some treatments were by telephone. By increasing convenience, and perhaps anxiety/resistance from daily diary monitoring, the drop out rate went from 75% to 15% and, by the end of the year, 25% were cigarette abstinent. That outcome is not so different from Russell's simple "stop smoking" advice in the UK study of medical advice as a change effector. While Martin and Prue (1985) see the diary and visit effects as specific change effecting variables, it is quite possible that one is seeing here an equivalent of the famous "Hawthorne (Western Electric) effect" (Roethlisberger and Dickson, 1946). In the 1920's, industrial engineers set about to improve production by changing workers' environmental conditions. Each time they added more lighting, for example, production went up, but as they reduced lighting, production again went up. Over time it was learned that almost any change that workers saw as well intentioned and facilitating led to increments in production. It is a kind of placebo effect.

The value of personal contact depends on how those experiencing it assess it. Consider that Grossarth-Maticek (1984) found that psychotherapy extended survival time for women with breast cancer and, when combined with chemotherapy, had a synergistic survival effect. We believe this effect is subsumed under Goldberg and Tull's (1983, and citing also Weisman and Worden) finding that terminal cancer patients with cooperating and mutually responsive interpersonal relationships live longer than those without, particularly if the latter have destructive relations. Data from Dyk and Sutherland (1956) studying women with colostomies suggest that enjoying sustaining versus destructive post-ostomy marital relationships can be predicted prior to disease on the basis of the warmth, trust, interdependency, and good sexuality in the marriage. Recall Chapter 9 and the finding that adherence in medication programs is poor when provided by physicians who are aggressive and ambitious, or self-effacing, and best under those aware, thoughtful, and nurturant. We believe this is another example of quality of contact at work in improving health self care.

Let us turn to a few examples from health promoting programs. Algert et al. (1985), treating obese women with gestational diabetes under conditions of dietary instruction, keeping a diet diary, and weekly counseling, showed that these women gained less weight during pregnancy than untreated lean diabetic women and non-diabetic non-obese women. One inference allowed (if the obese are not already simply at their "set point"), is that the counselor did the job well by being warm and supportive. Heinrich and Schag (1985) offered a special program of information and stress activity management for cancer patients and their spouses, compared to a control group of patients and spouses with normal care, all seen by the investigators over time. Although information levels went up more in the experimental group, the experimentals and controls did not differ in outcomes measured by psychosocial adjustment. Both groups improved in adjustment, an effect that can be interpreted as arising from constituting patient-spouse groups for the study and contact itself, which controls also experienced. The investigators note that many subjects in both groups said how pleased they were that someone was finally interested in what was happening to them, and further, they felt good about sharing their experiences in a way that might be useful to others in the group. Others working with women depressed after gynecological cancer surgery, and seeing moods lifting, hear these women say, "How wonderful it is simply to have someone knowledgeable to talk to!"

Coppotelli and Orleans (1985) investigated the effects of naturally occurring partner support among newly abstinent married women smokers. The most important factor determining relapse or abstinence was whether or not the husband helped. Components contributing to his helping were the husband's having successfully stopped smoking, and his relation with his wife about her quitting, promoting her abstinence, rewarding it, monitoring her, being a stress buffer, and not putting punitive pressure on her or being dominating (we take this as the absence of self-righteous commanding).

One of the features which make it most difficult to give up smoking, demonstrated in work with pregnant women as well (Institute for Health Policy, 1985) is if the husband is a smoker. Consider the constant cues to smoke, perhaps his sabotage of her effort if she is able to stop and he is not. Does that not make her, in his eyes, the better and stronger person, and thereby, as is the case with us frail mortals, the object of envy and anger? Husband involvement is essential for smoking cessation among pregnant women and, happily, it can appeal to his better and stronger instincts as a father wanting a healthy child.

The pregnant woman is likely to be asked to make a number of changes in her conduct which carry over to post partum living, for example better nutrition, alcohol and drug control (during pregnancy, very low intake or abstinence), stress management, exercise, and attention to safety (seat belts, accidents, etc.). Some professionals worry that asking too many things at once is a discouraging burden of demand. On the other hand, if the woman herself is the willing goal setter for comprehensive change, she can focus on central self-image changes, confidence, and gaining control with these behaviors. In any event, with group counseling for those who have trouble with change, even with so difficult an addiction as cigarettes one can hope to maintain reductions in one-quarter to one-third of those who had previously not been able to help themselves. This is not any great record for "cure," but for those women with better habits, it will represent a significant reduction in disease risk, and eventual disease burden.

Maimon and Zapka (1985), also Gravell, Zapka, and Maimon (1985) have like Malamud, set up research groups to educate breast self-examination among college women. Controls received no such group program. One program goal was for these women also to get their mothers to do BSE. One correlate of the observed improvement in BSE frequency and proficiency was the encouraged but still spontaneous discussion with other women close to them. Mothers who were talked to by their daughters also improved BSE.

We take the foregoing to illustrate not simply the wide recognition and use of the provision of interpersonal situations and norm setting emotional support in health promotion treatments, but as evidence that such interpersonal support, as continued structured contact of a sympathetic kind, is important in achieving treatment goals across a range of health needs and conditions. Simple things can and should be done. Miller (1985) observes that "showing interest" and reminding, via personal phone calls or a personal letter (no photocopy signature or bulk rate postage, please), greatly increase the rate of return visits for continuing treatment programs. Not delaying treatment once a person comes in, or is brought in, matters, although coercion (as in employer or probation imposed requirements— alcohol, driving safety, drugs) versus voluntary treatment involvement does not. It is quite important, as part of giving the woman a sense of control, and helping to tailor treatments, to provide an alternative for treatment forms or schedules or goals, for example letting alcoholics set as their target either abstinence or controlled (social) drinking.

Convenience also accounts for staying in or dropping out of treatments. Having to travel far, at inconvenient times or finding one's own transportation if one does not have a car impinge on continuation in care. So does the extent to which self-esteem is enhanced, as opposed to techniques which further challenge the already fragile self-esteem found in so many people who are not in charge of their habits or lives. Occasional change of pace or novelty in treatment can also be an asset for program groups— remember the Westinghouse studies cited above? New approaches can include role playing and imaginary rehearsals of how to behave under stress or temptation (wasn't it Luther who said, "since temptation cannot be avoided, one must learn to resist it")? Indeed, rehearsing temptation resistance is a powerful element in trial preventative efforts among teenagers (or younger children) likely to be exposed to drug use invitations from their, usually a bit older, peers. Here rehearsal in saying "no" and in being rewarded for that in the training group (usually in school) is a widely applied preparatory practice method. Such role playing sessions can be quite effective for bringing about change as well. Janis (1984) describes how in their anti-smoking clinic a heavy smoker would be told to play the role of herself, dramatized as in psychodrama, at the moment she is receiving the news that she has lung cancer. This was so upsetting that some, for the very first time, admitted that they *could* get cancer. This is an example of a destructive illusion— that one is invulnerable— being scuttled by a self-involving challenge, i.e., an "insult" to the defensive illusion.

Don't hurry. When change in complex behaviors comes too quickly it is not likely to last. Examples include strong appeals, some kind of office theater of threat or magnetism, or indeed anything which smacks of the vanity of the professional relying on the emotional components of the relationship ("transference" in psychoanalysis) to produce a quick "miracle cure" of conformity. Rosenthal cites Rozensky and Bellack to the effect that those patients most reponsive most quickly to health behavior program effects have the greatest relapse rate. Implied is the need for the woman herself to decide what she is going to do (remember Janis on "vigilance"), set her goals, and take the small regular steps toward these, integrating them bit by bit with what often must be quite major changes in her responses to situations, feelings of competence, commitment to change. One is, after all, aiming at self-regulation— even in something so minor as adherence to medication— and not doing something (which can include lying) to please the physician, or being momentarily caught up, hypnotized in some treatments which we do not commend, by the professional as office Svengali or Pied Piper who leads the transfixed fervent faithful. But out of the office, back in her world, Svengali— or Rasputin— is no longer there. She is left to her own resources and goals, and those are what must be relied upon for real cooperation.

In most cases, adverse conduct is part of personality needs, situational realities, sensivitity to ongoing feelings. When it comes to enduring changes useful for health, these are likely to be linked to whole sets of rationalizations, pleasures, and customary ways of doing things with others in the same boat (as drinkers, the obese, the sexually active, fellow smokers, etc.) Indeed, in studies of the initiation into unusual drug use (Blum, 1964), younger women were found to begin their "bad habits" under persuasion from boyfriends or older male friends as part of being a pleasing, agreeable companion. It is a kind of "proof of love." When lifestyles become integral to social and interpersonal activities, habits, even if admitted as "not good for me," the professional's good advice is easily ignored. A person can become quite angry, as well as anxious, if she is told to "shape up."

Lifestyle is a convenient term, but do not think of it as a unitary variable for health behavior. Mechanic (1979) has shown, studying children over a period of 16 years, that there is little that predicts from childhood attitudes to young adult health conduct. Those traits with some carry over are risk taking, sickness proneness, not changing behavior when sick, and also not paying much attention to pain. There is no one unifying attitude or personality observable in childhood which endures to young adulthood and which is a core trait for health responsibility. Matarazzo (1984), discussing Mechanic's data, is mindful that some expected relationships do obtain. For example those who were early, and late, risk takers drank more as young adults and engaged in less preventive medical care. Females generally were more health responsible than males. Other work further demonstrates the non-unitary nature of what may too readily be called "lifestyle." Kirscht (1983) cites work of Harris and Guten on a normal sample of city adults. They found six separate group statistical factors in health protective behaviors: (a) health practices as such, (b) safety, (c) preventative health care, (d) environmental hazard avoidance, (e) harmful substance avoidance, and (f) exercise. There is no ("g") for general type of good health behavior, nor any one type of environment or person to go with that. Importantly implied as well is the diversity of those who are at the many kinds of risk, and diversity in ways of seeking to keep well.

When Is Success Not Enough?
And When Is Knowledge Not Enough?

What constitutes "success" is, of course, a function of one's values and expectations as well as valid measurements. For example, Syme (1986), reviewing the same MRFIT data about which LeEnfant and Schweizen were so pleased (that 10 year, $115 million study of 13,000 men with at least two risk factors, all of whom said they were motivated to change smoking, diet, blood pressure, etc.), considers the 40% reduction rate in smoking to be a failure. "It should have been closer to 100 percent." It has become Syme's position that self-change efforts are simply not enough, that one must change the environments that contribute to risk. Heart disease has been examined, for example, and now studying the hypertension high risk group of city bus drivers, Syme and his colleagues are trying to arrange changes of schedules, less strenuous work loads, more time for meals and rest, all so that the work environment of the bus driver does not load the driver with hypertensive conditions.

For the purposes of the health professional working with the high risk woman, these observations on varying definitions of "success," and on the need to understand the woman's environment and how it too must be changed when she may be unable to work that change by herself, are essential. The health professional begins to work initially with those other people in the environment who presumably care enough about the woman to want to become the change in her environment, as for example partners who themselves go to work on giving up their smoking or alcoholism, or attend family counseling if that is required. But it may well be that it is a job, or a dangerous work environment, or an unsafe neighborhood which is also a risk precipitator. Knowledge of these risks is necessary for understanding, but may not in fact lead to a solution. That was the old dilemma of social medicine, or of social engineering, and it is still the challenge of preventive medicine and public health concerned with women's risks. Perhaps we should adduce a new priciple (the B&H Law?), "Whatever it is, if a risk factor has been there a long time, its sources are built in, and it ain't a goin' to be easy to change."

The Problem Patient: Her Number Is Legion

Obviously the best health promotion is that which is not necessary, for it has already been self-generated on the basis of naturally feeling good, being an educated, aware, self-regulating woman, being and living with fortunate competent others. For those kinds of conduct where it is widely recognized by the public that there is risk, as with smoking, obesity, STDs, contraceptive failure, drinking too much, not appearing for prenatal care, etc., one must assume that those women who are not now already doing wisely for themselves are the problem cases. The others, doing wisely, have either grown up "lucky," i.e., have not been exposed to the major psychosocial health risk factors, or when exposed, have been fortunate enough to be protected by buffering features. These can include a "right kind" of stress, social supports, home education for competence, or genetically and psychophysiologically self-directed personalities even when surrounded by adverse influence. Alternatively, those who engaged in high risk conduct and then changed on their own are obviously also "lucky" with respect to the availability of necessary self-awareness, social resources, assistance from others, optimism, self-control, capability, and coping alternatives.

An intriguing finding arises from those studies (Epstein) showing that those patients who adhere to a placebo regimen in controlled treatment programs are more likely to show improvement than those who are irregular in adherence. In one study (Coronary Project, 1980) adherence, *not* medication versus placebo, was the variable identified as influencing CHD mortality. As a personal variable, the capacity for cooperative adherence is then also a trait marker associated with psychological hardiness, and, here, mortality. How it functions to protect against chronic disease remains to be learned. The 50% or so who do not cooperate in adherence would appear to be the women who require our greatest health promotion attention.

To Repeat, Reach Out!

The role of office health promotor will involve "reaching out" beyond traditional one-to-one, in-the-office contact, the she-visits-and-I-am-here-and-that-is-the-end-to-it. Instead family members are asked to join as helpers and, if they themselves are "co-conspirators" in bad habits, to commit themselves to be participants in habit change. Families often share the same bad habits, or sometimes choose one of their members to be their lightening rod or scapegoat as family dynamic studies of heroin abusers consistently show. To involve the family is "reaching out." So too is introducing, with prior discussion, two of one's patients with similar risk behavior and to supervise them in becoming intensively communicating partners or "buddies," each helping the other in new regimes.

The next step may be setting up a group of one's patients who have similar problems, including inability to initiate or maintain needed lifestyle changes. At this point one is not simply reaching out but arranging an intervention run by others when the physician or nurse does not have time, motivation or skill to do it. That is the usual case. At this point, reaching out for health promotion and related disease prevention means reliance upon professional and community resources. This is referral of the patient, or groups of similar patients, to existing programs in the community for the typical specific "bad habits" (obesity, smoking, alcohol, drug abuse, being sedentary) or for preparatory birth training (the women's physician will likely already have been doing this through various forms of antenatal "methods"). Training classes for diabetes self-management or stress management and relaxation are also available in most cities. Support groups of many kinds can also be used when locally available.

Reaching out begins with expansion of traditional inquiries to and communication with the patient to become a positive influence on adherence and cooperation. It moves, in turn, from that to the larger and necessary joint responsibility, both patient and doctor, for cooperation in care. It also means going beyond traditional relationships to invite family participation to assist in regimens or life change. Many women's health professionals routinely expect spouse/partner involvement prenatally and perinatally. It is no revolution to expand that routine familial emotional and social support and shared educative role to include those other areas of living which are part of family life.

The patient may need partner and family involvement to secure needed health behavior changes, or to provide resources (intimacy, encouragement, concern for what the other is doing in health care, assistance for the disabled), the absence of which is dangerous.

Another step in reaching out is to expand one's knowledge of community resources, including those in hospitals with which one is affiliated, over the full range of women's behavioral or psychosocial needs— including sometimes their families. One identifies helping resources from post mastectomy support groups, or hysterectomy presurgical preparation groups, or post-abortion groups (see Burnell, et al., 1972) through weight control or exercise classes, to learning of professionals who lead groups helping hypertensives, Type A executives, or diabetics. Referr to such groups *only after* discussion with trusted knowledgeable colleagues and community leaders to rule out the many, indeed rampant, exploitive cult-and-quack "we promise a cure" or "greed incorporated" offerings. Yet a further level of health promotional resource use (reaching out) is referral for individual longer term treatment in health psychology or behavioral medicine or for psychotherapy. Socially and financially disadvantaged women will require a competent social worker or guidance. Finally, there is that health promoting which the clinical care provider encourages and applauds but in which he or she may have no part: those programs which are at the institutional, neighborhood, or mass media, community level.

The Whole Woman and Whole Programs

For many women, particularly those gynecological or obstetrical patients with conditions that are syndromes (PMS is a a good example but so is the somatizer, ante-natal high risk woman, the repeat STD case, or the "functional" menstrual disorder), there is no one "problem" or "bad habit" to be addressed by referral any more than, as research cited has shown, there is a dominant single trait of health behavior. Many women will present a cluster of interrelated problems where, clinically, the etiology, expression, management task, and future risk are all part of the mix of personality, situation, medical history, bad habits, adherence cooperation, and psychophysiological maladaptive response. Patients evaluated as having significant psychosocial-behavioral risk, or expressing these in their body as complaints and illnesses, usually have a number of elements which trouble them, and which constitute the treatment challenge. There are of course predominant presenting problems, for example depression and sexual dysfunction in the cancer patient, or anxiety-smoking-drinking or pre-eclampsia in a high risk pregnancy or pain-fatigue-facilities overuse in the somatizing woman. If one is to treat the woman as a whole person, and to have her joining actively in that "wholistic" enterprise, the one-habit, one modality treatment program will not be the treatment of choice.[1] (Psychotherapy should be recommended as specific treatment when depression or other emotional disorder is severe.)

A good approach is to establish, after careful evaluation both by the referring physician, or nurse practitioner, and the professional referred to, a program which aims not simply at the dominant risk, but multiply at the range of difficulties which are likely risks and deficits in well being. The preferred treatment group then will be one which addresses the syndrome at hand in the context of all of the risk and health behavior problems present in the patient. That implies patient self-evaluation for a number of health areas—a profile—and her commitment to a variety of changes, over a long period of time. She sets the priorities in cooperation with her health professionals.

The advantage is that one does not have a PMS patient remarkably improve only to have her die a week later from having not used her seat belt in an auto accident, or a "successful" cancer surgery case commit suicide as a result of undiagnosed depression. Multiple health-wellness profiles improvement may allow a good deal more progress, and thus enhanced esteem and felt self-control, so the woman can tackle some of the easier "self-work" first.

The whole woman approach is of course the care design for all primary care and/or its application historically and at present to pregnancy. Women's health care, and the speciality of obstetrics-gynecology, have long been committed to the health profile evaluation of management. Health promotion, as we noted in Chapter 1, is simply the natural evolution of that wholistic approach that embraces new knowledge and methods. One sees this multiple approach typically in syndrome care programs. Again take PMS as an example. Norris in his well known clinic uses not simply progesterone (a physiologically active placebo which allows women to feel changed and to reinterpret these sensations as "less distress") but has his patients change their diets, reduce alcohol and drug consumption, use vitamins, exercise, and learn to manage stressful environments. In his clinic there are evaluations for stressful events, anxiety, and depression (treated separately). Relaxation techniques are employed, the spouse is involved, support groups are part of care, careful exercise programs are developed, caffeine and salt intake reduced, food disorders are treated, self-monitoring is conducted daily—in other words a complete program for risk reduction and wellness is used to treat one syndrome, PMS. His is the whole woman approach, primary care along with the secondary care, wellness, traditional OB/GYN model at work. He reports it does work well (whatever, we must insist, its placebo component). One sees that such a multiple effort takes time, requires staff and materials, is a dedication in and of itself. Lark's (1984) self-help approach to PMS advises many of these same "health living" ingredients.

Osofsky and Keppel (1985) employ dietary measures in their "psychiatric" approach to the treatment of PMS. These include a balanced diet, reducing refined sugars, encouraging exercise, reducing smoking and alcohol intake, vitamin supplements, and the control of environmental stressors. Noting, along with Gold (1985), that double blind studies of progesterone show it to be no better than a placebo, they do not strongly recommend hormone use. Their approach can also be seen to emphasize general health measures for the whole woman. Gold (citing Dennerstein) observes that when PMS includes depression, that psychotherapy with pharmacotherapy is more effective than drugs alone.

Finding Your Alter Ego

We believe the ideal approach is for those physicians who are in solo or small group practice to identify a health behavior specialist who shares this philosophy, and to whom they may refer—but not lose—patients. The woman remains the patient of the original physician, and communication continues between her and the health behavior professional dealing with these several problem areas, usually in groups.

The larger clinic, hospital, HMO, or PPO will wish to employ a health behavior professional. He or she becomes a colleague with whom one is in frequent communication as part of one's own support as well as referral network. Consultation can be about, or referral for, the full range of psychosocial risk behaviors, cooperation psychosomatics, psychodynamics, even litigation propensities if need be. This is not referral "out" but treatment "within." If possible, establish a special unit in the institution. The sine qua non for measuring effectiveness initially, once the person or facility is established as complementary-to-oneself in service, is one's readiness to use the unit, and continued contact with its staff about one's patients who are now a shared responsibility. One of our colleagues at Stanford, oncologist Sam Ballon, calls the job of that resource, "being the alter ego" for health promotion acting on behalf of the health specialist and for the patient.

Summary

Much that applies either to securing short term regimen adherence or long term change can be learned from research and clinical evaluations in behavioral health. Negotiation for formal agreements on goals, use of frequent reminders, rewarding progress, employing support groups, assuring continuing contact by making care convenient, assuring that the health professionals involved are sympathetic personalities, giving the woman time to consider a regimen and then proceeding in short steps with practical elements, and imparting a sense of control, are all part of what is to be done.

"Reaching out" to understand the woman's life, not simply risks and conduct but also the barriers and potential facilitators to regimen adherence, is part of office-based health promotion. Husbands, partners, mothers, grown children can all be brought in to assist as part of the concerned and supportive group, both in the clinic for group sessions and at home. The health professional must also know what community resources exist by way of self-help and health behavior programs. The physician, nurse practitioner, licensed midwife also need a network of helpful ties. It is proposed that a regular relationship be set up with a professional skilled in health behavior change, including psychodynamics. Since many women have more than one problem that is psychosocial-behavioral, the work to be done— always in close liaison— is often over a long period of time, and across a range of feeling, situation, and conduct problems. It must be a wholistic approach.

The referral is not "out" to a possibly competing or unsympathetic professional but "within" one's network of colleagues. Perhaps one will want that person or service as part of one's hospital, clinic,

HMO, PPO, etc. Just as continuing professional-patient contact is essential for the initiation of programs for self-help in health, continuing contact is also the hallmark of consultative and shared responsibility of the health behavior specialist and the women's obstetrical-gynecological or general medical specialist. Consider and use that person or facility as one's "alter ego" for health promotion.

11

Evaluating and Targeting for Change

This chapter addresses the evaluation of the woman for psychological and behavioral risk, whether as etiological for the presenting complaint, or as sequelae of the disease and its treatments. The evaluation which proceeds by history-taking, listening, and observing how the woman behaves becomes the basis for establishing a profile of the woman with respect to her background, situation, personal styles and feelings, and conduct affecting her future disease risk and her current status. Where risks and problems obviously appear, these become targets for that cooperative intervention, the means to which we have discussed in the preceding two chapters. We will discuss special instances for referral in the two following chapers. Many of the risk and problems identified through the very simple evaluation procedures (it is after all but an item checklist) can be addressed by an office-based health promotion program.

Factors affecting whether the women's health professional begins this promotion or opts for consultation or referral, will depend upon the judged seriousness of the present situation. A correlated judgement is of the immediacy of change required, and the signs (usually the immediate past history or present attitudes/apparent competence) that the woman can or cannot commit herself to the program of change desired. The decision to consult or refer will also depend upon the rapport between the professional and the patient, the professional's interest in doing health promotion and the time available. Whether one has found a suitable professional (health psychologist, psychiatrist competent in behavioral medicine, licensed nurse with a health education specialty, clinical social worker skilled lay group leader) will also affect the decision on how much to involve oneself in the health promoting effort. Do keep in mind that the decision to refer should not diminish one's own responsibility for either the office assessment, the use of the techniques for assuring cooperation in adherence, or for maintaining oneself as one of the primary health promotion professionals in the woman's life, regardless of who else may also be rendering health care.

Let us reconsider the uncertainty which surrounds work on risk factors so far identified and their "targeting", with the woman, for change. Recall the recurring discussions about both research deficiencies. The list of items in Tables III, IV, and V vary considerably in the carefulness of work which led to their identification, in their applicability across population groups, in the evidence for disease risk reduction even when there is a change in the risk factor, and whether or not they are outcome determinants in their own right or serve primarily as markers for correlated or subsumed processes. The items differ among themselves considerably with respect to their specificity for particular disease outcomes, or whether they operate to augment risk for a range of conditions. Given this uncertainty, one may wonder if one is justified in targeting anything for change.

Reflection yields a positive reply. Examples include decreased lung cancer risk as a function of elapsed time since a smoker has given up cigarettes, or the role of medication in controlling hypertension including preeclampsia if the woman takes her medication, or the reduction in STD risk if the woman requires her partner to use a condom (or select fewer partners more carefully), or if she uses contraception regularly to avoid elective abortion of an unwanted child. Obesity, nutrition, seat belt use— there are many factors in the "yes, it is worth it" category. Even for somewhat less certain matters (for example, whether or not dietary cholesterol reduction, or Type A behavior reduction, really does affect CHD risk), one asks the question, what are the costs of doing it if it may not matter, as opposed to the costs of not doing it if it does matter? We don't mean to imply a simple 50/50 chance— that rarely is the situation— for a discussion of the much more complex heuristics of decison making in medicine (for mammography, see Eddy, 1982). Costs include a sense of defeat for failure, disruption as a woman goes off to a support group and does not cook dinner those nights, economic problems for the insurer or paying family, or disease risk possibly associated with the change effort— the latter probably most typically limited to poor self-prescribed diet or nutrition by hypervitamin supplement programs. The woman and her health professional will certainly address these matters of uncertainty and cost before any program, including routine medication and its likely efficacy and side effects, is undertaken. A woman may well decide that if, statistically, for any one item (say, obesity) her relative risk is decreased but a few percentage points by change, it is not worth it. (See Robbins and Blankenbaker (1982) for a most elaborate set of tables to calculate individual risk as a function of behavior.)

Yet if that same woman has risks, none of which has previously been the target of successful change, then this item-by-item justification for doing nothing may be self-defeating not only for the cumulative relative health risk, but also because it denies her a chance to try to put herself more in control of her life; to develop confidence and competence which may very well have implications for a range of her health care decisions, somatizing, and self-care actions. Our argument is, then, that if there is reasonable evidence that a factor may play a role in predisposing, triggering, exaggerating some outcome of consequence to the woman, and if the change effort has low costs in itself, and if the change effort may have benefits unrelated to particular disease reduction, then one may commit oneself to introducing change. The calculation here is much like that in prescribing drugs, the ratio of effective to lethal doses— the narrower the safety margin the higher the stakes, the greater the needed liklihood of efficacy, before one prescribes. Examples of areas for intervention are cigarette smoking, accident proneness, seat belt use, overeating, exercise, poor nutrition, high stress vulnerability and self-exposure to stressors, heavy drinking, abusive drug use, erratic contraception, repeated STD exposure, chronic hostility, depression, or anxiety, being abused or medication regimen failures.

Whether or not there is a relative reduction in disease risk which is experienced by the woman as better health, most of the programs which target health change do have other benefits, even if they are not sustained. Any reduction in unnecessary consumption— alcohol, cigarettes, fast food fats, cocaine, chocolates— can save money. Participants enjoy programs which help them feel better for making friends, get things off their chest, not feel so alone, and think of themselves as helping and being helped by women like themselves.

Self-esteem, other coping abilities, learning more about how to talk to others to make them into a "social support," looking good, and just feeling better can be important by-products.

Getting the Information

Observe the sequence of our approach to evaluation: we began with the identification of potential risk factors and moved to conditions useful for securing better cooperation in regimen adherence, including change programs. Now we come to the health profile inquiry. The sequence reflects not simply the obvious, that one must know a range of potential risk factors for discerning inquiry, but that the conditions useful for securing the cooperative commitment in care may also apply to obtaining a better history/evaluation. Inquiry about pychosocial-behavioral features is a dialogue. It depends upon the woman's voluntary, self-assessed reports. One wants that reporting to be as accurate as possible. Accuracy is aided when defense mechanisms such as denying are absent and when disruptive emotions do not cloud the woman's judgement. The efficacy of the history taking procedure itself (relevant and necessary) rests upon rapport that encourages a trusting, self-disclosing exchange. One aims to get a situational commitment by the woman to the work of that cooperative, evaluative endeavour. The evaluation process is a microcosm of that which is necessary to health promotion per se.

Diagnostic discrepancies based on prevalence and reliability data in Chapter 3 show that history taking is by no means an assured art when it comes either to uncovering risk items, allowing correct conduct-related diagnosis, or planning health objectives. The first omission is the physician's when no inquiry is made, or when it is perfunctory. The second omission is quite likely to be the woman's, for memory is often unreliable, and people are very defensive about revealing bad habits or making self-esteem damaging admissions. Some women really are unable to describe what their life is like, how they feel, or what they are doing. Assume that many patients will be defensive, or fib about those conditions where there is a social norm and implicit admonition, about what is the right thing to do or feel. Do not assume that all misrepresentations are conscious; fibs, and some denial, are so automatic and psychologically necessary that they are unconscious. People also deceive to make themselves look better to the important person who is the physician or other health professional. And they lie in order not to face themseves, or to be challenged to abandon those bad habits which they cherish.

In history-taking the physician avoids the error of omission by reviewing the risk lists and and incorporating case relevant items, including a psychosocial problem history (past and present) in the routine interview. The physician cannot dispel defensiveness totally, but can ameliorate it by conveying in words as well as looks and gestures the supportive understanding that all of us mortals are frail, and all of us do things which are bad for us. We all feel bad in ways we wish we did not. Many of us live in circumstances we prefer were otherwise. There is much that we would like to change about ourselves that seems beyond our control. The physician as a philosopher, like Galen, generates an atmosphere of tolerance conducive to more accurate reporting. And of course, the habit and problem inquiry which asks concretely about yesterday and this last week specifically makes patient recollection easier.

For all of those conditions where pychosocial and behavior features appear as risks, one also inquires to see if there are also concomitants such that a syndrome is present. Whether the complaints are diffused, or of pain unsubstantiated organically, or are functional/psychosomatic in terms of the loading of components, or whether demonstrably organic, one will also want to inquire about and record as part of the constellation of distress and illness conduct how the woman feels about it, and what she is doing in response to her complaints and associated emotions. One should learn how her family and friends are reacting to her condition. We noted earlier the possible utility of a tri-axial diagnostic system; organic, psychological, social. Such a system is not yet in operation as formal diagnosis, but these current features are to be entered as part of the record and physician's understanding of what is happening now, i. e., the complaint or disease as the intrusive distressing reality (or a useful excuse or manipulative device) in the woman's life.

As a matter of routine, given the proposed additional focus on conditions shown by prevalence data to be common, but rarely diagnosed, one would expect the women's health professional now to be alert to discover, whether in maternity care, gynocological office visits or surgical preparation, considerably more of these underdiagnosed consequential psychosocial behavior risks and reactions. For example, expect to inquire after the presence of anxiety, depression, fatigue, sexual dysfunction, and felt helplessness/hopelessness, or to be able to infer massive denial/repression (i.e., "everything is just fine"). Be sensitive to hostility and negative affect. Also expect to find, upon direct inquiry, much more than conventionally recorded heavy use of alcohol, use of illicit drugs, chronic use of prescribed sedatives and tranquilizers (often obtained by having several "regular" physicians, each prescribing for her); heavier smoking than initially reported, and for those with weight problems, fluctuations in weight in a diet-binge pattern (see Polivy and Herman, 1985). Among some patients will be found health food and vitamin overdosing, sexual activity with STD risk, self-destructive actions observable in repeated work or home accidents or other non-habit related self-harm or compulsive risk-taking measured by speeding tickets and auto accidents or for that matter, walking at night in dangerous areas, or frequenting bars alone, inviting exposure to attack.

For those in whom problem areas are identified, it is important to ask about prior control or treatment efforts. Many women may well have tried, for example, weight control classes or Alcoholics Anonymous and have dropped out. Dropping out is important to know about since, as Henderson et al. (1982) in a review report, it is a good predictor of subsequent failures. Keep in mind that a typical history of risk behaviors is not of steady state behavior. Not only is there predictable change with age (alcohol consumption usually declines, as does also exercise and hypertension; and weight and depression increase as does loneliness among the elderly) but over weeks and months considerable fluctuations occurs. Heroin addicts typically "dry out" on their own for long periods, whereas for drinking and obesity one can see binge and abstinence periods. What one wishes to establish then, for the patient's risk exposure, is not a simple recollected average, but high and low extremes, patterns over time and the life situations and feelings moods which trigger increased risk conduct or, happily, self-control efforts. The women's care provider will already be familiar with the fluctuation PMS, but even here a diary will allow differential diagnosis between "true" PMS (cyclical, regular, periods of no distress) and chronic distress exacerbated in the luteal phase.

If the women's professionals are to attend to potential disease and trauma which they could be called to attend, particularly if a specialist appreciates their role in primary care— then one does not limit one's traditional concerns. Seat belt use is not a typical inquiry area, but since prevalence of failure is high, and is directly associated with risk of trauma and death in highway accidents, it is entirely appropriate that it be part of the inquiry. So too with home accidents, rape exposure, or casual sex or drugs as "recreational," or contraceptive failure so as to feel "spontaneous" or "blameless" as part of denied sexuality.

If risk factors are found, the next inquiry step is to document the evolution and nature of the risk factor itself. One learns its onset time and circumstances, intensity of expression or presence, and its meaning to the woman in the life context in which it occurs. That knowledge helps to shape an estimate of the magnitude of risk for those behaviors or psychosocial conditions with linear or other gradient relations to outcomes. Cigarettes, alcohol, cocaine, and promiscuity are examples. Earlier onset, greater use, continuing use uninterrupted, each appears to constitute a greater obstetrical, or CHD and cancer danger. Cigarette smoking occurring as part of a cluster where there is also anxiety, heavy drinking, other smoking (cannabis), or other drug use is likely a more severe risk. Because it is embedded in a matrix of many bad habits likely set in family contexts, it/they will also be the more difficult to alter. One may formulate, conceptualize, that greater difficulty in change in several ways. For example, these can be mutually triggering cues to habit initiation. Behavior may be seen as compulsions or addictions, or as aspects of social deficits in rearing and environment. One can also find risk behavior as expressions of present personality problems, or as the psychological "choice" of a problem by a whole family as part of their dynamics. Each such formulation calls attention to a different aspect of the risk feature's interrelatedness to living. Each reminds us that health habit changes, for those who have not already initiated change by the time they see a professional, will involve the context of living, being by no means a mechanical reform.

Let us make a minimal list of psychosocial and behavioral conditions which should be inquired about when considering risk, and for understanding the woman's life. Many items are no doubt already matters of inquiry; consider them reminders. For a different approach to risk inquiry, a form for the woman to use herself for computer risk processing, see Robbins and Blankenbaker (1982). In the same text (whose editors teach family and community medicine) will be found detailed discussions of the requirements for, assessments of, and planning for patient self-help practices in the areas of nutrition, weight control, exercise, alcohol use, tobacco control, appropriate use of drugs, rest and sleep, and stress management.

The reminder list below can be reproduced for convenience as a history taking checklist and patient file document without copyright permission. It can be converted, amended, we hope constantly revised and updated as the professional wishes, so that the woman herself can complete it while waiting in the office. If so, make the questions clear and simple and be sure her written replies are reviewed. The goal here is dialogue and understanding, not record keeping for its own sake. It is presumed this evaluation will follow medical work-up.

Psychosocial Behavior Risk Profile Inquiry: A History Taking and Evaluation Reminder List

Name

Life Situation And Diagnostic Status
Present Complaints and Current Diagnosis/Diagnoses: How long has she been experiencing this condition before deciding to make this visit to you as a health care provider? Does reference to Tables III, IV, V, or other data, suggest the condition may have psychosocial-behavioral components in its etiology? As having adverse emotion/adjustment consequences generating further health risk? As having adverse emotional/adjustment consequences which, if unattended, will unnecessarily diminish quality of life? (Complete this item only after the conclusion of this evaluation.) What is going on in the woman's life now which may have contributed to her decision to seek professional care at this time?

BACKGROUND AND SITUATION: Age   Race/ethnicity

Highest educational level achieved: Employed:
                                           Part time   Full time

Can she read English? (Test with a simple test.)
(If she cannot, and perhaps one-third of American adults are functional illiterates, how can she read prescription labels, self-care instruction, or directions to find her way to the specialist she has been referred to?

Current occupation: Does job match education
                                       (if not, what inconsistency)

If employed, what work place risks for injury, toxin exposure:

"   " is strenuous physical effort required: yes/no

"   " is the boss helpful, friendly: yes/no

"   " are there any friendly, helpful colleagues: yes/no

MARITAL STATUS:
Single Married (how long)

Separated/divorced   Widowed (how recently)
(how recently)

If unmarried, is there a continuing, sexually intimate relationship with a partner?

If married, is the relationship with husband warm and supportive?

Any children?   How many at home?

WORK BURDEN PER WEEK:
Employment hours   Housework hours

Obligated shopping &
family meal preparation   Childcare hours

Care of ill/disabled persons   Other duties/compulsory activities

Commuting, child transport hours   Sum of hours for all work
(weekly average)

Hours per month for all
medical visits

Leisure: Sum of hours (weekly average) leisure, entertainment, fun, relaxation, hobbies, sport-for-pleasure, "other" for oneself:

Passive: (TV, movies, drinking) hours as %

ESTIMATED SOCIO-ECONOMIC LEVEL:[1]
Very poor and exremely disadvantaged

Below average income with severely limited resources

Normal range American middle and working class

Unusually high SEC

RESIDENCE SITUATIONS:
How many people living in the same household unit?

How many square feet (approx.) for them: estimate density from extremely crowded to uncrowded.

If living alone, isolated, lonely?

Household safety: fire extinguisher in the kitchen?

Smoke detectors?   where are poisons, garden chemicals, household chemicals stored?

Has there been a fire at home in recent years? Circumstances?

When was the last accident at home requiring medical attention for any resident there?

HOME MEDICINE CHEST:
What OTCs are regularly kept at home?

What OTCs are used on the average once a week or more?

What prescriptions are on hand in medicine chest/cabinets?

Last time expiration dates checked?

Any requiring cold or dark storage?

Any injectibles requiring sterile procedure?

What prescriptions are in current use?

What current prescriptions are not being used as directed? Why not?

Can children reach any stored medicines? Poisons?

If pregnant, any with teralogenic risk? (explore, evaluate)

NEIGHBORHOOD RISKS:
High or low for mugging, rape, other violence?

Home or community water supply: ground water contamination from high tech or chemical industries?

Are hand guns kept in the house: loaded? locked up?

VEHICLE SAFETY:
How many trips yesterday?

How often was the seat belt used?

Driven over 50,000 miles each year?

How often in six months have you been a passenger with a driver who had three or more drinks within two hours before driving (driver weight 110-150 lbs, or four or more drinks with body weight 150-190)?

When was the last time the woman herself drove after having three drinks within two hours before driving (body weight 110-150, or two drinks with body weight 90-110)?

Does she ride or is she a passenger on a motorcycle?

When was the last speeding ticket? How many over the last three years?

Last vehicular accident and circumstances?

Accident frequency over last three years?

SOCIAL NETWORKS:
Any club or group memberships where meetings are regularly attended?

Frequent church attendance?

How well acquainted in the community?

Any close friends "I can really talk to" ?

Anyone to count on in case of need, trouble?

(Keep in mind replies to earlier query on isolation in living and presence/absence of close ties with a sexual partner)

HEALTH CARE NETWORKS, AVAILABILITY, USE, DISSATISFACTION:
How many different physicians seen over the last 12 months?

How many of these were according to her, helpful and competent?

Other healers seen during the last year (naturopath, unlicensed midwives, herbalists, chiropractors, religious healers, etc.)

Mental health care: psychiatrist or psychologist?   Why?

Last time to a dentist or dental technician?

Health insurance?   Is it adequate?

What, if any, health care needs are so budget bustingly expensive that she has delayed, worried about, or not sought care?

What problems of inconvenience exist with respect to going to a doctor (baby sitters, distance, no auto available, no bus line, conflict with work demands, and opposed employer, personal disability makes travel difficult, too sick to go, husband/partner opposed, etc.)

DISABILITIES, CHRONIC ILLNESS, OTHER LIMITING CONDITIONS:
What impact do these have on her self care, morbidity risk?

What effect on her sexual, work, family life?

How adequately can she cope?

How does she feel about herself?

Do outside supportive or change-assisting resources need to be utilized?

(From the physicians own medical record: visits other than than antenatal care this last year. Estimated sum of all healer visits for bodily complaints, excluding mental health care.)

At home is there a home medical advisor book on hand?

(If not, the professional may wish to recommend one. For example, for the educated woman, the 1984 *Complete Health Care Advisor* (Berman, NY St. Martins Press) and *The New Body Ourselves*, 1984 (NY Simon and Schuster).

PERSONAL HEALTH HABITS AND LIFE STYLES
Cigarettes smoked: How many daily?

Marijuana smoked: How many joints weekly?

Alcohol: How many drinks last week (each drink defined as one shot of hard liquor, one bottle of beer, one glass of wine)?

On the average, over 40 drinks per week?

10-40 drinks per week?

Less than 10 drinks per week?

On the average, drinks only with evening meals and in company of others? Or?

Within the last year experienced in association with drinking: passing out, blackouts (not remembering), accident, violent arguments, arrest, fired from job for drinking, drinking in the morning, not being able to stop when she wanted, going to a clinic AA or hospital because of drinking, being told by others she had an alcohol problem....?

Is husband or partner a problem drinker?

Has she ever been beaten, abused by a drunken partner? Other abuse victimization?

Last time? What were the consequences?

Other drugs used "recreationally" as a habit or compulsively:

cocaine   amphetamines   heroin   "designer drugs"   PCP

If intravenous drug use, explore hazards and treatment resistance.

LSD   others

How often have tranquilizers, sedatives been used this last month to help sleep, reduce tension, improve mood, alter feelings?

Exercise:

Walking   jogging   climbing stairs   swimming   at work

weekly health club work-out   exercise machine   aerobics class

Sum active hours per week?

Or sedentary: (Walking less than half a mile, climbing no more than six flights of stairs daily, with no supplemental exercise)

How many hours sleep on the average night?

If now experiencing sleeplessness, or needing sleep aids, what is disturbing?

DIET AND NUTRITION:
Present weight/height

Overweight (to what degree)

Any binge eating, vomiting (bulemia)?

Pre-anorexic food-avoiding preoccupations (anorexic)?

Crash diets?

On a slimming program? What one?

Underweight (to what degree)

Review menus for recent meals.

Is there evidence for a responsible balance of green and or yellow vegetables, fruits, fibers, vitamins and mineral rich foods, fish or chicken, low fat dairy products, whole grain breads/cereals and other complete carbohydrates?

In view of the woman's weight, circulating lipids, possible "hospital malnutrition" arising from chemotherapy, pregnancy, other malnutrition in association with poverty, common inadequate nutrition among the aged even when not impoverished, common low hemoglobin among women—iron intake is often insufficient—calcium needs when there is osteoporosis risk, concurrent disease status, (diabetes, hypertension, vitamin deficiencies) are there dietary changes that are required? If the woman appears to need general information on nutrition and is literate, one may wish to give her a copy—a supply of which should be on hand—of Dietary Guidelines for Americans (USDA - DHHS, 1985). A copy capable of being photocopied can be obtained from the USDA Office of Government and Public Affairs, Washington DC 20250.
Is she now adequately making:

An effort to control sugar intake   How?

An effort to control salt intake   How?

An effort to assure fiber intake   How?

An effort to control fat intake   How?

Any minerals regularly? (special attention to calcium intake levels preferably above ADR)

Any vitamins regularly? (special inquiry as to A beta carotine, and C as per American Cancer Society recommendations) Aware of hypervitaminosis risks?

Habits for cooked food storage for bacterial control: how long typically are cooked foods left unrefrigerated?

When there is ground water contamination from high tech or chemical industries affecting city or private water supply are bottled waters used?

TRAVEL PRECAUTIONS AND INNOCULATION STATUS:
For those planning travel to Asia, Africa, Mexico, what precautions are understood as necessary with regard to drinking water, ice in drinks, brushing teeth, eating salads or uncooked vegetables, water contact in schistosomiasis regions.

What innoculations are planned?   Anti-malaria medication?

Present innoculation status: tetanus   typhoids   polio
rubella   influenza

DENTAL:
How often are teeth brushed? flossed?

How often is denticator or equivalent gum conditioner used?

SEX AND FERTILITY:
Contraceptives: if fertile and control desired, what is used?

Any problems in use? How often forgotten?

Sexual preference: hetero   bisexual   lesbian

Felt sexual satisfaction/dysfunction: pain orgasmic?

What sexual sources of worry, or distress, depression?

How many different partners this last year?

If several partners, awareness of the range of "available" STDs?

How well are partners known?   Is her husband or partner promiscuous?

If she is sexually active, and/or if her partners are, does she require that condoms be used?

For the women at STD risk, when was the last check for chlamydia?   Herpes?

Any unncessary anxieties about rash, AIDS, non-bacterial discharge?

If very active, are partners found in bars and/or does conduct expose her to risk of rape, or other harm?

If young, does she hitchhike, walk or bicycle alone at night, pick up hitchhikers?

SPORTS RISK:
If a skiier, does she exercise to become fit before skiing?

Take a day or two for high altitude adjustment?

Swim in chlorinated water with cystitis recurrence, increased URI or conjunctivitis experienced?

Sunbathe with resulting strong cancer risk if white?

Jog with experienced orthopedic problems; back, knees, feet?
Aware of jogging risks?

If dangerous sports (parachuting, horse jumping/hunting, polo, mountain climbing, hang gliding, racing) are risks denied (counter phobia) or understood and accepted as worth it?

REPRODUCTIVE SYSTEM: SELF-CARE

How often does she do breast self-examinations?

Is her BSE procedure competent? (demonstrate)

Pap smears how often?

Has she ever failed to respond to a recall for further examination/testing for any lab result?

What vaginal sprays, douches, employed?

If she plans to become pregnant again, are there any apparent psychosocial-behavioral risk factors of which she and her birth attendants should be aware (review Table III, for example, age, parity, prior abortion history, hypertension, STD, cigarettes, single status, own ambivalence, opposed husband, adverse event stress vulnerability, work place exertion, teratogens (Review Table III)).

SELF-CARE FOR CURRENT MEDICAL PROBLEMS:

As examples: adherence to hypertension medication, diabetes diet and medication, cystitis hygiene, caffeine control for fibrocystic disease of the breast. Review all illnesses for which control is sought, and review what she is doing. Any psychosomatic? What implications?

Does she believe the physician is in charge of her health and will do all that needs doing (i.e., passivity with risk of reduced self-care, poor outcomes, disappointment)?

Does she confidently request, or aggressively demand—if that is what it takes—information about her illness, her medication, ways of making her care more satisfactory to her?

STRESS EXPOSURE AND RESPONSE:

Does she feel she is under a lot of stress? If yes, what?

If Type A with often angry, hostile, enraged feelings, has she considered either stress management or psychotherapy attendance?

Evaluating and Targeting for Change 291

How many change events in the last two years does she consider to have been difficult to adjust to or cope with?

Does she feel there are many daily hassles?

Does she feel she is "in charge", "managing well", and that most things go the way she wants them to?

When things do go wrong, does she feel she knows what to do, has resources she can use, and has been through troubles before so she knows she can manage?

Is life unpredictable and out of control?

Low energy, fatigue, exhaustion, worn out?

EMERGENCIES:
At home are telephone numbers visible and immediately at hand by the phone for medical care, police, fire?

If there are family members with illness problems or risks portending emergency, are family members prepared to act and not delay (e.g., CHD, in pregnancy for eclampsia or ectopic hemorraging, etc.) Does she know who in the neighborhood is competent in cardiopulmonary resuscitation?

Do her children know where to go for first aid?

CURRENT WARNING SIGNS ABOUT PSYCHOLOGICAL CONDITIONS THAT DETRACT FROM WELLNESS, MAY SIGNAL DISEASE RISK, AND CAN BENEFIT FROM TIMELY INTERVENTION:
High levels of diffuse or changing complaints not substantiated by physical findings

Chronic anxiety:[2] (tense, worried, trembling, fearful, sense of impending doom, palpitations, nightmares, palms sweating, phobias, sleeplessness, things out of control).

Depression:[3] (moody, blue, down in the dumps, nothing to look forward to, nothing to live for, miserable feeling, appetite loss, sleepless, not wanting to get up in the morning, no energy, prefer to be dead, hating oneself, guilt ridden, crying jags, nothing goes right, so many things wrong that are all her fault, thinks of suicide or wants to die).

Hostility:[4] is she chronically angry, acid tongued, demeaning and disparaging of others, finding fault, intolerant, unforgiving, cruel, vengeful, bitter, grim, punitive, neither gentle, nurturant or loving? (Does she make you feel ill at ease and afraid? One's own intuitive reactions, if one is oneself both emotionally balanced and sensitive, are wisely attended to).

Dominance and confidence:[5] is she "in charge" of herself and her life, confortably in command, dominant when necessary, resourceful and sure of herself, optimistic? Or is she on the deficit and disadvantaged side with respect to these important personal traits?

What is her overall health rating: does she rate her overall health as poor?

Does she suffer from chronic fatigue? Low energy levels?

Hopelessness/helplessness (likely overlaps depression and fatigue and stress vulnerability) includes response to situational and life circumstances where one has or feels no resources at hand to lean on, no options or choices, nothing one can do, nothing seems to work, no self-confidence, inability to cope, overwhelmed, being weak in a hostile world.

Accident prone: refer to history of recent accidents or near misses probe for preoccupations, acute anxiety, depression, use of alcohol or other drugs, medication CNS or cardiovascular side effects, anger, self-destructiveness, diminished sensory-motor capabilities possibly associated with disease onset.

Other risk factors from Tables III, IV, V depending on present status (pregnancy, familial history-genetic liability, medical history and current status or exposure.) Review as appropriate.

PRIOR EFFORTS AT SELF-CHANGE OR IMPROVED SELF-CARE:
Has she ever sought to gain better control of her life, habits, unhappy feelings, fitness (e.g., programs for weight control, smoking, drinking, exercise, stress

management, self-realization, counseling, inquiries about marital, illness or surgery support, infertility support, help for battered woman or rape)?

What is the "track record" for change as desired, partial change, relapse, felt failure?

What settings, programs, and change areas work best for her?

What are the worst obstacles, barriers?

THE PRESENT:
Is there anything she would like to change about herself[6] and her life?

Where do we go together from here; making the plan for health promotion?

Is any problem/goal so difficult, severe, time consuming that referral to a health behavior specialist, support group, residential care "time out", counselor or psychotherapist, behavior control program, seems in order?

The Professional Themselves

Here is a different set of risk factors, ones not to be reviewed with the woman (except perhaps to ask her what she would like to see changed in the care her physician, nurse, other care-giver antenatal program or hospital provide). These items are matters of reflection for the health professional himself or herself.

The physician, nurse, or midwife enjoying too much responsibility: accepting patient passivity, and self-care disinterest, enjoying a self-image as a very powerful, very important person. Doing too much, seeing too many patients, playing God.

An insufficient professional network not encouraging patient use of consultation, not asking one's colleague about difficult or unclear diagnostic/treatment problems, not continuing with serious professional education. This shown by not reading the journals and not going to meetings, reading Medical Economics instead of the serious journals, relying on the detail man for knowledge of pharmacotherapeutics, not referring the patient one cannot handle to another professional, not referring the psychologically disturbed patient for counseling/psychotherapy or psychiatric evaluation.

Not doing all one can to engage in office-based health promotion: there is no fault in not having done that before, for the field is new and neither medical school, residency, nor nurse training has paid attention to the matter of risks "out there" and the woman's role in taking charge of her health. It is the case that broader efforts at health education have, until recently, produced empirical evidence that was discouraging. But one knows now that behavioral intervention can work. Hemminki and Starfield (1978), working in perinatal mortality, attribute lack of health promotion in the office to the physician's until-now exclusion of these nonconventional areas from the definition of medical responsibility.

The Hospital Where One Practices

The annual findings from the Joint Commission on the Accreditation of Hospitals on one's own institution will often contain reminders about the things that people do, and are not doing, as organizational members, that adversely affect the health of women and their babies in the hospital. While the thrust of this monograph attends to what can be done in the office, or away from it by way of affecting the woman as she lives, we do not wish to ignore the likelihood that most institutions can be improved with respect to the quality of care rendered. These too are "people factors."

Our own earlier work (Blum, 1958) on hospital features associated with malpractice risk, and quality of care, showed remarkable variability among institutions. Credentialing work supervision and work quality review, how staff got along with one another, staff equipment adequacy, how competently and sensitively the institution is managed, and standards of both practice and human decency all make for differences in malpractice suits, rates, quality of care, and patient satisfaction.

In Obstetrics Particularly

Given the "obstetrical battleground" over the new technology and the woman and her family's voice in delivery where satisfaction is an outcome criterion (see Table III) along with morbidity/mortality, standards for practice as a concensus, and means of tissue and medical audit and department supervision, are essential matters. These interact with patient decision factors as well, as for example in anesthetics administered perinatally, for caesarean, in the presence of husband and family or other support figures in labor.

In the Hospital or Medical School

Recall a John Hopkins study (Chapter 9) showing that training the physician for cooperation makes an immediate, subsequent difference in the patient's level of cooperation in care. We have seen that education to date has been, for obstetrical-gynecological specialists, sadly lacking. Professionals' attitudes as well as skills are shaped by the educational content and millieu. The school or hospital teaching thrusts do affect the risk of illness and felt "wellness" of the woman. What is the atmosphere in your institution?

As with health behavior and psychosocial change for the woman patient, so with the institutions of medicine and its practitioners. A new goal has been enunciated, techniques for its achievement suggested, and criteria for evaluation of the process and its effects exist. But change is difficult for all humans when it comes to habits and life settings. Medical and allied professionals must also learn new attitudes, a new reponsibility, new confidence, new ways of doing things, and must make repeated self-assessments. That occurs slowly and is best done with social support. The course for health promotion in medicine will be similar to other "lifestyle" changes.

Summary

Given the number of psychosocial and behavioral risk factors identified as consequential predictors, and components of the complaints and illnesses of women, it is important for the women's health professional to be attentive to the social situation, lifestyles, habits, and relevant feelings, traits, and attitudes of his or her patients. History taking and the subsequent domain of professional concern must be expanded to include risk factor assessment. It is an allowable inference from the epidemiological data that history taking, and attention to preventive needs, has often been inadequate for women's health care.

One wants to know the range and history of risks: onset, intensity, how expressed, and in what life context. Given risk factors present in a patient, one is also attuned diagnostically to the greater probability of the presence or emergence of those pathologocial conditions with which they have been found associated.

A sample inquiry list is presented. It is a guide only.

The physician will be alert to the possible presence of one or more of the possible pathological outcomes for which current conditions are a risk. If no such pathology is yet present the physician will be reminded that these illnesses are now more likely for his/her patient, even if still unlikely as outcomes when true population prevalence for a woman of that age, parity, etc., is low. As she ages, the pathological outcome for the major "killer" diseases becomes more likely. With or without change in her behavior, or other risk conditions, should new symptoms be presented which present a differential diagnostic challenge, the risks history could be helpful in arriving at a diagnosis.

One may also find that the woman's awareness of her self-help need may be greater than the professional's; she may report a history of self-change effort failures or relapses, the circumstances of which are of utmost consequence to the professional participant, or the agent referred to the lifestyle change endeavor. Such knowledge coupled with recognition that health education per se has been generally unsuccessful, and that intensive, active, complex health promotion— including behavioral medicine and health psychological interventions— are not assured successes, will assist both the professional and his/her patient to be realistic as well as enterprising.

It is very likely that those women with the most enduring, severe, and multiple risks are probably least likely to be responsive either to sophisticated efforts on the health provider's part to secure adherence to safer living or to attending support groups or other treatment efforts. She may very well have already given up on self-help and be discouraged. Even when she cannot change readily, the professional continues to offer encouragement and reward for any signs of progress. And one does not further hazard an already possibly present sense of despair or low self-esteem by now futile warning or criticism, or that insult which is too readily conveyed by the wise and wealthy to the poor and perplexed. People live their lives as best they can. Once the patient, the support group, specialists, and community agencies have done all there is to do, there is a time for patience, acceptance, hope for spontaneous change. Health promotion is not a religion of exhortation or condemnation. Its aim is to help.

Most of those now practicing medicine will not have been trained for helping women to keep themselves well. Innovation in practice is required. As with all of us seeking self-change, assuming further responsibility and adding new dimensions of skill are difficult challenges. One is glad for the effort and for small steps forward. It is the same with the major organizations which are centers for care. Hospitals and medical schools come slowly to change, especially when the arenas of health promotion, preventive medicine, and public health, as capable of being practiced from the office, are not ordinarily viewed as "the cutting edge" of science. These efforts do not enjoy those substantial gratifications from technology, prestige, and income which accompany the "high tech," readily incorporated advances. Nevertheless, since the medical and allied professions can contribute greatly to disease reduction and enhanced felt well-being of women by initiating changes in institutional training, expected standards of care, and the allocation of time and facilities, health promotion is the business of medical and allied institutions. Here too, even slow change is welcome.

Footnotes

1. Sociologists traditionally (after Hollingshead) distinguish five classes, from greatly disadvantaged to very well off. Household income (or personal income for those living alone) is a significant component, as are level of education, prestige and responsibility of occupation, comfort and size of housing and class of neighborhood, class level of social acquaintances. Income is the biggest item, but some low income persons can be in higher classes, e.g., students at college, military personnel enjoying perks of housing, clothing, food; elderly living with well off children. Rough estimates suffice here to establish risk levels associated with extreme poverty/disadvantage or being below average in household income with lower level employment, etc. For health risk purposes, one is here dealing with resources (personal and external), adverse event exposure and events, environmental control capabilities and life choice options, probable genetic components (physique, stature, maternal obstetrical history, intelligence), childhood nutrition, and disease history. For income-based categorization, note that in 1984, about 14% (Bureau of Census, 1985) of the U.S. population had a household income for a family of four below $10,609 (the poverty line). About half of U.S. households have incomes between $10,000 and $35,000. Note too that when a woman is the single head of a household in which there are children, the average income is less than half,

$11,000. The average is $23,000 for married couples with children. The single woman with children will be seen to be bearing the burdens of poverty, work, and childcare (Statistical Abstracts of the U.S., 1985). Her further obstetrical risk is obvious.

2. Research indicates a number of psychological tests which can be reliably used for assessing a wide variety of traits, behaviors, and attitudes. If there is anything about the patient which suggests the need for a more formal psychological appraisal, the health behavior specialist suggested as being part of your practice setting/network and "alter ego" should be able to conduct, or arrange for, such testing and interpretive work up. If the patient appears psychiatrically ill, as for example with disorders of affect or thinking, direct referral to a mental health specialist is in order.

3. Ibid.

4. Ibid.

5. Ibid.

6. Currie and Beasley (1982) offer a health goal checklist which includes "feeling good about myself," relaxing, getting closer to the family, being less tired, hobby, a better sex life, better time management, stopping smoking, more work satisfaction, avoiding heart attack, losing weight, lowering blood pressure, handling stress, sleeping soundly, avoiding alcohol problems, avoiding cancer, getting rid of pain, more exercise, a more healthful diet, dealing better with illness of self or family, a better spiritual life, injury risk reduction.

12

Negotiating Diagnoses Through Referral: A Simple Health Behavior

This chapter addresses the happy probability that large numbers of women can be helped to feel better through relatively short, simple counseling interventions. The groups to be assisted are those with and without organic disease, whose worries about illness put an additional burden of anxiety upon them, or whose high levels of organically unsubstantiated complaints reflect other concerns that they can talk about but have not. In this group will be those who have, over a long period of time, been presenting complaints to the physician—often "making the rounds" of healers when not in a prepaid HMO. Most of these women are recognized as somatizers but some bear more profound diagnoses such as (undocumented) angina. Many are on irrelevant medication regimes, and their diagnosis has been a matter of somewhat awkward negotiation. It is awkward because neither the diagnosis nor the treatment addresses the woman's sensitivity to her life circumstances as etiological, and awkward because the physician, while accepting the diagnosis, is by no means smiling over a differential diagnostic tour de force.

The treatment which is likely to be effective is brief psychotherapy offered, perhaps over a few months by a competent health oriented professional. Remember the prevalence and complaint risk data of Chapters 3 and 4? There it was shown that symptoms in everyday life are the rule, that the concerns of the woman when she comes to the physician are not judged to be "real," organic illnesses—although medications are readily prescribed—that many "real" syndromes such as PMS or menopausal distress carry strong affective tension and personal stress, and that symptom levels do vary predictably.

The first point to be made is one that most women's health care providers would agree upon. Nevertheless, for physicians who may be technically oriented, pushed for time, and uncertain what to do about the great mass of somatizing complaints neither explicable nor treatable, it is a "fact" disregarded as annoying. The "fact" accepted is that all complaints are "legitimate" in the sense that they represent how the woman best characterizes her situation, feelings, self, body, or needs at the moment. Her provisional definition of what is wrong is referred to or being expressed by bodily symptoms: headache, abdominal pain, pruritis, dysparenuia, and fatigue (See Table V). Psychosomaticists, or workers interested in psychophysiology such as Barskey (1979), reviewing how symptoms are "amplified" as a function of other features in living, or personal psychodynamic history; or workers in social medicine such as Eisenberg (1984) have all driven the point home to the women's health professional. All complaints are "real," representing something felt and said in body language.

Eisenberg (1984) has remarked, "the experience of illness always results from interactions between soma and psyche" and further, "... behavior is the final common pathway in many chains of disease causation"; after all, schistosomiasis depends upon "how humans dispose of waste and use water." With our caveat that behavior must be included in Eisenberg's psychosomatic formulations, Eisenberg states, "all disease is psychosomatic in the sense that both psychosocial and somatic forces enter into the genesis of the clinical conditions from which patients seek relief." Whether or not that disease is "real" is, Eisenberg contends, subject only to current organic diagnostic standards. He discusses placebo effects shown to alter white blood count, peptic ulcer, pupil diameter, circulating lipoproteins, and steroids, and cites Wolf's study showing that patient expectations could reverse the ordinary drug effects of ipicac, or lead to atropine mimicking prostigmine.

Eisenberg goes on to cite work by Gath et al. (1982) showing that hysterectomy benefitted women with organic or psychiatric menorrhagia, these diagnoses were inferred from bleeding rated as organic or dysfunctional on the basis of pathologist's examination of the uterine specimen. The work of Martin et al. (1980) is cited showing that for hysterical patients (Briquet's syndrome, somatoform disorder) with multiple gynecological complaints, hysterectomy is to no avail. Eisenberg offers Gath et al.'s interpretation that psychiatric disorder is more likely in women made vulnerable by the discomforts of dysfunctional menorrhagia. The data we have reviewed would suggest much more—that emotional disorder may be any of the following: primary, etiological, precipitating, concomitant, responsive or, for we must always be sensitive to methodological error, misdiagnosed.

Some complaints of illness burden seen by the physician express diffuse maladaption or distress, those "general symtoms" of the NCHS reports (in Table II) of GP diagnosis. For some patients, this will be a prodromal stage before vulnerability to continued distress and organ system perturbation, and dysregulation. This is finally expressed in organic form such that traditional medical diagnosis becomes appropriate, as for example Appel's (1983) "emotional drain" and neuroticism diagnosed the year prior to myocardial infarction, or Craig and Brown (1984) describing the temporal sequence of stress-depression-physical pathology. The physician's search for a diagnosable disorder, "a disease doctors know," began with the initial frank confession qua reassurance to the effect that "there's nothing I can find wrong." This can be unresponsive to how the woman "really" feels.

As Balint (1957) observed, this mutually unsatisfactory conflict between the woman's feeling and the medical diagnostic systems may generate a process of (mutually unrecognized) negotiation where the patient presents a variety of complaints over time, "proposing" these, until the doctor and patient agree on a respectable, justifying diagnosis. In a parallel way, the repeat prescription was found by Balint and his colleagues to represent an agreement to not closely examine what is wrong in the patient's life, but instead to substitute the prescription for "something the patient needs from his environment," or in her life. The repeat prescription in the absence of demonstrable efficacy serves then to maintain a distant, cordial but fragile doctor-patient relationship where treatment does not attend to those personal and environmental factors which have produced the state of need partially satisfied by medication. In essence the patient is allowed to say, "my symptoms are real, the doctor says so, what is wrong with me is not in my life but outside me, a disease." For a review of the phenomenon of patient preference for attribution of cause to something "not me," see Janis and Rodin (1982), and Haan (1982), citing Herzlich (1975). The latter cite, for example, is a study by Storms and Nisbet where insomniacs were given placebos described to them as being capable of producing the symptoms of arousal typical of insomnia—rapid pulse, etc. The investigators' expectation was that those patients able to blame their excited condition on the pill and not their own emotions, would be relieved and would go to sleep faster than controls receiving a placebo not characterized as arousing. So it was. We believe that the "it's a disease, not me," displacement of distress is a serious barrier to that assumption of responsibility for oneself, including insight into sources of distress, which successful health promotion requires.

Insofar as the woman responding to problems with diffuse distress expressed as somatic complaints and emotionality is given, in traditional office visit fashion, "reassurance" that her symptoms are "not serious", she will continue to search for a diagnosis, a new physician, or another healer who will confirm her inner reality, i.e., that she is and "has a right" to be "feeling bad."

That there is a tendency for physician and patient eventually to arrive at a negotiated, justifying diagnosis may be inferred from the work of Costa, Fleg, McCrae, and Lakatta, cited by Costa and McCrae (1985). Using archival data, four groups of men were categorized: one developing anginal complaints and ECG signs of coronary artery disease (CAD), another with angina complaints but no ECG signs of ischemia over a period of 5 to 11 years, a group with ECG ischemic signs but no reported chest pain over 5-15 years, and a fourth group age matched, with neither anginal complaints nor CAD over 10 to 20 years. Those who were diagnosed as having angina pectoris but had no ECG signs were higher in neuroticism than those with no pain but ECG ischemic signs. We infer that their formal diagnosis was the response of the physician to the continued patient "proposal" of an illness. Costa and McCrae also cite work by Ostfeld et al. studying men over a four year period where it was observed that neuroticism predicted that diagnosis of angina pectoris which was without objective signs of myocardial infarction. Since neuroticism, symptoms reporting, and medical visits are correlated, one would expect the diagnosis to be a "negotiated" one. Costa and McCrae argue that it is because the cardiovascular system is expressive of emotion (and immediately responsive to stressors) that neuroticism qua higher stress as emotionality involves patient awareness of and worry focused on the patient's own cardiovascular responsivity. This association of stress responsibility, anxiety, and felt vulnerability "clouds the diagnosis of cardiovascular disease."

At the very least, such findings suggest the utility of that recommended evaluation (see Chapter 11) which attends to psychological symptoms and to social problems, both as warnings as to predilection to high symptom reporting, and as cues as to where precipitating stressors are to be found. A simple treatment found efficacious is a brief series of 40 or 50 minute "talking" sessions, whether directly psychotherapeutic (talking about feelings and their origins), or problem-oriented counseling focusing on resources and coping. Typically any brief counseling series brings considerable relief from anxiety or reactive depression (Rosenthal and Frank, 1956; Frank, 1973). A counseling series can promote real life coping solutions that can relieve worry or despair accompanying organic disease. Both strategies are responses to that "call for help" which symptoms so often represent, and for which sympathetic, sensible counseling or supportive referral is a good response (Hall, 1983).

Whatever the components in the ameliorative process, one finds that it is an effective means for reducing the use of medical services: the "medical cost offset" phenomenon. Mumford et al. (1984) review that literature using meta analysis to combine results from 58 studies. In modest interventions where patients receive information relevant to their condition and care, and emotional support, there is reduction in both inpatient hospital days and outpatient service use. Post heart attack patients who were given such simple treatments experienced an average two days less hospitalization. For chronically ill patients, six psychotherapy visits yield a cost offset—what Mumford terms a dose response relationship for psychotherapy. Relying on five experimental studies, the average reduction in outpatient service utilization was about 23%, and 73% for inpatient services. Reductions are greater for persons over the age of 55.

Mumford points out that the elderly (using age 65 as a cut off) constitute 11% of the population but account for 29% of all health expenditures. On the other hand, they receive only 2-4% of outpatient mental health services. This implies significant underservice. A national survey found 8% of those over 65 with "no one to talk to," vs. 5% for those under 65. Recall that SEC status is likely to fall with age, that risk of loss through bereavement and subsequent reduced social supports is high, that life change (moving, income loss, disability) is common, and that symptom reporting as well as diagnosable illnesses are greater for the elderly. Regrettably, physicians spend less time with their elderly patients than others (Mumford, citing Keeler). Mumford also observes that those few elders who are treated psychiatrically have greater chronic organic disease than the untreated, so that the observed reduction in service utilization suggests a genuinely powerful impact on a high risk group. It is possible that elders without family to care for them, perhaps understandably frightened by their isolation, may be more often admitted, or kept longer in the hospital. Because psychotherapy/counseling provides a buffer against exacerbation of disorders (some latent or present), admissions would also be reduced. Patients may present their symptoms as being less acute or disabling in order to decrease their sense of distress and produce more sense of control and self-confidence. This may also relieve neuroticism and situational distress response. It also shapes a medical judgment from the physician that few or no hospital days are necessary. If a correlate of psychotherapy is more self-help behavior (some via therapist direct guidance), then acute illness exacerbating features could also be moderated, i.e., improved regimen adherence.

The work of Budmen et al. (1984), whose patients were self-referred for emotional distress but not functional somatic complaint, indicates that duration of counseling past six visits does not predict greater change in use of medical services. Also, "insight" (understanding some of the repressed origin of or reasons for somatic feeling) was not a therapeutic result related to change in utilization levels. Nor is it always the case that counseling yields lower medical service utilization. Budman reviews a study, citing McHugh et al., of underserved Mexican Americans who began to use medical services more often, and by implication more appropriately, for their health needs after mental health counseling.

France and Robson (1984) worked in the UK with patients presenting personal problems or coping with organic diseases such as multiple sclerosis or cancer. These sessions were spread out over several weeks, and the treatment goal was to enhance feelings of well-being and self-reliance. The focus was on real life problems, how to cope with them, and how to find practical solutions. Counseled patients, in contrast with controls treated only medically, showed more rapid improvement, medicine costs cut in half, and a 50% reduction in care utilization.

More didactic approaches seem not to help. Clymer et al. (1984) review work (they cite Moore, LoGerfo, and Inui) on the evaluation of a self-care program using the book, *TAKE CARE OF YOURSELF* by Vickery and Fries (Addison-Wesley, 1976). The book, suggesting when to visit a physician and when to do home care, was provided along with instructions (to HMO members) to keep a symptom diary. There were three groups: a no book control, a book plus simultaneous seminar option group, and one that promised a $50 bonus if by year's end, using the book, they reduced physician visits by 3% from the prior year. All three groups reduced their utilization rates, but no one group significantly more than another. Neither self-care, book, nor money incentive are as effective as intensive "human touch" counseling sensitive to the symptomatic woman.

The most dramatic example of such effects is reported by Cummings (1985) with HMO patients where, from among 100,000 HMO patients, those somatacizing (somatizing) were identified: the heavy users of services without substantiated chronic illnesses. Although a computer was used for selections, Cumming notes that a perfectly good screening device would be a chart weight coupled with a range of diffuse diagnoses on the notes inside. Somatizers were assigned to brief psychotherapy or control over five years. Initial findings indicate that unecessary service utilization dropped by almost half, and that costs to the HMO would be cut by $16 million.

The positive effects on medical care utilization rates produced by psychotherapeutic interventions (note that in some studies cited, interventions had not intended to have that effect) generate the speculation that utilization in patients with serious illness may affect some of the same mechanisms which are identified etiologically in women's specific morbidity risk, and are shown to be related to symptom reporting levels. These mechanisms include social support, coping strategies and implied sense of self-confidence, control, predictability, reduced helplessness/hopelessness, anxiety, and depression as stress-of-disease reactions. There is no evidence that we have found which suggests reduced "real" mordibity risk following such interventions, but that is a measure easily confounded by the differential availability of patients for diagnostic recording.

Cohen and Lazarus (1982) in their specific discussion of coping with illness report that the literature is inconsistent with respect to psychotherapeutic effects. Postsurgical recovery does not seem much affected (although some studies show it is predicted by presurgical anxiety levels), whereas for myocardial infarction patients there is speedier recovery and fewer cardiac incidents in hospital. Nevertheless, improved coping does affect confidence and social functions, i.e., some kinds of "wellness." Cohen and Lazarus refer to the work of Engel and of Adolph Meyer, a founder of American psychiatry, as consonant with this self-help goal. For those preoccupied, sensitive, neurotic, stressed, or desperate women whose symptom reporting and medical care use is lessened by brief psychotherapy, one assumes that what has happened is amelioration of their felt distress, reduction in its somatic displacement, the redefinition of terms away from inappropriate body language. These are all a part of the routine counseling work of focusing on feelings and what life is really like in the world of the high symptom level woman.

A New, Simple, Health Behavior for Somatizers

This work suggests that those with high levels of symptoms, or with illness coping struggles, can engage in important health behavior with direct effects on wellness. Consider that the Mumford data indicate that those most affected by health counseling or psychotherapy are older and at high risk of experiences shown to be psychosocial risk factors, and concurrent or co-morbid high serious, multiple, chronic, and life endangering disease. A change in one health behavior such as seeing a mental health professional (e.g., a specialist in health psychology, psychotherapy, behavioral medicine) can work to improve felt well-being and self-perceived health as measured by care utilization levels. The woman's health professional continues to monitor her state of wellness in cooperation with her counselor.

Summary Comment

An important concern of the woman's health professional is helping her maintain wellness, and preventing or responding to those conditions which diminish that. Much of the diminished wellness of women is never brought to the attention of the physician or other health professional, but is suffered and self-treated at home. When a medical visit does occur, many of the complaints will not be capable of characterization as physical disease or obvious biochemical perturbation. Much that diminishes the woman's wellness will consist of high diffuse or changing symptoms, pains, fatigue, complaints or syndromes with mood, and emotional or "I can't cope" components. The epidemiological and etiological research demonstrates that rates of reporting for the relatively non-specific expressions of distress vary remarkably in association with social, life event, and psychological conduct features, including a woman's skills in coping with life and health problems.

In many cases, physiological, family, and interpersonal events operate over time to lead to more specific "medicalized" diagnoses. These may be negotiated agreements between doctor and patient giving an acceptable name to psychobiological distress, and sometimes resulting in repeat prescriptions. A chain of events may also occur where psychosocial-behavioral features affect bodily regulatory systems so that over time, tissue pathology, or discrete patterns of physiosocial dysfunction become observable.

Short term counseling interventions show a high rate of success in reducing complaint levels as measured by utilization of medical facilities. Such interventions also work to reduce utilization where there is a major disorder and recovery— apparently in cases where insufficient personal resources (including coping skills) or perhaps anxieties, initially limit the patient's ability or confidence to be as responsibly self-directing as the physical conditions would in fact permit. It is recommended that such patients be referred for short term counseling. Good outcome means reduced cost, feeling better, clearer patient self-descriptions as to what is wrong and "where it hurts," as well as good practice in the woman taking charge of her own life as much as possible.

13

Referral for Serious Biopsychological Concomitants of Reproductive System Conditions

In this chapter we advocate referral for specialized treatment of women suffering conditions commonly associated with serious reproductive system disorder or disease. The conditions include severe anxiety, chronic depression, chronic (unaccountable) pelvic pain, chronic sexual dysfunction and physical syndromes with etiology and expression where emotional features are consequential, as for example PMS and other menstrual disorders. Some patients facing surgery will also require special psychological preparation. Some treatments are so profound in their effects as to warrant special post operative intervention. For the most part the foregoing special conditions are distressing and disabling, hazard medical management, and predispose the patient to further disorder.

The suggestion to refer presumes that these conditions are not optimally treated through the brief office based methods ordinarily available to the women's health professional, for example the dialogue recommended in Chapter 9 and 10 as basic to cooperation in regimen adherence. Very disruptive conditions are not likely to benefit initially by routine self-help life management programs. To the contrary, these serious emotional and psychophysiologically reactive disorders (as in sexual dysfunction) are likely so profound as to prevent more education assisted self-help programs. In this sense, health psychotherapeutic interventions in this gynecological-obstetrical ill population are necessary pre-treatments before the woman is able to fully participate in and benefit from life style or habit changes which are more rational in their emphasis. For a discussion of the range of illness patients possibly benefitting from referrals to improve their and their families' ability to cope with the illness, see Roback (1984).

It is the case that formal treatment methods, employed upon referral, employ some of the same "generic" assets that are represented in working toward cooperation for adherence. These could include treatment occurring within a group which is supportive, aiming toward a feeling of confidence on the part of the woman to not feel alone in her distress, clarity of definition with respect to pain and what causes it, developing resources and coping methods, moving her toward a greater sense of predictability of life, and of self-control. These are treatment goals, whether the treatment uses the new methods of behavioral medicine, or the modern versions of psychotherapy, sometimes with concomitant pharmacotherapy. The research results, especially "meta-analysis" studies of outcomes which combine findings from many studies, show that interpersonal interventions professionally conducted are likely to be useful. And, when medication for moods or emotion is indicated, outcomes are better (more comprehensive, enduring) when interpersonal treatments are also provided.

Under no circumstances is the obvious presence of serious emotional distress of chronic disability to be taken as an indicator that the woman is "only functional." Recall the much higher "downstream" physical illness risk associated with depression, or hostility, the role of anxiety as a strong obstetrical complication indicator, or the presence of "emotional drain" in the year before myocardial infarction. The psychobiological model, which we find useful, warns against the "either/or" mind body dichotomy. Certainly the thrust of risk studies and those of the disease process, such as stress on neuroendocrinimmunemodulation, stands in evidence. As Mozley (1980) stated in his discussion of infertility, "intrapsychic mechanisms affect all body physiology."

With respect to chronic fatigue and depression, one must keep in mind the contribution to risk prediction made by work on myocardial infarction (MI) suggesting the high prevalence of complaints summarized in the characterization of "emotional drain," or "vital exhaustion and depression" (Appels and Mulder 1984) found just prior to MI. Such summary terms may not be offered by the patient because the language employed to describe feelings or body states is learned in the family as well as through prior experience with physicians. The woman may not say "emotional drain," but when the history and symptoms fit, and the woman has not been recently examined by an internist/cardiologist, an MI risk exists which is possibly undetectable in advance by EKG. The prevalence of fatigue, plus anxiety symptoms referred to cardiovascular function in gynecological populations with a lower true prevalence of MI, means that the efficiency of emotional drain as an indicator is quite poor. For example, alertness to emotional drain as a possible MI risk will mean that those patients examined, or referred for possible cardiovascular disease, will be found illness free. Given MI risk without positive prior signs, the group with latent pathology is also subject to the false negative error. Attention to fatigue/emotional drain, while a necessary caution, may provide a sensitive but by no means specific screening device in populations where cardiovascular disease true prevalence is low.

Cancer: Sexual Dysfunction and Depression

Both Greer and Hesse (1982) and Nadelson (1978) describe the range of gynecological disease conditions which affect female sexuality. Anderson and Hacker (1983) and Anderson and Jochinsen (1985) describe the frequent adverse effects of gynecological cancer on sexuality, including its negative impact on marital adjustment and self esteem. Lieber (cited by Anderson, 1983), in a survey of recently treated surviving patients with cancers of many sites, found that females were most likely to be depressed with a decline of sexual desire— 67% in women as opposed to 27% in men. For patients given radiation therapy, one-half showed sexual dysfunction eight months or more post cancer treatment. Without psychological intervention that dysfunction continued through the follow-up of two years. Nadelson (1978) reported that 75% of women treated by radiation for cervical cancer experience sexual dysfunction.

Hurney and Holland (1985) review sequelae in cancer surgeries resulting in ostomies, including pelvic exenteration. All patients suffer reproductive and vaginal lubricative loss, and most lose sexual drive early and orgasm post operatively. They review Sutherland's early work observing common impairment after colostomy, of social and sexual function with depression, anxiety, and felt isolation as sequelae. Reducing these adverse outcomes was the presence of a supportive family, and the ability of a spouse to cope with the ostomy. Hurney and Holland present a typical course postoperatively: initially physically preoccupied with pain, adjustment, survival, but as physical health and functioning improves, a decline psychologically to low morale and depression. Many women feel they cannot admit to "bad feelings," thinking this might, as stress, precipitate further disease (recall Chapter 2 and victim self-blaming). Anxiety continues to rise postoperatively, probably in association with adjustment problems, sexual dysfunction, and fears of recurrent disease. Studies show that the spouse becomes even more anxious than the patient and both may engage in desperate efforts to gain control over the situation. As for sexuality, here as elsewhere "Patients don't ask and doctors don't tell," so that for those with the physical possibility of full or partial return to orgasmic sex, intimate sexuality of any kind—being touched and held which is so important to those vulnerable and suffering—recovery may unnecessarily fail. The authors cite the conclusion to a U.K. study on ileostomy patients who did ask their physicians about sexual problems. Physician replies were "unhelpful." Sexual dysfunction is another one of those "diseases the doctors don't know."

Hurney and Holland discuss corrective measures, crediting Duke in the U.K. as first, in 1947, to propose counseling—including sexual counseling—by adjusted "expert" recovered patients, matched for age and social class to the new colostomy patient. Self-help groups and one-to-one "veteran" patient visits (pre and post surgery) are successful programs under the auspices of the American Cancer Society. Beyond post operative information, both patient and spouse may also require attention and direct discussion of emotions and sexuality, "immediate referral to . . . experts . . . when emotional or sexual function is impaired . . . but cannot be handled by the family physician" (p. 179). Certainly such emotions can be powerful. The authors describe patients who refuse surgery for life threatening cancer because they fear subsequent sexual incompetence and would prefer not to live without sex. Clearly, the assurance of at least partial recovery and thorough counseling is in order. There is not much information about women with respect to postoperative sexuality and its correlates because, as Hurney and Holland say, "less attention has been paid" to women. This echoes our own criticism that women are underserved by research in the psychosocial behavioral arena with respect to risk studies and for evaluated treatments.

Other work confirms the disruption associated with cancer and its treatments, including the sense of loss and grief, along with anger and denial. Fear of cancer contagion through sexual intercourse can affect both partners (Good and Capone, 1980). Cheek (1976) studied women with cancer of the vulva undergoing pelvic exenteration, and all were severely disturbed in their emotions and social relations. Chapman et al. (1979) show that emotional distress and sexual dysfunction are common following chemotherapy (cases of Hodgkins disease), with disruption in family and friendships. Siebel et al. (1980) report cervical cancer patients undergoing irradiation have marital disruption and reduced orgasmic capacity: a finding taken strongly to indicate the need for counseling. Anderson and Hacker (1983) followed vulvar surgery patients and reported continuing sexual dysfunction as the most common sequela. Krouse and Krouse (1981) compared gynecological oncology surgery patients with mastectomy cases and found more severe depression among the former. Depression is, of course, associated with a variety of dysfunctions: sexual, physiological, and interpersonal.

Counseling treatments have not been extensively evaluated except in sex therapies per se (Kaplan, 1983) but do appear to work for the woman cancer patient. In one of the few studies (other than the major American Cancer Society programs) informally evaluated by Hurney and Holland and Lamong et al. (1978), found that two-thirds did benefit from sexual counseling. Capone (1980) and Krant (1981) affirm the value of psychotherapy. Forester et al. (1985) show that psychotherapy administered during radiotherapy, for disease at any site, led to less severe physical symptoms and emotional distress in treated patients versus controls. The treatments administered were brief, simple, and only once a week. Benefits were attributed to the widespread need of these patients for a professional "to whom they could turn at this difficult time . . . patients felt they were in a fearful situation alone."

Weisman (1984, p. 108) emphasizes a point made by Cullen, Fox, and Isen in 1976 to the effect that "successful cancer treatment (often) has exacted a price that damages a patient's quality of life and therefore undermines the concept of comprehensive cancer care." He cites his and other investigations to the effect that psychological factors not only affect the quality of the terminal period, but also may lengthen life. Again, the intimate relationship and social support variable is operative.

Lazarus (1983) discusses what may be a fundamental problem in the work of health care providers. He refers to the "trivialization of distress." This process emphasizes the stiff upper lip, technological intervention, and excludes the whole person. Lazarus cites the work of Welisch et al. (1983) concerning a large number of cancer patients in the hospital but homebound. While pain was their primary immediate problem, matters of emotion (depression, suicidal tendencies, anxiety, guilt, fears of death and disability) were ranked second. Welisch et al. propose that the medical audit—that peer review for quality of care assessment—include appraisal of the provider's attention to these aspects of illness. Their review of audits showed that there was no attention at all to these facets of diagnosis and treatment in 70%. He argues that it is because of disregard and trivialization of real-life related illness components. In one study, over half of internists' patients were distressed by over work, financial, and/or sexual components of their illness situation, and 10% were considering suicide. These serious problems must be kept in mind as one plans the care of the cancer patient, and indeed any patient seriously or life disruptingly ill.

Avery, in Moos (1984) calls attention to another consequential problem with the health care provider treating the cancer patient. It is "burnout," and Avery argues that not only is it bad for caregivers directly but may also result in a further emotional burden being placed upon the patient. Avoidance and withdrawal from the patient, as well as anger, may be aspects of the emotional state of the caregiver. Moos gives examples of an anger repressing nurse who secretly added weights to a patient's traction, and another who intentionally gave injections in a painful manner.

Good and Capone (1980) consider the cancer diagnosis-treatment-recovery period as one of crisis, where social support and help toward adaptation is as important as any other rehabilitation effort. Specific goals are reduction of psychological distress, restoration of self-image, and maximizing sexual capabilities. To accomplish this, counseling works to mobilize resources, reduce guilt of self-blame for illness (attributed typically to recrudescence in adults of childhood learned prohibitions against masturbation, abortion, promiscuity, adultery, etc.), differentiate whenever possible between probable real dangers and worse fantasized fears of death (worst for patients who have had parents or friends die from similar cancers), and to learn and work through the personal meaning of cancer for the woman. Typically, the spouse is to be involved in the treatment because both parties are suffering.

Drug Regimes

By no means is sexual dysfunction limited to oncological disease. One is aware of the debilitating effects in males of diabetes, of activity reductions associated with cardiovascular disease, arthritis, neuropathy, indeed a range of disabling conditions. This includes those who experience genital organ pain or incompetence, or emotional reactions such as shame, fear, and self-doubt. In the same way, a range of medications may have an effect on sexuality or produce adverse emotional reactions. With others, one may wish upon learning of, say, depression, to check if a medication may be implicated. Watt (1982) for example reviews hypertension medications with potential impact on sexuality (diuretics, propanalol, spironolactone, clonidine, reserpine). Compounds targeted on the CNS, from tranquilizers to barbiturates, lithium carbonate, or self-administered drugs such as alcohol or heroin, may have specific effects. Induced changes may be interpreted in such a way psychologically as to affect function. Antihistamines and anticholinergics may have sexual function impact. Oral contraceptives may produce reactions of reduced sexuality, particularly in association with depression, as reported by Wenderlein (1980). Depression may be also produced by anti-hypertensives, CNS compounds, alcohol, hormones, etc.

There are a number of simple principles associated with pharmacotherapy and self-administered (recreational, addictive, self-medicating) drug use. These are as follows: (a) placebo effects are common, may take many forms, may be guided not only by physician expectations but also by the characteristics of the setting and behavior of others, and by the patient's (or self-administered user's) mood or expectations (see Blum, 1968). All placebo effects are not positive (b) any compound efficacious enough pharmacodynamically to produce a desired effect will have potential for adverse "side effects" (c) since almost any compound is pharmokinetically systemic, some side effects will be experienced as CNS effects on emotions, mentation, motor, or other behavioral capabilities (d) the range of individual sensitivities to drugs is considerable, and is augmented by the individual meanings which may be assigned to awareness of psychological or physiologic change. Thus, active placebo effects are likely to occur for any drug.

With respect to health promoting interventions, the foregoing imply that (e) when the health promotional intervention is aimed at achieving better adherence for medication regimen cooperation, one must assess both the "real" pharmacodynamic effects of medications being rejected and such "meanings" that are part of significant interpersonal activities (f) when the intervention is with patients following medication regimens essential to their health care, it may be difficult to distinguish the pharmacodynamic effects of the medication from those of the disease process. A useful approach in treatment is self-monitoring to distinguish specific from general drug effects, and to explore possible reasons for illness— from loneliness and fear to punishment and guilt. Potentially helpful feelings of control can be introduced by assisting the woman to know more about herself— to learn more about direct versus interpreted medication reactions (g) when the intervention is with women experiencing syndromes where medication may be used, but where its role as an active placebo is of great consequence (typically hormone therapies for reproductive disorders), it is important to structure a variety of influences. These may include setting, other's expectations, teaching a "proper interpretation" of pharmacodynamic effects, and other fitness- enhancing activities, all to enhance such placebo effects as may occur (h) when women are experiencing serious adverse reactions in direct consequence of essential medication regimens, especially when these entail emotional distress (and presuming that full disclosure and discussion to assure informed consent as part of a cooperative treatment decision to accept such suffering has occurred), the physician will wish to consider referral to support groups and/or health behavior specialists. These can provide assistance in coping with pain, nausea, dysfunction, or disability. Generally the "mood overlay" in such treatments is great enough that support groups and/or counseling— using methods noted earlier such as imaging, "positive talk," shared feelings, encouraging knowledge for control, developing alternative skills as coping— will produce a "feeling better" outcome.

Infertility

Mahlstedt (1985) in a sympathetic review calls attention to the widespread depression, as well as other severe distress reflected in marital relationships and self-esteem, which occurs among infertile couples. She discusses the profound sense of loss associated, helplessness, hopelessness, the reduction in sexual spontaneity, the destruction of felt sexual identity and pride, the sense of social isolation, the devastation of the sense of control. As a stress experience Mahlstedt contends infertility is comparable to death or divorce, with medical treatments themselves powerfully stressful. Guilt and anger may also occur, along with a self-consciousness which reflects itself in a reluctance to reveal their distress. And when they do, medical personnel are reported to respond inadequately by virtue of insufficient psychological training, lack of time for discussion, and among an unknown number, devaluations of despair as consequential to the woman and her husband. Such rejections are incompatible with the work of grieving which must be allowed to occur along with the development of new identities not dependent upon fertility. Couples are to learn sympathy, for listening to each other's anguish, to take time for fun with each other, and communicating openly to those who will listen. For this purpose support groups are recommended, particularly since these bypass the problems of the untrained, time pressed or sometimes anti psychological health professional. The national movement Resolve appears to work well to provide a couples-run remedy.

Lalos et al. (1984) also investigates the situation of the infertile couple and, while attributing infertility itself to psychological factors in less than 20% of cases (Mozley, 1980, reduces that to 5%), also describes severe emotional and social effects; grief, guilt, depression, inferiority feelings, disrupted sexuality and marriage, and isolation or distancing from friends and relatives typically unable to be supportive. All couples in their studies have expressed the need for professional support and counseling. For that probably small proportion where psychological features are primary determinants of infertility, as for example where intercourse is rare or ejaculation is not achieved, where there is vaginismus or functional dyspareunia, and where the fertility wish is genuine (beware: Mozley cites Sandler with cases of successful fertility induction leading to suicide when infertility was an unconcious psychodynamic defense against pregnancy and motherhood), counseling is in order. Mann (1956) reported a reduction in the rate of habitual abortion in a program which included counseling, along with medical measures. In communities without Resolve, one seeks to establish it or its equivalent.

Pelvic Pain

Melamed, working on pelvic pain (1983) without substantiated tissue pathology, calls attention to the now thoroughly established relationship with its etiology in psychosocial processes. Recall that Taylor (1949), and Duncan and Taylor (1952) considered such pelvic pain as arising from local vascular congestion as a function of emotional distress. This followed the work of Henker (1979) and many others, of the possible responsiveness of such pain to counseling intervention. (Recall that success is less when there is secondary gain, i.e., when one is receiving disability payments based on the pain complaint.) Duration of pain, number of prior surgical procedures, and level of drug dependency and subjective pain levels are also treatment success predictors. (See Maruta et al., 1979). There are a number of pain, or pain and stress treatment centers, many part of teaching or general hospital programs. One recommends referral of the chronic pain patient there.

Hysterectomy

Roeske (1980) calls attention to the psychological risks of hysterectomy. She reports work to the effect that post hysterectomy women, more than post cholecystectomy ones, require more prescriptions for depression, and receive more psychiatric referrals. When hospitalized post surgically, they stay longer than cholecystectomy comparison groups (although the hysterectomy-psychiatric hospitalization group also have a more frequent family history of psychiatric disorder). Depression prevalence rates vary considerably with the population; in studies she reviews from 7 to 70%, whereas in Youngs and Wise (1980), disturbance ranges by group from 30% to 80%. Norris (1983) confirms depression and, further, sees exaggerated PMS as a postoperative risk. Youngs and Wise (1980) report post surgical comparison studies, again hysterectomy vs. cholecystectomy, finding psychological distress at a rate of three to one.

Risk features (see Table IV) affecting rate variability include high or absent pre operative anxiety, SEC (educated women do better), work status (employed do better), age (older do better), husband's response (men in cultures which value women for fertility are a adverse influence). Women with esteem derived from other than womanhood-fertility sources, and those experiencing post surgical relief from physical distress or cancer dangers do better. Menzer is cited, by Youngs and Wise, with respect to the role of confidence in femininity, prior experience with loss and more coping skills, and enjoying better interpersonal care in hospital. Serious marital problems, absence of tissue pathology (i.e., patients realize the procedure was not necessary), and prior psychiatric difficulties are adverse indicators.

That severe depression may occur is not a surprise, for the loss of an organ central to self-image, reproductive function, and marital relationship (in the fertility oriented class or culture) must indeed be a loss. Thus for those with threatened loss, recovery may depend both upon the ability to mourn loss, reestablish roles and identities, and restructure intimate relationships. To facilitate these, preoperative and postoperative counseling can be of assistance.

Surgical Abortion, Perinatal Loss

Both Adler (1980) and Nadelson (1978) offer reviews and comment with respect to psychosocial abortion recovery. Strong adverse reactions are rare, but are more common among those young— and among adolescents, those youngest who identify with the to-be-destroyed infant rather than mothering role in therapeutic abortion, with those unmarried, Catholic, with prior mental illness, interpersonally immature, with unstable and conflict ridden relations with partner, negative relations with the mother, ambivalence toward the child, and opposing religious and cultural values in self and/or partner. Surgical stress also affects outcome, with least ill effects from dilation and evacuation as opposed to saline and prostaglandin instillation. Counseling outcomes show best effects among those younger where group treatments are in order. As age increases individual counseling appears more in order; for older women, the limited data suggest counseling may be ineffective.

Jorensen et al. (1985) report on the reactions of women aborted surgically because of ultrasound diagnosed (in the second trimester) fetal malfunction. We presume their findings can be generalized to other women undergoing abortion in response to medical advice with respect to fetal malformation. Severe psychological trauma, sometimes long-lasting, was universal in a small Swedish sample. Half were considered so disabled as to be unable to cope and readjust—a reaction comparable to parents experiencing perinatal death. Supportive contacts for both pregancy and perinatal loss are seen as required. In the case of the selective abortion, guilt feelings may be stronger, and anger toward the medical attendants may also be present. While the authors argue for sympathetic, active psychological support forthcoming from the physician, one can anticipate circumstances where the physician, after initial sympathy but otherwise lacking time or inclination, and where grief seems unabating, would refer for counseling.

Lewis (1984) also considers the mourning process after stillbirth or neonatal death. He emphasizes the importance of not allowing the idealization of the dead baby, and of cautioning parents about rushing into another pregnancy before the mourning process is complete.

Any perinatal loss can be expected to be a profound psychological trauma which will, or should, set in motion the grieving process. Grief by itself does not necessarily need professional assistance beyond sympathy and support which any health professional might be expected, professionally and humanly, to render. The situation is complicated by the possiblility that the physician or midwife responsible for pregnancy care/delivery may himself/herself be feeling so upset about the event (be feeling unable to deal with the parents' emotions), that emotional withdrawal, rather than support, is the reaction. Bourne (1968) compared physicians reactions to stillbirths versus live births, concluding that the physician was likely to respond with unconscious alienation, as reflected upon retrospective inquiry by refusals to discuss the case, forgetting details, and being abrupt. Assuming this risk, one estimates the potential disruption or support for the parents if the physician is, in fact, worried about some actual malpractice or, in these litigious days, if the parental grief is transformed into anger, blame adds the threat of lawsuit. Perinatal death then may not be simply a tragic event which one expects the responsible physician or midwife to handle as best he or she can. Required is self-assessment for withdrawal, or felt inadequacy, or malpractice suit related anxieties and angers. When there is a human deficiency in an already inevitably difficult circumstance, referral to some other professional, including pastoral counseling for the religious parent, is indeed in order.

PMS

There is continuing debate about the nature, multiplicity, prevalence, and best treatment for premenstrual syndrome. Norris (1983) contends that 40% of all menstruating women experience some symptoms, and that five to ten percent will suffer severe and properly diagnosable PMS. Others (see Osofsky and Kappel 1985) offer a similar range. Whether or not progesterone therapy is employed—as an active placebo (controlled blend trials indicate it is only that—O'Brien (1985), Osofsky and Kappel (1985))—the existence and popularity of PMS support groups demonstrate the value of women sharing their distress, information about it, and methods for alleviation. Whether or not PMS is complicated or triggered by eating disorders, alcoholism, severe depression, or stress, "whole woman" health enhancing PMS programs appear to do well when multiply targeted, as for example assistance to maintain recommended diets, exercise, smoking and alcohol reduction, and stress management.

The evaluation of PMS treatments is limited by the very diversity of complaints, and the particularly high and variable placebo effects recorded. Youngs and Works-Lind (1985), for example, review studies to the effect that 80% of PMS women may experience placebo benefits. It is sensible to assume that placebo effects may be maximized and best directed where multiple activities and influences arouse positive expectations and felt fitness, and produce sensations capable of being interpreted as "being changed and feeling better." Hormone therapy, as for example progesterone, may best be interpreted as allowing that effect.

When PMS treatments are office based, not part of multiple program clinics, the high incidence of psychopathological etiology among women diagnosed as PMS (see Table V) suggests the value of referral for psychotherpay per se, or for those health behavior treatments by professionals whose methods employ similar techniques. When severe depression is found, whether in the PMS or any other sample, psychiatric referral for probably drug therapy is simultaneous with psychological interventions. Youngs and Works-Lind (1985) discuss the problems of differential diagnoses, PMS as a "pure" syndrome, the general course of a range of treatments, and generally good results obtained including for that subsample referred for psychotherapy.

Other Precipitating States: The Woman's Reproductive System As An Illness Site Particularly Sensitive to Emotion

Any reproductive system condition which has a personal meaning which is deeply threatening to the woman, where disruptive perturbations in physiological function are occurring, where traumatic medical treatments or condition outcomes (e.g., neonatal death) are involved, or where the illness episode or recovery period is hazarded by the need to make major readjustments compels our attention. The readjustment may need to occur (a) in self-image and confidence (following organ loss, mutilation), (b) physical functioning (associated with disabling, organ loss, reduced energy, medication effects), (c) accommodation to pain, or (d) sexual, family, or work adjustments which can be stressful for any woman, however "invulnerable" she might appear. Indeed by no means must all of these elements in the foregoing (a) through (d) "gang of four stressor" be present to produce adverse and continuing negative affect and/or serious disability in the woman. As we have seen in our review of risk factors, reproductive system condition diseases are more likely to occur when there are preexisting vulnerabilities (defined as a stress vulnerable history or as emotional, personal, social disorders and deficits). And when reproduction related diseases/disorders do occur, these seem more likely than many other diseases to be accompanied, in women, by adverse psychological reactions. Thus any disease/disorder affecting the reproductive system may not only partly originate in, but most surely become associated with severe reactions of depression or anxiety. Typically these reactions do not respond to the physician's or nurse's necessarily limited office based brief efforts at amelioration. Again, consultation and referral may be in order.

Well known to women's health professionals, based simply on prevalence, are the post partum conditions of "the blues," post partum depression or psychosis per se. There can be problems of borderline diagnoses here, but the former is quite common, self-limiting, and is not extreme whereas the latter is the more severe, extended but happily, infrequent. Post partum psychoses are anticipated and readily recognized by those doing obstetrical work, and are routinely referred for psychiatric care which, with anti depressive medication and psychotherapy, yield good results. One will also see psychotic states triggered during pregnancy, or by menopause, with a greater risk presumed for those women with prior histories of emotional disorder, including being currently in remission from severe disorders. These major changes in bodily state can readily be seen as triggering events in those whose history demonstrates vulnerability as predisposition.

Misery without Referral

Misery is part of the human condition. It is certainly understandable as reaction to serious illness, role disability, dying, loss, depriving conditions such as infertility, felt "shameful" diseases such as STD, or mutilating states which may be repugnant to self and others such as follow exenteration or radical mastectomy, or ostomy. Even when one is not seriously ill, we have seen from Chapter 4 that the ordinary woman's sensitive condition is one of rather high levels of felt unwellness, including of course distress associated with reproductive life and monthly cycles. Is the health professional to evaluate all despair as now to be "medicalized," requiring either one's own intervention, or if that impossible or failing, consultation or referral?

The question is a fundamental one. Bearing on the reply are the following subsidiary questions: Is the reaction or condition one which thorough evaluation research has shown can be alleviated through intervention at a rate (and with a probability of improved feeling/function/wellness) greater than if there were no intervention? One does not know for any individual case that the best statistical prediction will apply, but one uses that statistical prediction (generally to the effect that treated emotional disorders and behavioral malfunction do improve, and do it more quickly, fully, with rather than without treatment). Secondly, is the time span consequential, i.e., is the period of disability likely to be a long one unless treatment is rendered? Generally there is risk as a function of duration, as people become hopeless, or find manipulative satisfactions as substitutes for full functioning, or as the probability itself for further disorder magnifies. What is "long"? It probably depends on tolerance and cost/benefit estimates. Acute anxiety for a week feels a month's worth, but is hardly worth referring since recovery will occur before or just as the woman is seen. Acute depression extending for two weeks may justify treatment because one cannot know that it is not becoming chronic, or because suicide may be a risk (whenever in doubt ask the woman if she is thinking about it). For the deep depression extending itself the question is, is the depression more severe than the news or condition warrants, or more intense than one normally sees under similar conditions? If these answers are not clear, it is good to refer to a mental health professional for consultation and diagnostic evaluation.

One also asks practical questions as to cost and convenience, for example, is it worth it to the woman to go to a support group or counseling where there is a good probability of feeling better— never a certainty— as against the certain costs of inconvenience, and personal expenditure if her insurance program is inadequate with respect to such reimbursements? Another adverse cost question, this time when there are third party payers, is whether conventional medical care utilization expenses which are a function of depression and future disease risk, or somatizing (somaticizing) should be allowed to continue, be reimbursed, when there is evidence that they can markedly be reduced by short term counseling intervention. Perhaps carriers should demand psychotherapy for somatizers.

The issue of how much psychosocial misery to be suffered for how long, given a reasonable estimate that this woman's misery is (a) treatable, (b) treatment affordable, or sometimes a criterion, (c) is lasting longer than "normal" self-limiting misery for women with similar "objective" reproductive disorders or states, is embedded in expectations. At the personal and related culture group membership level, these are of the same order that affect expressing complaints about pain: "stiff upper lip" as a personal value versus "help whenever possible." The woman who demands or is angry about her present misery can easily persuade the physician, nurse practitioner, or midwife that referral is in order. The woman who suffers silently, deprecates herself as not deserving treatment or insists— a culturally admired response— that one must "grin and bear it" may be seen as not needing or wanting remedy. At this point the same dialogue is required as in discussion of treatment regimens already recommended; one must find out what she really feels and wants at a level of discourse more revealing than that of the conventional, self-minimizing, stoical comment.

The context of aspirations for wellness as part of changing standards as to "quality of life" will also bear on referral decisions. In 1900 high infant mortality rates were accepted as the norm (although the rich and well nourished have always fared well above the norm); today one aims at very low infant mortality as a "right" as well as a standard. With regard to "wellness," with its correlated subjective characterizations of "being happy," "self-realization," "enjoying good health," and "being fulfilled," we currently see the raising of popular aspirations. This is part of the experience of and demand for social and health advances generally. Wellness is certainly an aspect of the health promotion thrust and the women's health movement. Expanding aspirations are reflected in the growth of service industries generally; medical, psychotherapeutic, behavior-change, governmentally in welfare support, but also in hot tubs, convenience foods, the three television household, cosmetics; a thousand ways in which a secular society explores means presumed to make life here-and-now enriched and enjoyable. Obviously many of these are superficial, others are expensive fashion, some are disasters (those that are selfish, impulsive, and impose community burdens, e.g., cocaine, promiscuity associated with AIDS risk, unplanned babies born to those mothers without the maturity or resources to nurture them.

What level of aspiration to set for the treatment of the psychosocial miseries of the woman will depend upon how the woman and her health care professional together define what is possible, practical, and desirable. Keep in mind that that which is desirable may be sought as an experiment in what might be. For women who are suffering, who accept suffering, who expect nothing more, those who "idealize unhappiness," there are good reasons to open the door to health promotional treatments as new experiments in living.

Resistance

Some women will not want to go to support groups, health counseling or that intensive personal care that may be necessary for severe depressions. If the referral is to a psychiatrist, resistance may be immediate and powerful (BMJ editorial, 1978). Some women's specialists, or other physicians and allied practitioners may themselves be reluctant to make such referral, either for fear of "insulting" their patients by the implied illegitimacy of complaints or stigma associated with emotional distress (Do you think I'm crazy?!) out of an inability to feel comfortable handling discussions of the women's being miserable and needing other care, or out of a fear of "losing" their patient to another practitioner.

Depending upon the seriousness of the condition, including the risk it poses for disease management and future risk, the professional will make a decision as to whether to treat the resistance as one of the same order of magnitude as other failures to follow recommended treatments. The same procedures for enhancement apply here as were set forth in Chapter 9: establishing a milieu for dialogue, reaching for sympathetic understanding of the sources for non cooperation, examining these collaboratively and respectfully with the woman, reaching out to her family for assistance in securing cooperation. If, as before discussed, the barrier to change is within the health professional (recall some providers do not want informed, self-reliant patients), that is likely to be immediately perceived by the woman, and if she is herself in doubt, will be put to use by her as a defense against charge. Essentially, "I agree with you, doctor (or nurse, or midwife), I will live with what I have and not try some new treatment method." As with other commitments to health promotion, the health professional must examine his or her own position and determine if that is in the best interests of the woman, and compatible with emerging standards for care in disease prevention, distress amelioration, and enhanced wellness.

Networks Again

We suggested earlier that referral for consultation and/or health behavior treatment is easier if the health behavior professional is part of the immediate practice network of the women's medical health professional. Referral to someone who is part of one's own clinic, hospital, or practice group is not referral "out," not rejection, not acting out the mind/body dichotomy, but referral within the network of colleagues, for specific assistance, for help with problems that are part of the reproductive biological status of being a woman. The reproductive medical specialist maintains responsibility for reproductive system and perhaps primary care, and maintains communication with the professional to whom referral is made so as to be kept informed of needs, progress, and future health care implications.

Thus, we again recommend affiliation of a health promotion or health behavior specialist trained in both risk prevention and emotion-behavior treatments as part of the internal referral system of any modern practice group. How that competent specialist came to be, i.e., whether from psychiatry to gynecology-obstetrics to psychosomatics, or from training in psychology to behavioral medicine or nurse-practitioner counseling to health promotion probably does not matter. Variations in theoretical emphasis in practice do not matter. What does matter is that the specialist for referral is knowledgeable in the fields here reviewed.

When it is not possible for a direct and continuing affiliation of the sort that makes daily or weekly informal consultations easy, the alternative is to be sure that the health professional does have the wider contact network required. A list of available support groups in the community from post mastectomy or ostomy through infertility, PMS, and the battered woman, to classes and programs targeted on behavior specifics: smoking, obesity, alcohol, other drugs, exercise, stress management, and relaxation, diabetes, etc., is essential.

If the community is fortunate, there may also be programs not so specifically targeted which address the whole woman and her range of emotional disturbances, illness managing, behavior changing needs, and self-control enhancing needs. Some of these are "Wellness" programs; others go under titles such as "Taking Charge of Your Life" or "Women's Health Self-Help."

Legitimizing A Holistic Approach

In California where we practice, teach, and do research, "holistic" medicine is a good idea soured by the characteristics of some of those claiming to practice it. There are gurus, self-styled "shamans," "good witches," spiritualists," and quacks of all shapes and persuasions. A glance at a recent popular "holistic health" book shows chapters ranging from extremely sensible to the, in our opinion, utterly pernicious or lunatic. We hope it is not too late to retrieve the term on behalf of sensible folk, whether as "wholistic" or "holistic." One recognizes that today's reasonable work in women's health is that which works within the context of the woman's life, does attend to her experiences and actions, and seeks a psychobiological integration for the understanding of her illness risk and capacity for change. One aims for coordinated treatment of the various concomitants and sensitivities of being a woman at hazard. One builds on her hardiness where it is found. One uses the collaborative model for achieving sensible self-help for disease risk reduction and a sense of well being. One takes the task as a life-long one, for risk and sensitivity are continuous, and disorder recurrently and diversely expresses itself.

It is likely that the typical evaluation of a woman showing herself to be at risk for consequential illness, or trauma, or whose present condition has serious emotion or behavioral concomitants, or sequelae will not be a "single problem" woman defined in terms of just smoking too much, being "just PMS", or only not attending antenatal care. Problems are likely presented in clusters; troubles accumulate and recruit one another, like muscle spasms. The plan one addresses with the woman may initially focus on the conduct and feeling most critical for current care, but will at an appropriate time consider all that she might want to do, over time and slowly, step by step, to make life longer and more worth living with respect to health, fitness, and "feeling good." For this reason, single target programs, while often essential and complete (whether postmastectomy group, Resolve, or alcoholism treatment) must be considered in terms of the possible wider range of women's health and wellness risks and needs. The women's health professional, and some of the groups in which the woman may participate, including for example, regular neighborhood "women's health" assemblies, may be envisioned as a series of contact opportunities to be employed, perhaps infrequently but nevertheless over a period of years. The model here is exactly that which is primary care itself, or the continuing accessibility of the women's health professional. It is now extended to that aspect of both primary and specialized secondary and tertiary reproductive system care needs that incorporate health promotion treatments.

Summary

Some psychological conditions are severely disabling and distressing to women, psychophysiologically may involve sexual dysfunction, and commonly accompany serious illness and its treatments, or reproductive conditions or cyclical episodes. Adverse reactions of this sort are most often associated with gynecological cancer and its treatments. However, some women with hysterectomies or following abortion, some with chronic pain, some infertile, some on medication regimens, some with PMS or other menstrual or menopausal disorder, and some during or after pregnancy, will be equally severely affected. The foregoing are not exclusive response risk groups, for any conditions where "the gang of four" stressors operate may have serious long term disruptive effects. The stressors to which we refer are condition-derived personal meanings and self-images which are deeply threatening; disruptive physiological perturbations; traumatic medical treatments or condition outcomes; and illness and/or recovery period hazarded by need to make major readjustments in such areas as physical functioning, accommodation to pain, and sexual-family-work adjustments.

These adverse responses are not simply distressing in themselves, extending that to family members, but also may carry risk of further future disease risk with need for hazard management. For these reasons, referral to health psychological-behavioral medicine, counseling or psychotherapy professionals, to support groups, and in some instances successful mastering patients as expert advisors, is in order. All of these should be part of the professional network of the women's health professional, i.e., one should know how such groups, expert patient advisors, and health professionals may be found and referred to. It is particularly useful if there is set up within one's own immediate collegial practice group (whether clinic, hospital, HMO, PPO, etc.) a professional facility which can provide consultation and treatment services as alter ego for the medical professional responsible for women's reproductive system care.

Resistance to referral can occur, arising from attitudes and anxieties or resource limitations within the woman and her circumstances. The approach to resistance is via a dialogue with the woman. One aims to sympathetically identify problems, generate her self-awareness, reward positive signs, and collaboratively to consider solutions. One acknowledges that "solutions" will only be partial since life is difficult, disease is common, and loss and pain and death are inevitable.

Resistance may also occur within the health professional. Again it is ordinarily a function of training, attitudes, group standards and institutional pressures, individual fears, and resource limitations. When it arises and is recognized by the individual one hopes the women's health professional will reflect upon incompatibilities between that bias, resistance, and women's health and wellness needs. We trust such resistance among professionals will become less frequent as medical institutions themselves embrace the changes implicit in disease prevention, health promotion, and the "wellness" concept. In the long run, one is talking as much about philosophy as medicine or psychology. In the Old Greek sense, philosophy was a matter of decision and ideology about how, in the face of opportunity, chance, knowledge, and consistent adversity, to go as gracefully and as wisely as possible about the business of living and dying.

14

Future Directions

This chapter proposes some areas for investigation. Our purpose is to illustrate and to stimulate relevant work in consequential areas, ones which may prove interesting, particularly to investigators—including clinicians—newly making a commitment to women's wellness and disease prevention.

Systematization in Obstetrical Risk Prediction

In Chapter 6 we emphasized the need to improve obstetrical risk scales through the testing of hypothesized relevant psychosocial behavioral variables now identified as having general predictive value for wellness, but not yet incorporated into obstetrical scales. Additional methodological work on item analysis, and more careful delineation of outcome criteria including improved subscale specificity are all needs that have been discussed. Because there must be great emphasis on prevention of low birth weight, it is apposite to combine that prevention intervention effort with risk scale development. Work on obstetrical risk scales merits high priority.

Search for Underlying Covariance in Gynecological Illness

Psychosocial prevention in gynecology will benefit from sophisticated descriptive studies of a prognostic nature. We have elsewhere

(Blum et al., 1984) presented a need and model for such work. It anticipates interaction among traits, biosocial status, conduct, family and social situation, perception of medical care, community support networks, and experienced stress all as contributing to factors, syndromes, or underlying "typologies" capable of identification through LISREL analysis of covariance methods. We expect such factors to be found associated with the incidence of a range of and complaints referrable to the reproductive system.

Working on "Best Test" Consensus

The number of psychological instruments employed to measure traits hypothesized as relevant to health risk is astonishing. The instruments themselves range from the carefully developed to the casual ad hoc assembly of "hunch" items. Widespread current problems of trait or construct definition, lack of replicability of findings, and unreliability in measurement all stem, in part, from the variations in psychometric quality and test choice in work on risk etiology. In gynecological psychosomatics and obstetrical risk, for example, it is particularly evident that those developing instruments have not enjoyed good psychometric advice.

Required as one remedy are efforts to improve trait identification (criterion measurement of independent personality variables) through major screening programs for "best tests" that may then be used as standard instruments by psychosomatic and other reproductive biology workers who are not themselves in the test construction business. (For similar needs expressed for psychotherapy evaluation work, see Williams and Spitzer, 1984.) One conceives here of a programmatic need to apply to large heterogeneous, stratified populations a range of instruments to identify which are efficient and reliable, tests with demonstrable concept validity. Results would be disseminated to non-psychometric research workers as a manual on best tests to use given work needs x, y, or z. The problem is one that any biologist recognizes for assays or for diagnostic procedures using equipment. When the characteristic of interest is known and measurable, one uses a reliable test. Psychosocial studies are no different.

Table VI below presents tests which have been used in studies reviewed for this monograph. These represent only a fraction of those available, as reference to test catalogues or a recent Buros MENTAL

MEASUREMENTS YEARBOOK will show. Our categories for what is measured are sometimes arbitrary. A glance at the table shows that there is considerable overlap, for example, tests of sexual function or marital intimacy may both tap similar universes of function and experience. Tests of sexual intimacy, family relations, and social support may be tapping similar universes. Personality as affect, premenstrual or menstrual mood, postpartum scales and subscales of general personality tests will all be picking up negative affect and neuroticism. Symptom inventories may also be used epidemiologically as measurements for neuroticism or other personality disturbance. Probably related stress vulnerability as measured on a life events or "hassles" scale might be expected to correlate with symptom levels, trait anxiety, or neuroticism, as a measure of vulnerability. One speculates that ill populations compared to well ones, whether defined by medical or psychological criteria, might well show cross correlations on many of the scales, however separate-appearing may be the categories.

A great service will be performed when work of the sort reported in McReynolds (1981), McReynolds and Christenson (1984), and for neonatal assessment by J. Osofsky (1979) and her colleagues, is systematized in a handbook for research workers in the psychosocial health risk field so that one has for ready reference (a) particulars about the utility and weakness of the tests used in psychosocial disease relationship studies including the evaluation of such tests, questionnaires, and rating scales when used for specific to specific prediction, i.e., to demonstrate etiological roles for specific diseases (b) recommendations as to best tests for widely used trait/state measures such as depression, anxiety, and negative affect and (c) a list of places to go for test purchase, administration directions, and computer scoring capabilities. For now, a good resource is the Health Instrument File, c/o School of Nursing, Universtiy of Pittsburgh, Pennsylvania.

Table VI
Psychological Tests Used in Risk Assessment, Self-Report Health Status, Psychosomatic Research, and Illness Impact Studies

Self-Administered

INTELLIGENCE
WAIS Verbal
Mill Hill Test of Verbal
   Intelligence

FAMILY AND/OR MARITAL RELATIONS
Short Marital Adjustment Scale
Lock Wallace Marital Adjustment
   Scale
Inventory of Family Feelings
Family Environment Scale
Waring Intimacy Questionnaire
Precursor Study Family Attitudes
   Scale

AUTONOMIC SENSITIVITY
Autonomic Perception Questionnaire

ILLNESS COPING, IMPACT
Psychosocial Adjustment to
   Illness Scale
Ways of Coping Checklist
Sickness impact profile
   (Am. Heart Ass., Bargner)

PERCEIVED SELF-CONTROL
Rotter Locus of Control
Multidimension Health Locus
   of Control
Leverson-Miller Locus of Control
McReynolds Preference for Control
   Scale

STRESSFUL EXPERIENCE, LIFE
EVENTS, EVENT VULNERABILITY
Elliot Eisdorfer Stressful Events
Daily Hassles Scale
Life Experience Survey
Schedule of Recent Experiences
Recent Life Change Questionnaire
Social Readjustment Rating Scale
Life Events Inventory
Schedule of Daily Experiences
Beford College Life Events and
   Difficulties Scale

CAPACITY TO SUSTAIN
ATTENTION
Continuous Performance Test

PERSONALITY: General
(pathology, multiple dimensions or
   traits)
Minnesota Multiphasic
   Personality Inventory (MMPI)
California Personality Inventory

PERSONALITY: Rigidity, dogmatism
Rokeach Dogmatism Scale

PERSONALITY: Mood
Kellner Symptom Resting Test
 (measures felt inadequacy)
Kellner Symptom Questionnaire
Rubinow Visual Analog Scales
Aitken Visual Analog
Profile of Mood States
Nowlis Mood Adjective Checklist

PERSONALITY: Type A
Jenkins Activity Survey
Vickers Scale
Framingham Scale
Bortner Scale

PERSONALITY: Affect
Beck Depression Inventory
NIMH Trait Anxiety Scale
NIMH Depression Scale
Differential Emotion Scale
Spielberger State Anxiety
Free Anxiety Subscale: Middlesex
 Hospital
Taylor Manifest Anxiety
Grimm Psychology Tension Inventory
Zung Self-Rating Depression Scale
Zung Self-Rating Anxiety Scale
IPAT Anxiety Scale

OPTIMISM
Life Orientation Test (LOT)

PERSONALITY: Transcendence
Self-Transcendence Scale

Mental Health Inventory
Eysenck EPG
Catel 16PF Test
Edwards Personal Preference
 Inventory
NIMH Diagnostic Interview Schedule
 (DIS) for Psychiatric Disorders
Research Diagnostic Criteria
 (Spitzer)
Type A Structured Interview
 (ATBP SI)
DSM III (nomenclature and
 standards for all psychiatric
 disorders)

VITAL EXHAUSTION AND
DEPRESSION AND
EMOTIONAL DRAIN
Maastricht Myocardial Infarction
 Risk Questionnaire

PERSONALITY: Repression-
 expression
Stimulus Screening Scale
Goldstein Repression-Threat Denial
Byrnes Repression-Sensitization
 Scale
Stimulus Screening Scale
Marlowe Crowne Social Desirability
 Scale
Self-Consciousness Scale

PERSONALITY: SOMATIZATION
 (Psychiatric for hysteria)
Screening Test for Somatization
 (Othner and DeSouza)
Checklist for Somatization Disorder
 (DSM III)

SYMPTOMS, SELF-REPORTED
HEALTH COMPLAINT LEVELS
 (Simultaneously used to identify
 emotional disturbance and
 psychiatric disorder)

PERSONALITY: Hostility
Cook-Medley Ho MMPI Subscale
Caine & Foulds Hostility &
  Direction of Hostility
  Questionnaire
Rosenzweig Pictures
  Frustration Test

PREGNANCY ATTITUDES
Attitude to Pregnancy Scale
Parental Attitudes Research
  Inventory
Pregnancy Research Questionnaire
Life Event Scale for Obstetrical Patients
HIP Pregnancy Questionnaire
Blau Maternal Attitudes to
  Pregnancy Scale
Adaptive Potential for Pregnancy
  Scale
ZAR Pregnancy Attitude Scale
Burnstein Pregnancy Anxiety Test

SOCIAL SUPPORT
Surtees Index of Social Support
Older American Resources and
  Services Questionnaire
Social Support Questionnaire
Perceived Social Support
Personal Assessment of Intimacy
  in Relationships Scale
Miller Social Intimacy Scale
UCLA Loneliness Scale
Berle Social Support Index

PHYSICIAN-PATIENT RELATIONSHIP
DOQ: Doctor Opinion Questionnaire
PAT: Patient Attitude Test
PCT: Patient Cooperativeness Test

Brief Symptom Inventory
Cohen/Hoberman Symptom
  Checklist
Cornell Medical Index
MacMillan HOS
Hopkins Symptom Checklist
  SCL 90R
Health Status Questionnaire
Pennebaker PILL
Wahler Physical Symptoms
  Inventory
General Well Being Scale
Daily Hassles Scale
Christensen Health History
Life Satisfaction Index Z
Kellner Symptom Questionnaire

HUMOR
Situational Humor Response
  Test
Sense of Humor Questionnaire

ALCOHOLISM
Michigan Alcoholism Screening Test

POSTPARTUM
Postpartum Emotional Disorders
Braverman-Roux Postpartum
  Depression Scale

SEXUAL FUNCTION
Byrne Sex Information Questionnaire
Derogatis Sexual Function Inventory

WORK SITUATION &
ADJUSTMENT
Job-Related Tension Index
Work Environment Scale

PAIN
McGill Pain Questionnaire

FAMILY HISTORY
Family History Diagnostic
　Criterion (Andreasen)

NEONATAL ASSESSMENT
Apgar
Brazelton Neonatal Behavior
　Assessment Scale
Dubowitz Assessment of
　Gestational Age
Prechtl and Beintema
　Neurological Examination
Parmalee Neurological Examination
Gesell Developmental Schedules
Griffiths's Mental Development Scale
Graham Behavior Test and
　Graham-Rosenblith Tests
Bayley Scales of Infant Development
Cattell Infant Intelligence Scale
Einstein Scales of Sensormotor
　Intelligence (Escalona & Cormon)
Uzgiris and Hunt Assessment Procedure

MENSTRUATION (mood)
Moose Menstrual Distress Scale
Halbreich Premenstrual Assessment

OTHER
Lykken Activity Preference
　Questionnaire

Individual Administration

PERSONALITY
Thematic Apperception Test
Rorschach
Field Dependency
Paykel Interview for Recent Life Events
Psychiatric Epidemiology Research Interview
Archetypical AT 9 Alexithymea Test
Hamilton Rating Scale for Depression

SICKNESS IMPACT
Karnofsky Performance Status Scale

Etiological Mechanisms

In earlier chapters we have discussed the necessity for the understanding of disease prevention, or wellness, to move beyond risk factors as trait markers to specification of the events which induce physiological changes which, in turn, as continuing perturbation lead to signs and symptoms, syndromes, and the emergence of pathology. We noted some of the major paths such research has taken historically, as for example in psychosomatics and psychophysiology. The scientific literature is currently occupied with exciting classes of such mechanisms or effects, as for example those associated with suppression of NK killer cell immune response, the differential production of one or another group of endorphins, the production and effects of the stress endocrines; catecholamines and the possible modulators of cortisol; immune system variables such as interleukin 1 as mediator of host response to infection and inflammation, interleukin 2 which appears responsible for immune system T lymphocyte production (mitosis), and monocyte derived macrophages in procoagulation activity sensitive to perturbation as a component in immune response. Work is also being done (Ruff et al., 1985) on circulating monocytes chemotaxically influenced by peripheral benzodiazepam receptors. The postulated link between neuropeptides as humoral mediators of felt mood states and reactions, and as communicating to monocytes with subsequent possible effects on the immune system, possibly in interaction with prostaglandins or beta endorphins, is indeed provocative.

The foregoing illustrations are of possible intermediate events which provide a measurable dependent variable testable against hypothesized risk variables, buffers, interacting "constitutional" or personal features, and stressor levels and kinds to describe a possible ordered array of such variables acting to enhance or suppress immune function, inflammation, circulation, tissue repair. It is work on mechanisms which is required to join epidemiological risk prediction to the understanding of the "choice" and course of a psychobiological event culminating in diagnosable disease. Our bets are on this area of work as an extremely productive one.

Locating and Learning Acceptable Complaints

Distressed women may express their felt non-wellness by focused complaint, but the avenue for determining that focus in the absence of substantiating tissue pathology or in the presence of multiple transient biochemical perturbations is unknown. Work on the processs of self-location of illness is in order. We suspect it will be shown related to physiological response specificities, vulnerable organ systems, perturbed recovery sequences after stress, childhood family values specifying acceptable styles of complaint, locations significant for personal meaning, and that learning which has taken place in medical care. One bet is that a critical learning period is menarche as an adolescent "becoming" a woman.

Too Much Medication: Is There a Way Out?

Recall the data in Chapter 2 showing that women even when receiving no diagnosis on an office visit may very well receive a prescription. Recall too that while it is depression that is so widespread, and as yet inexplicable among women— along with, we suspect, correlated felt fatigue— that tranquilizers are the medicine they are often given even though the ubiquitious diazepam may itself have a depressing effect. Prescription studies allow a conclusion that both patient and doctor living up to high tech pharmacological fashion "better living through chemistry" give and take more drugs than are necessary, but consider that surfeit as good and proper.

It is a costly non-solution; medication is expensive, the side effects risks (including dependency) from useless medication are real and avoidable, the continuing agreement to address the wrong issue through needless prescriptions affronts good quality of care and blunts acumen, and one wonders if easy pill popping is compatible with the difficult task of self-responsibility for the complex business of discipline for lifestyles, or achieving joy. Our hypothesis is that those women most involved in repeat prescriptions and the high turnover medicine cabinet will be resistant to other self-change, and that their like-minded prescription-production-line physicians will also be adverse to the hard work of health promotion. If so, such symbolic twosomes are impediments to improved health.

Needed: research on changing the needless prescription habit. Prospective studies, for example, on adolescent females do offer such an opportunity. One wants to link the learning of complaints and medicines with girls' ideas as to how the body works, and is affected. For classes of disorders such as PMS, some dysmenorrheas, pruritis, and chronic pelvic pain, such studies may well suggest optimal points in time for education prior to the crystallization of the complaint and prescription habit and when its emotional components may, as in crisis intervention, best be alleviated. One thinks immediately of the alexithymic patient, unable to verbalize and apparently at more at risk for chronic pain and post-traumatic stress disorder. Would it be possible to identify this group at age 12 and to facilitate (e.g., through imagery practice, hypnosis, and reward for verbalizations) their other-than-somatic expression, thus making them—one hypothesizes—amenable to better self-assessment and "working through" as better coping or stress response at an other than somatic level?

More Attention to Sleep Disorder

Abnormal sleeping patterns were early on (but not later) in the Alameda study, morbidity/mortality predictors. One asks, however, if these may not also be symptomatic of earlier observable temperament irregularities which are an early expression of distress reflecting reverberating physiologic perturbation as disease precursor? Given evidence to the effect that sleep following experience is consolidating for learning, may it not also be the case that those patients suffering sleep disturbance, including nightmares as reported during REM (rapid eye movement) awakening, that following counseling or group support, would show no or reduced recovery even when initially matched for symptom and life dysfunction severity? One might also seek to measure counseling treatment efficacy by the degree of sleep disruption induced by it. Would sleep quality provide a measure, following medical visits, to predict to the degree of initial cooperation (compliance) following instruction in life style change, as for example, when unhealthy lifestyles are so closely integrated into needs that their disruption is threatening?

Sleep disturbance is common enough under felt stress (see Winters, 1985), when in pain, and when depressed; yet it does not appear as a study variable either in obstetrical risk prediction or in gynecological complaint incidence prediction. Does it deserve testing?

Mother-Daughter Pairs and Prediction

Again, the obvious. Reported are correlates between mother's physique and obstetrical risk and her daughter when daughter becomes pregnant. Demonstrable are genetic components in some "lifestyle" disorders such as alcoholism, and in conditions/illnesses such as schizophrenia, some depression, hypertension and CHD risk, and diabetes. All in turn are obstetrical risk predictors. When low SEC is maintained by mother and daughter, i.e., when there is no class mobility between the generations, one also expects positive correlations in early sexual activity, age of first conception, contraception behavior which in turn should be associated with cervical cancer onset, abortion, STD. Transgenerational experiences (beliefs, problem solving, self-concepts) also appear to play a role in the ability of families to cope with lifestyle problems, as for example, alcoholism or other drug risk. Obviously daughters learn from and model themselves after, as well as inherit from, mothers and grandmothers.

We have seen no research which uses either grandmother or mother and the degree of (concordat) rated problem and risk in daughter now pregnant. One wishes to test if those risks duplicated over family generations are potentiating, "synergistic" as far as risk weights are concerned. Are such items of special predictive value when entered into risk prediction matrices, as for example, for contraception failure, STD risk, obstetrical risk, sexual dysfunction or gynecological complaints as well as for hypertension and CHD?

A testable "hunch": where there is a familial history of obstetrical risk and complications, the pregnant primiparous daughter of the same SEC, even in the absence of physical risk indicators, will have a greater obstetrical complication rate, and that at a magnitude expressing the multiplicity and severity of risks in mother and grandmother. Also, duplicated risk cross-generationally will show potiention, defined as more than additive weights for discriminant analysis in OB risk prediction. These are examples of a search for unexplained variance in present OB risk.

Not Yet a Whole Picture

It astonishes us that so little is known about the health behavior profiles of women. The knowledge deficiency is closely related to that earlier discussed with respect to unknown covariance that might allow the generation of typologies to understand the risk of gynecological disease incidence. Yet even in pregnancy where there is frequent observation, one does not even know what crude clusters may exist with respect to the range of now identified obstetrical risk, psychosocial-behavioral, and correlated physical disease variables. One does not even know, for nationally representative populations, how many women with what biosocial characteristics drink how much alcohol during what periods of pregnancy. Nor do we know what clusters exist tying drinking to smoking to cocaine to nutrition to anxiety to STD, etc. One can find out for the individual patient, one could do profiles of one's own clinic patients, but does one know how these compare to other women in the community, to these same women when not pregnant, to these same women after referral for behavioral treatments, for example in programs designed to reduce low birth weights? At the very simplest level, descriptive research, and inferential constructs derived from it as to origins and effects, is missing.

Placebo Main Effect

There are dozens of hunches to be followed in any of these areas. Our bet, for example, based on the statistical main effect found for placebo compliance, that across a group of women showing desired reductions in risk behavior antenatally, derived from low birth weight prevention programs; those women who maintain better self care one year postpartum will be found, looking back at birth weight data, to have infants of higher birth weights, with all other known risk factors controlled.

Fatigue or Low Energy

We have seen (Chapter 3) how common it is for women to feel "below par" or, with PMS, irritable and "out of sorts." These expressions may usually be taken as summary statements for being overburdened by challenge and demand (stress) or chronic psychopathological overlay for reproductive cycle exacerbation of negative feelings. In PMS, one finds remarkably too little attention paid to the possible physiological correlates as differentiating expressions of high and low fatigue levels. What for example if one were to examine the primitive hypothesis that fatigue itself will be found, "out there" in an epidemiological study (not restricted to PMS self-referred patients) to be cyclical with the ovarian cycle and another biorhythm such as REM-sleep induced variations in depression analogues with greater fatigue expression upon awakening than are found at mid-day periods? What if one further tested for non-depression fatigue as a subliminal "stress" response postulated to be reflected in correlated levels of glucose, growth hormone, prolactin, cortisol, or interleukins, as examples? One controls, of course, for biosocial status, concurrent disease, anemia, work exertion as part of life circumstance, simultaneous experience of individuals in the living group, sleep disturbance, etc. We propose such tests not with confidence as to the excellence of such hunches, but simply by way of trying to stimulate work which looks at common problems of women in the environments where they live, to begin to distinguish (just as PMS work is doing) subsets of intercorrelated complaints, and to test for psychophysiological correlates and, thence, mechanisms.

Given current work on the importance of circulatory/coagulation function, one might, by way of speculation turned into observation, test the proposition that one group of chronically fatigued women of reproductive age will be those where the luteal phase of the cycle or the menstruation period is stress defined by higher levels of macrophages, interleukins, etc., in plasma, the uterus, or peritoneal fluid using an own-control design as well as cross comparisons. In the same way one might wish to test for monocyte and macrophage concentrations or prostaglandin products, or indeed the ratios thereof, comparing "true" PMS to the "psychological" PMS group at menstruation, again as a function of an expected relationship between stress expressed as felt bodily disturbance and perturbation or indeed environmental events responded to as trauma. Implied is dysregulation in immune system function(s). One might wish to go on to complicate the foregoing primitive model by suggesting that beta endorphin levels will be found higher among those women with low complaint but high macrophage levels. Implied is that neuroendocrine stress responses "work" when endogenous pain suppression mechanisms come into play simultaneous with immune system activation, providing there is a speedy return to baseline (non stress pre-menstruation) hormone levels, i.e., that dysregulation is transient not chronic.

Again with respect to fatigue, recall that symptom sensitivity is greater in women with the more autonomic CNS lability. One might well postulate in a prospective study of teenage girls for pre-PMS risk, that those with greater autonomic lability, and internal state and symptom sensitivity, will be more at risk of PMS. Implied: PMS severity is an aspect of sensitivity to internal change, and that there is a correlate between reproductive system complaints and CNS lability. With any positive findings, one would wish to test the stability and extensiveness of that lability associated with reproductive cycle self-sensitivity. Could such ability be, like other psychophysiological patterns, a CNS trait first remarkable in childhood, or indeed as a function of a Gessel developmental rating in infancy as unstable temperament? Be that so, what concordance is to be found in twin, or other familial studies? And if present, concerning oneself now with the great quest for lifetime pathways for disease expression, could there be a subgroup of unstable temperament babies becoming the autonomic CNS labile children becoming early post menarche dysmenorrhea become PMS who are also children of "hot" cardiovascular, hypertensive stress stimuli reactors and themselves then also "hot" reactors? When primiparous, are these women at higher risk for preeclampsia and anxiety with subsequent higher rate of complications? Are those also the first, comparatively, to develop CHD morbidity? And when comparing the early unstable, self-sensitive labile—were there to be any such—would the low morbidity subgroup within the larger set be those enjoying by adolescence some of the psychosocial features elsewhere found associated with reduced risk, e.g., better self-control for diet, internal locus of control, more and closer family/social relations, and resourcefulness.

It is past time for long range prospective studies using large female populations, where formal hypotheses are set forth in advance, where careful measures are made along the way. The longitudinal development studies, such as those long underway at Berkeley (Institute for Personality Assessment and Research or at the Fels Institute) offer models with which psychosomatic work is to be incorporated.

Classifying Somatizers

The state of our diagnosis and logic with respect to that large general class of women termed somatizers is entirely unsatisfactory.

Future Directions

Within that mix are the healthy, wealthy over-utilizers of services, the self-rated "poor health" group some of whom are chronically ill, the elderly at high mortality risk, hysterics now confusingly enshrined in DSM III (the official psychiatric diagnostic system) as "somatizers" (people cannot even agree on spelling, whether "somatizer" or "somaticizer"), the psychosomatic group whose physical illness is understood as the expression of specific psychodynamic or psychophysiological states (ulcers, allergy, hypertension), the many women with complaints referrable to the reproductive system who are found without organic basis, some called "functional." Among these, often with initial diffuse distress, a subset may have "negotiated" diagnoses from angina to PMS. Included as well are many women whose complaint is their chronic local resident demon; headache, chronic pain, pruritis, etc.

That psychological factors contribute greatly is evident; refer to Tables II, III, IV, and V. That overlap with depression and neuroticism particularly is great is also clear from the data. As we have discussed, the selfsame tests are used, both epidemiolgically and clinically, to garner self-reports of physical and "functional" symptoms and to infer psychiatric disorder/psychological disease. Thirteen instruments capable of that dual use are listed in Table VI. But it is also the case that high symptom levels, for a subset, represent a mortality risk, for example "emotional drain" presaging myocardial infarct.

Chapters 3 and 4 presenting discrete influences on symptom levels or "choice," suggest the possibility of a great number of "syndromes," i.e., of clusters of symptoms, psychosocial-behavioral characteristics, psychophysiological components, sometimes emerging disease processes, or as noted, immediate mortality risk. One regrets the absence of epidemiological data which better define subgroups, use their characteristics to construct risk estimates, and require the development of instruments and diagnostic criteria much more specific than the symptom counters used (validly) to infer psychiatric status, including other than "true" PMS. The work to be done is descriptive, but strenously requires knowledge of the complaint-correlate data, of development in psychosomatics, health psychology and substrate psychophysiology and neuropharmacology. Given the immense burden of now essentially undesignated disorder, where there are almost no guides to differential diagnosis or risk prediction, work in this arena deserves a high priority.

Reexamining Roles and Institutions

Research proceeds not simply on the basis of a chain of findings and derived hypothesis, or intuitive hunches, and from the developing intellectual construction of organizing theory, but also from attitudinal frameworks which may be implicit and contain contemporary value positions with respect to how nature "really works." Kuhn (1970) in his work on the history of science, argues that theories persist in spite of accumulating incompatible, and thus rejected and disbelieved data until, rather like an earthquake, sudden revisions in the accepted structures of knowledge take place. Work on the sociology of knowledge shows how there is an interpenetration of ways of thinking such that scientific inquiry is dependent not simply on the available techniques, but on available ideas, and images as well. Today's analogous thinking about brain qua computer is an example.

One already knows that there are value conflicts, strains, which affect viewpoints with respect to health promotion. Some of these are considered in Chapters 1 and 2, for example, on the changing social role of the physician vis-a-vis the patient over the last four decades. One transition, with conflict, is from the more to the less authoritarian doctor and from the passive to active and skeptical patient roles. The shift is expressed in health promotion from unilateral to shared responsibility, and is seen in its language, for example, "compliance" versus "cooperation."

This is no revolutionary change, seen in terms of the history of science or medical practice, but can be a disconcerting one for the professional with traditional habits of practice. One research question arises which asks if there is a relationship between willingness to undertake preventive medical efforts, including the emerging professional role in health promotion and descriptive measures of the professional's work setting, self-identification, or confidence in dealing with new and ambiguous challenges. Are women's specialists who pride themselves as surgeons more likely than others to be disinterested on prevention via lifestyle and outreach? Are training settings which reward for technical skill and do not emphasize interpersonal relations, psychosomatics, or which send residents out on family visits more likely to attract and groom physicians uninterested in prevention as measured by what they really say and do with patients? How do measurably competent and active professionals involved in health promotion differ from those least so by way of background, training, patient load characteristics, or their own personalities? Is the malpractice suit record of the non-prevention oriented physician more peppered with lawsuits? Is it still the case, as it was in the California Medical Association research of the late 1950's, that the malpractice suit prone physician avoids communication, is authoritarian, encourages patient passivity, wants ego-feeding gratitude, will have more personal psychopathology?

If one accepts the arguments for prevention and one finds current efforts in the training of physicians inadequate, how does one innovate successfully? The problem of changing the teaching styles entrenched in medical school would surely be no easier than that of changing lifestyles for individuals. Consider that the recent American College of Obstetrics and Gynecology (1985) report earlier cited to the effect that residents are given very little real training in prevention, including the relevant fields of public health psychosomatics and health psychology. To correct this, what institutional experiments in innovation can be undertaken? Certainly one knows that there is resistance to that innovation which intrudes upon established belief, practice, interests, and reward systems.

One also is aware of the major positive curricula change in some medical schools. Nevertheless, one study (Blum, 1964) indicates that one way to avoid sabotage, resistance, in a medical institution is to start new services rather than to try to force change in old ones. Indeed, in that study (although we did not publish this portion of the data), there was evidence that the forced change method (brute power by the administrator) not only disorganized a service but may have been a health risk for resisting employees. Among a small staff, several of those experiencing forced change suffered heart attacks. Other "control" service staff did not. At what costs then does one wish to compel change on those rare occasions one has to power to do so? Or to resist it?

Reexamining Values Affecting Concept Choices for Research: Is There, Should There Be, a Perfect Low-Risk Woman?

The risk factors known to us from research play little role in theory, except for models such as those offered for CHD or within a sphere, as for example Lazarus' (1980) work on stress, or social supports. There has been little examination of risk factors in the aggregrate except insofar as the aggregate is itself a broad category such as SE or graphic conceptual schemes—the schematic wiring diagrams, cubes, etc., in interacting etiological conceptual models.

Thus, there has been no theory building at the personality-and -health level which incorporates a range of psychosocial factors. We are by no means prepared to perform such a task here, but we suspect that one way to initiate it is to see what is provoked simply if we combine reliably identified risk factors to construct a picture of the lowest risk, admirably well, woman. That sketch is necessarily an insufficient "biography" because it can only be composed of currently identified risk elements. Nevertheless, what emerges is a worrisome portrait, for it raises in our minds the question as to whether there are hidden values which have powered research in health psychology so as to produce such definitions of and implied demands for health behavior perfection. Is she a straw woman we have drawn, or is there some real problem in the value system which defines her? You will see, she is not quite human.

Begin with the fact the perfected low risk woman is under age 55 (for obstetrical risk, and depending on the scale in use, not over 35), lives in an uncrowded middle or upper class setting, is slim, exercises daily, has an admirable health history, and enjoys a secure, adequate family income. She is wise in her diet, neither binging nor crashing nor quailing undisciplined in the face of chocolates. Nutritional balance is her aim for her family's meals, and she assures herself complex carbohydrates, cruciform vegetables, and other fibers. Attentive to awesome details of food safety, the family barbeque is used carefully, courting neither parasites, from raw fish, pork or beef or carcinogens. She serves cooked sea fish twice weekly, drives carefully, and always with her seat belt fastened. She has a sexually satisfying and emotionally intimate relationship with her husband, is contraceptively diligent, and while bearing the characteristic sensivity of a woman to her inward self, being sensitive to rhythms and change, she neither under nor over uses medical care. She is cautious in using OTC preparations and does not seek out prescriptions.

She has a wide circle of friends, regularly goes to church, is part of and enjoys being a member of a stable, well- integrated social group with enduring rock hard values. These allow her to feel good in and to be a real part of, as well as to make sense of her (even if it is an organized illusion) coherent world. She has had enough experience with normal hardship to have accumulated self-confidence and a reservoir of techniques for dealing with troubles; she knows and has access to multiple resources outside herself. Furthermore, she feels her world to be, in daily life, under her control. As part of that she is comfortably dominant socially, although rarely must she be aggressive, and is saved ugly hostility since her status and authority as wife, mother, civic person, and manager at work, are respectfully acknowledged by those around her. She experiences very little life change in terms of surprising events, and avoids daily hassles because she regulates her life, lives in a routine world, and is not easily threatened by normal problems. Hers is a strong, optimistic personality with a placid and stable temperament. She has been fortunate in that untimely deaths in her family, or divorce, have not occurred; she lives in that region of a technologically advanced nation which suffers neither war, migration, economic depression, nor political crises.

Her mental health is excellent, and while she has her ups and downs as everyone does, added the propensity to depression to which women are more prone than men, the emotions she has are appropriate to her world and in themselves satisfying for the most part. She can be anxious, but that is useful in mobilizing her to action. She does ignore that which she cannot change but she does not entirely repress her feelings. Should she feel "symptomatic" she is insightful enough to know that the felt stress, including occasional physiological malfunction, may speak in any body system, but she does not complain of bodily symptomatology as a misplaced referrent for her distress. If something does go askew in life so that occasional headache and dysmenorrhea ensue, she is initially tolerant of her symptoms, understanding these are part of living. On one occasion, however, during a take over bid for the company in which her husband was an executive, she began to suffer that which her friends told her must be PMS. Through her gynecologist she was referred to behavioral therapy. She responded well to biofeedback training, and found she could use her imagery (planting a new garden) to block irritability and that "swollen" feeling. She was, as garden club president, delighted with her mantra recitation ("om ne pad me chrysanthemum").

She drinks wine in moderation, does not smoke, visits her peridontist twice yearly, looks up material from *The New, Our Bodies Ourselves* or the PDR, as necessary, and engages her physician in a mature, fully communicative relationship. She does not forget the doctor's advice, while her doctor is ever mindful that she will insist on sharing important decisions about her care with that physician. A skeptic, she rightly does not trust her physician to make only correct judgements. He does not really enjoy her sharp questions but realizes her attitude is a health care advantage for her.

She is born of parents who are also healthy, emotionally stable, and financially well-off. There was no genetic risk or burden transmitted, and her parents, like her, are well- proportioned and well-muscled. Our woman has been loved and well-cared for as a child. She maintains her good interpersonal relations partly because of these learned and also temperamentally bio-programmed social skills and capacities for warmth and trust. Yet, when really threatened, she is dangerous. As befits our species, a territorial, aggressive, yet social predatory omnivore, hers is modernly adaptive.

She works at a managerial level in a safe, toxin free environment. Her superiors appreciate her, the company offers complete medical insurance as well as a wide range of programs for exercise, stress management, relaxation, meditation. Because she is from a good family and well-schooled, there is no danger of status inconsistency or discrepant class mobility as she moves upward in management in her company. She has had occasional love affairs with male executive colleagues, but only with affection and excitement, no HP viruses are transmitted. Nowadays, having attended to TV AIDS reports, she would probably require a condom be used for any intercourse, whether oral, anal, or vaginal, with any new lover, at least until she has assured herself absolutely as to his freedom from STD. It would be reassuring if, feeling romantic after such loving interludes, she not only dreams lovely dreams, but is moved to write poetry. Unfortunately there are no data showing either tender dreams or poetry as reducing health risk.

ENOUGH! This construction of a person which uses identified low risk features as its building blocks has become satire. Is something awry with current features which, when amalgamated as the composite low-risk woman, yield a television stereotype of a 1960's elite women's college graduate? Can anyone be so conforming to middle class American values? So health conscious? Should they be? Can we find no relief in the risk literature allowing us also to advocate love, humor (Martin and Lefcourt, 1983), forms of delightful madness (maybe a zany hobby of growing red worms for fishing in a pit in her backyard?), flexibility, religious feeling, wisdom, gentleness, womanhood conscious of its intrinsic powers? Of course such items are not excluded from any biography, but since much of what people are or do is unreported or irrelevant to health, it is irrelevant here.

An advocate of progress and evolutionary technology may propose that this perfected woman demonstrates that western civilization—or Japan as counterpart enjoying even greater conforming moral and social integration—has been generating its ideal forms (as presented, for example, in Redbook or New Woman magazine, not by Plato) in a Darwinian fashion. Has it not established as ideal social norms and lifestyles, long before health psychological research existed, those which now turn out to maximize wellness as well as comfort and competitive advantage? In other words, the respectable woman living the successful conventional life is also following the fittest, known today, prescription for good health. If so, it has come to pass, with Candide, that middle and upper class America (or indeed wealthy, urban, anywhere) is the best of all present possible worlds.

A small difficulty arises if one seeks to reconcile the social Darwinian model exalting comfortable community norms of post-industrial society as best-for-health with the alternative dictums sometimes offered for lifestyle health to the effect that one should not stray for health's sake from the recent evolutionary history of man as hunter-gatherer. That advice, with echoes of Rousseau the romantic, is often found in text and magazine and argues that what is bad for humans in their conduct or ingestion is to stray from those habits compatible with body and mind as adapted in recent evolution, one presumes Cro Magnon, for the primitive life. Since hunter-gathers did not have refined sugars, processed fats, dirty air, cigarettes (with the exception of American Indians) or distilled alcohol, and did exercise, live in close groups, practice natural childbirth, etc., some seek a naturalistic fit between evolved body design and chosen healthiest lifestyle. Such advice also claims a Darwinian justification and is compatible with much in today's anti-rational, California "holistic" longing for natural health food and "good witches" as their midwives. That ideology overlooks the 40 years expected life span for hunter-gather tribes but it need not worry about that when the "holistic" health practices are imbedded in the well-protected life of the metropolitan woman who differs little in fact from the one we have just constructed, except for her romantic anti-rational and anti-technological medicine idealism.

Yet the elements pieced together for our contruction of the perfected low risk woman allow a suggestion other than manifest Darwinian destiny as explanatory of her fit with contemporary values as well as her adaptable fitness. It may be that the gestalt which constitutes that portrait derives its elements from the conventional values of a generation of investigators whose tested risk factors are cultural virtues believed, in any event, to represent the wise and the good, balance the Apollonian middle way as ideal. One may not claim that the findings with respect to the pragmatic value for wellness of restraint, responsibility, mental health, success, control, rationalism, etc., are incorrect; only that the process which has led to the focus in research on these socially approved traits— as opposed to others more frivolous— may have its origins in pervasive cultural values.

Certainly one does not discount findings of effects so consistently adverse to health as heavy and continuing cigarette smoking, poor nutrition, wild driving or heroin injection with a dirty needle. One may, however, pause over the too hurried embrace of generalized teetotalling morality derived from observation of the quite rare fetal alcoholism syndrome which would rule out all maternal wine sipping. There was quick acceptance in the late 1960's of claimed teratogenic effects of LSD based on findings in a group of troubled, low SEC mothers. Our own research found no such effects. To the contrary, flower children's babies were well and precocious in spite of psychadelic dosing (see Blum et al., 1972). Today there is elevation of the cult of youthful dieting and exercise to the point where amenorrhea, if not anorexia, orthopedic injury, and arthritis take over.

In the portrait of the perfected low risk woman we discern a potpourri of cultural themes: rationalism, the Protestant ethic, Puritan energy and discipline, that conformity which is so American that de Tocqueville branded it in the 1820's as our ubiquitous flaw; and that alertness to fashions and illusion in health and health care which characterize our high tech "aware" society. Do these themes prove out in health risk prediction because they are central aspects of our culture so that adherence, their expression by an individual, reflects an underlying harmony, the fit of a person in society? That too would be capable of a Darwinian gloss; the fittest are those who fit in, adapt to their surroundings as ecological niche. Or, alternatively, have research workers been examining church attendance but not spirituality, self-control but not the altered consciousness states of poetry, capacity to predict via routine rather than to respond by laughing in surprise, amount of alcohol consumed but not preference for a Gevry Chambertin 1971 over a 1985 Virginia Dare jug wine dare, because these are our cultural legacy as to the hierarchy of what is "really important"?

There are many studies on children's health beliefs. Some of them show how when children become ill, they place that alien event in a moral context, asking, "What did I do wrong that made me sick?" or "Why is God punishing me?" Are we as research workers carrying over some of this health-as-morality equivalence? Most people by now have rejected the prejudiced notion that the poor are poor only because they want to be, yet one does hear that the chronically sick are ill because they are irresponsible.

As a result of the questions raised by the coincidence of finding as good for us what our culture already believes in, one must recommend that studies relevant to health risk embrace the anthropological, sociological, philosphical issues which illuminate how we come to select our psychosocial research topics.

Our manufactured portrait of the low risk woman suggests a conservative person. In our own research on the family etiology of youthful drug risk (Blum et al., 1972), family conservatism was indeed a powerful correlate, and in multiple discriminant analysis a statistical predictor— of low or no problem outcome risk. As social animals we do create institutional structures which meet our needs (as with other primates) for affiliation and interdependency, and we do generate values in support of those gratifying institutions to which belongingness is so important, be that for God, queen, and country; or Marx, motherland, and the proletariat. It is our impression that the more conservative aspects of societies, when translated into individual conduct and lifestyle, emerge overall as predictors for better health. After all, the ability to control and predict, caution in action, the absence of any environmental perturbation, firm in-place social networks, no discrepant individual social mobility or migration, are hardly prescriptions for change. Perhaps, after all, that stability as regularity and coherence, a well fed status quo is in fact is best for health. But one may not exclude the possiblility of a co-existing bias to the effect that health educators or promotion research workers may also be selecting concepts to test, and methods of proof which adhere to the central tendency of a society itself becoming perhaps more conservative. Indeed, the selection process whereby one comes to be in a position to advocate health policy or receive support for health research may bias in favor of those sound and trustworthy folk with histories of institutional loyalty, sage pronouncements, disciplined publication, and prudent fiscal management. Could it be otherwise? We would like to think such bias is not too great a blemish, since we ourselves have reported findings favoring "conservative" health habits and family styles, i.e., we are guilty of the charges. But again, we argue for the value of reflection, self-criticism (the Great Leap somewhere...) for our alert participation in the ongoing process of medical care improvement.

Research on Diversity for Wellness Is Needed

Whatever accounts for the present picture (critics may hold we are simply being unfair), we believe it is apparent that the composite low disease risk, high wellness woman is sucessful, rational, conventional, and very lucky. But she is not the person, if she exists at all anywhere, to whom the health promotional effort must address itself. What the disease prevention field must address is all the rest of womankind who are not so lucky, or conservative and well placed, and who suffer what appear to be the normal human condition of multiple potentiating, possible early latent, risks. Surely it is unlikely that risk prevention would be able to turn everyone into someone much resembling our composite model. One asks then if there are not other ways of living, being, which allow for reasonable health and longevity, and which are biologically tolerant of diversity? What one needs to look at is what keeps the rest of us—with our adverse life and health histories, depressed if we are sensitive, suffering crises day to day, straying from balance and caution, never coping quite as we should—reasonably healthy?

Henry and Stephens (1977) propose for good health a combination of primate needs satisfied, coupled with a religious capacity culminating in a set of rules to live by, that they call the "cultural canon." Antonovsky (1980), inspecting the range of pathogens, incompetencies, life catastophes most of us experience, asks how it is that any of us stay alive? Or want to? He proposes that it is because of a cohesive sense of things as part of cohesive group membership, values. These are appealing summary concepts, and can be diversely held, expressed from group to group. Pluralism among small cohesive groups would allow health. One does not know if these are adequate summary concepts. It is a major research task to address the question of health maintainance in diverse groups, "pluralism" in health promotion. One asks if there are unconventional, i.e., not conforming but change responsive lifestyles, personalities, values which also constitute health maintaining patterns? How do those, whether in Bohemian groups or eccentric, iconoclastic, autonomous individuals— ever survive to venerable years?

With respect to population diversity, will there be found subgroups with high wellness, whose characteristics are quite different from the controlling successful conforming model woman which our reading of the contemporary data generates? One hopes that there will be found not simply such groups, but the elements in them which are easily cultivated through health promotion— as for example the appeal to fun or effervescent good feeling already known to be found through exercise— that tranquility attainable through meditation or an inbred "philosophy of life." We do believe it would be helpful to seek, through innovation and evaluation, ways to reduce risk in those myriad subgroups— many already at social-economic or personal disadvantage— who will not aspire to or have the stomach for yuppie or middle class virtue and chic as their health modality, and whose development of health self-direction, self-responsibility might better be molded in ways germaine to their own lives and group values. The research task then is to search within the disadvantaged or unconventional population for variables not yet identified which work, within those life contexts, to reduce risk and which appear to have the potential of being modifiable through one or another health promotional effort.

Testing Interventions

There have been three major modalities employed for change in health behavior: the behavioral-cognitive group methods so similiar in efforts against targeted behaviors such as obesity, smoking, alcoholism; the range of conventional, more psychodynamic therapies, whether individual or group, to deal with psychological features; and finally, health education, the latter as the major institutional and community approach. There are, of course, modifications, the more complex schemes of Farquhar for communities, the expert ex-patient counseling methods of the American Cancer Society, or training for BSE, or the "say no" role rehearsals for training adolescents to resist their friends' illicit drug overtures. When evaluation shows anti smoking programs for pregnant women to yield only 25% abstinence, or PMS treatment success entirely attributable to placebo effects, it is evident that there is considerable room for experimental treatments carefully evaluated as to recruitment, process, and outcome.

Since so much of risk for ob-gyn disease is associated with low SEC and few personality resources, one might well posit that social competence is a central variable. Yet how can one be competent if illiterate, or demoralized by disadvantage as an important minority of Americans, or in the UK, the Asian immigrants, are? A good test would be random assignment of large numbers of women, a heterogenous sample, all with profiles of conduct laden with risk, to several kinds of treatments, one of which might be not behavioral health as traditionally offered, but simply literacy education in the local library. Another might be assertiveness and training for direct self-esteem bolstering. Our bet is that illiterate women with initially poor health habits will, after literacy training, show an improvement in health behavior, but one equal to the specific health training for matched control groups only after several years have elapsed. One cannot assume that literacy equals health; one may propose that women become literate become more self-confident, do have a new resource allowing them to read medicine labels and find their way to the medical clinic, and out of pride become assertive enough to defend themselves against some of the societal onslaught which is stress. Assumed, that the same tough, persevering women who, at middle age, take literacy courses when offered would do the same "quick study" learning for health classes as such. We posit a class of disadvantaged ambitious, self-improving women who will benefit from whatever opportunities their restrictive environments offer.

The generation and evaluation of community health promotion methods relying on neighborhood networks, rather than formal groups and mass communication, is also to be recommended. This is, for health promotion, but an aspect of the older community development concept. It seem well worthwhile to compare neighborhoods, providing leadership to create at the street or block level women's health groups, these compared to no intervention controls. Such data as are relevant suggest it is a worthy experiment and much overdue.

Needed: Nourishment

We earlier concluded and complained that research attending to wellness and disease prevention for women is undernourished, not thriving. We are convinced there are thousands of dedicated women's health professionals who appreciate the need and would wish further knowledge in the field. Where are they to find the encouragement for that work within their own institutions if those institutions are, as is typical, offering approval and promotion for high tech surgical developments, or research on molecular biology and genetics with little attention to less reductionistic concepts applicable to obstetrical and gynecological risk prediction or treatment evaluation? And where will they find financial support? In these days of reduced support by most governments for most science, pity women's health enterprises so low on the totem pole.

We take as base line evidence for undernourishment the cultural-political values represented by insurance payments under the U.S. Federal insurance, Medicare. It is an outlandishly bad example. Reimbursement for many psychosocial-behavioral interventions is either disallowed or so insufficient as to be disallowing. The recommendations of the Institute of Medicine low birthweight prevention study took note of this deficiency. Happily, some improvement in reimbursement has followed. Nevertheless, with Medicare as the friendly standard for Federal health care support, who, as the saying goes, needs enemies? Until pilot studies of the adequacy of these revised payment systems and outcomes are undertaken, studies also attentive to the payment system risk from greedy health providers who drive up costs and from competing HMOs interested in saving money at the patient's expense, one holds our entire payments system for presentation suspect of gross inadequacy.

We are heartened by the health promotion movement and in particular by the recommendations, cited in Chapter 1, by, in the U.S., the Institute of Medicine and the Surgeon General, in the U.K. by the Health Education Council, and in Canada by the Quebec provincial authorities. Perhaps the time has come when that research will be supported which holds forth a reasonable promise to improve women's health and wellness.

Summary

Research activities bearing on disease prevention and wellness for women are insufficient and undersupported.

We have nevertheless noted several topics which may prove attractive to those new investigators who one hopes will enter the field. There is much to be done to expand the scientific basis for health promotion through the identification of risk factors and disease course, the systematization of diagnosis and prediction, and the evaluation and practice of innovative interventions at community, group, or individual levels. Please join us in the effort.

Bibliography

Abbott, B.B., Schoen, L.S. and Badia, P.   Predictable and unpredictable shock: behavioral measures of aversion and physiological measures of stress. *Psycho. Bull.* 96:45-71 (1984).

Adamson, K., Mueller-Heubach, E. and Myers, R.E.   Production of fetal asphyxia in the rhesus monkey by administration of catecholamines to the mother. *Am. J. Obstet. & Gynecol.* 109:249 (1971).

Ader, R.   Psychosomatic and psychoimmunological research. *Psychosom. Med.* 42:307-322 (1980).

Ader, R. (ed.).   *Psychoneuroimmunology.* New York: Academic Press, 1981.

Adler, N.   Psychosocial issues of therapeutic abortion. In: Youngs and Ehrhardt (eds.), *Psychosomatic Obstetrics and Gynecology*, New York: Appleton-Century-Crofts, 1980, 159-177.

Adler-Stortholz, K., et al.   A prospective study of herpes simplex virus infection in a defined population in Houston, Texas. *Am. J. Obstet. & Gynecol.* 151:582-585 (1985).

Affonson, D.   "Missing pieces"—A study of postpartum feelings. *Birth and Fam. J.* 4(4):159-164 (1977).

Ahmed, P. (ed.).   *Pregnancy, Childbirth and Parenthood: Coping with Medical Issues.* New York: Elsevier, 1981.

Ahmed, P. and Kolker, A.   Pregnancy in modern society. In: *Pregnancy, Childbirth and Parenthood: Coping with Medical Issues.* P. Ahmed (ed.), New York: Elsevier, 1981.

Ainsworth, M. S.   The development of infant-mothering attachment. In: *Review of Child Development Research* (Vol. 3)., B. Caldwell and H. Ricciuti (eds.), Chicago: University of Chicago Press, 1973.

Ainsworth, M. S. Infant-mother attachment and social development: Socialization as a product of reciprocal responsiveness to signals. In: *The Integration of the Child into the Social World.* M. Richards (ed.), Cambridge: Cambridge University Press, 1974.

Akhtan, T. and Sehgal, N. Prognostic value of a prepartum and intrapartum risk-scoring method. *Southern Med. J.* 73:411-414 (1980).

Alagna, S.W. and Redd, D.M. Predictors of proficient technique and successful lesion detection in breast self-examination. *Health Psychol.* 3:113-127 (1984).

Alberman, E. Facts and Figures. In: Chard & Richards (eds.), *Benefits and Hazards of the New Obstetrics,* London: Heinemann, 1977,

Alberman, E. Low Birthweight. In: *Perinatal Epidemiology.* M.B. Bracken (ed.), New York and London: Oxford University Press, 1984.

Alder, E.M. and Cox, J.L. Breast feeding and post-natal depression, *J. Psychosom. Res.,* 139-144 (1983).

Aldrich, C.K. A case of recurrent pseudocyesis. *Perspect. Biol. Mod.* 16:11 (1972).

Algert, S., Shragg, P. and Hollingsworth, P.R. Moderate caloric restriction in obese women with gestational diabetes. *Ob. Gyn.* 65:487-491 (1985).

Alter, M. Anencephalus, Hydrocephalus and Spinal Bifida. In: *Perinatal Epidemiology.* New York and London: Oxford University Press, 1984.

American Academy of Pediatrics Committee on Fetus and Newborn. *Standards and Recommendations for Hospital Care of Newborn Infants (5th ed.).* Evanston: American Academy of Pediatrics.

American Cancer Society. *Facts and Figures.* (February, 1985).

American College of Obstetricians and Gynecologists. News release. January 4, 1978.

American College of Obstetricians and Gynecologists. *Preventive Health Care in Obstetrics - Gynecology Residency Training.* Washington, D.C.: Department of Health and Human Services, 1985.

American College of Obstetricians and Gynecologists. *Standards for Obstetrical and Gynecological Services.* Chicago: 1974.

American Psychologist 712-719 (June 1986). Comment: letters by Deutsch; Green, Lazarus, and Folkman; Dohrenwend and Shrout, Cohen.

American Public Health Association. Position paper 7924: Alternatives in maternity care. *Am. Journal of Public Health* 70(3):310-312 (1980).

American Public Health Association. Position paper on guidelines for licensing and regulating birth centers (3rd draft). Chicago: 1982.

Amias, A.G. Sexual life after gynaecological operations. *Br. Med. J.* 2(5971):608-609 (1975) and 5972:680-681 (1975).

Ammala, P. and Kariniemi, V. Short term variability of fetal heart rate during pregnancy complicated by hypertension. *Brit. J. Obs. and Gynaecol.* 90:705-709 (1983).

Ammon, G. and Schibalstii, A.K. On the psychodynamics of premature birth and psychosomatic illness. *Dynamische Psychiat.* 10:346-359 (1977).
Angel, J.L. Human biology, health and history. Greece from first settlement until now. In: *Report to the American Philosophical Society, Year Book*, 168-172 (1954).
Andersen, B.L. Psychological Aspects of Gynaecological Cancer. In: *Psychology and Gynaecological Problems*. A. Broome and L. Wallace (eds.), London: Tavistock, 1984.
Andersen, B.L. and Hacker, N.F. Psychosexual adjustment after vulvar surgery. *Ob.-Gyn.* 62(4):457-62 (1983).
Andersen, B.L. and Hacker, N.F. Treatment for gynecologic cancer: a review of the effects on female sexuality. *Health Psychol.* 2(2):203-331 (1983).
Andersen, B.L., Karlsson, J.A., Andersen, B. and Tewfik, H.H. Anxiety and cancer treatment: response to stressful radiotherapy. *Health Psychol.* 3:535-551 (1984).
Andersen, B.L. and Jochinsen, P.R. Sexual functioning among breast cancer, gynecological cancer and healthy women. *J. Consult. Clin. Psychol.* 53 (1985).
Andersen, D.E. Behavioral stress and experimental hypertension. In: T.M. Field, P.M. McCabe, and N. Schneiderman (eds.), *Stress and Coping*, Hillsdale, N.J.: Erlbaum, 1985, 117-133.
Andersen, S.F. and Brower, L.J. A scientific survey of siblings at birth. In: D. Steward and L. Steward (eds.), *Compulsory Hospitalization* (Vol. 3). Marble Hill, Mo.: Banner Press, (1979), 877-898.
Anderson, K.O., et al. Rheumatoid arthritis: review of psychological factors related to etiology, effects and treatment. *Psychol. Bull.* 98:358-387 (1985).
Andiman, W.A and Horstmann, D.M. Congenital and Perinatal Viral Infections. In: *Perinatal Epidemiology*. M.B. Bracken (ed.), New York and London: Oxford University Press, 1984.
Andrew, G., et al. Life event stress, social support, coping style and risk of psychological impairment. *J. Nerv. Ment. Dis.* 166:307-316 (1978).
Anisman, H. and Sklar, L.S. Psychological insult and pathology: contribution of neurochemical, hormonal and immunological mechanisms. In: Steptoe and Mathews, *Health Care and Human Behavior*, New York and London: Academic Press, 1984, 1113-1146.
Antonovsky, A. *Health, Stress and Coping*. San Francisco: Jossey-Bass, 1980.
Apfel, R.J. and Sifneos, P.F. Alexithymea: concept and measurement. *Psychother. Psychosom.* 32:180-190 (1979).
Appels, A. and Mulder, P. Imminent myocardial infarction: a psychological study. *J. Human Stress* 129-134 (Fall 1984).

Appels, A. The year before myocardial infarction. In: T.M. Dembrowski, T.H. Schmidt and G. Blunchen (eds.), *Biobehavioral Bases of Coronary Heart Disease: Karger Biobehavioral Medicine Series 2.*, Basel: Karger, 1983, 18-38.

Aral, S.O., et al. Genital herpes: does knowledge lead to action? *Am. J. of Public Health* 75:69-72 (1985).

Aral, S.O., Mosher, W.D. and Cates, W. Self-reported pelvic inflammatory disease in the U.S. *Am. J. Pub. Health* 75:1216-1218 (1985).

Arms, S. *Immaculate Deception: A New Look at Women and Childbirth in America.* Boston: Houghton Mifflin, 1975.

Aro, T. Maternal diseases, alcohol consumption and smoking during pregnancy associated with reduction limb defects. *Early Hum. Dev.* 9(1):49-57 (1983).

Ashford, J.R. Policies for maternity care in England and Wales. In: S. Kitzinger and J.A. Davis (eds.), *The Place of Birth*, Oxford: Oxford University Press, 1978, 14-43.

Assaf, A.R., Cummings, M.K., Graham, S., Mettlin, C. and Marshall, J.R. Comparison of three methods of teaching women how to perform breast self examination. *Health Ed. Quart.* 12:259-272.

Assessment of the adaptive potential of the mother-infant system. *Seminars on Perinatology* (Vol. 3). New York: Grune & Stratton, 1979.

Aubrey, R.H. American College of Obstetricians and Gynecologists: Standards for safe childbearing. In: D. Steward and L. Steward (eds.), *21st Century Obstetrics Now*, Chapel Hill: National Association of Parents and Professionals for Safe Alternatives in childbirth, 1977, 15-26.

Aubrey, R.H. and Pennington, J.C. Identification and evaluation of high-risk pregnancy: the perinatal concept. *Clinical Ob.-Gyn.* 16:3-27 (1973).

Aubrey, R.H. Identification of the high risk perinatal patient. In: *Perinatal Intensive Care*, S. Aladjem and A.K. Brown (eds.), St. Louis: C.V. Mosby, 1978.

Axelrod, J. and Reisine, T.D. Stress hormones: their interaction and regulation. *Science* 224:452-459 (1984).

Backstrom, T. and Mattson, B. Correlation of symptoms in pre-menstrual tension to oestrogen and progesterone concentrations in blood plasma. *Neuro-psychobiology*, 1:80-86 (1975).

Baider, L. Time limited thematic group with post-mastectomy patients. *J. Psychosom. Res.* 28:323-330 (1984).

Bailar, J.C. Mammographic screening: a reappraisal of benefits and risks. *Clin. Ob-Gyn.* 21:1-14 (1978).

Baird, D.D. and Wilcox, A.J. Cigarette smoking and delayed conception. *JAMA* 253:2979-2983 (1985).

Baker, A.A., Morrison, M., Game, J.A., Thorpe, J.G. Admitting schizophrenic mothers with their babies. *Lancet* 2:237-239 (1961).

Baker, L.J., Dearborn, J., Hastings, J.E. and Hamburger, K. Type A behavior in women: a review. *Health Psychol.* 3:477-497 (1984).
Baker, M., Dorzab, J., Winokur, G. and Cadoret, R. Depressive disease: the effect of the postpartum state. *Biol. Psychiatry* 3:357-365 (1971).
Bakketeig, L.S.: Perinatal mortality by birth order within cohorts based on sibship size. *Br. Med. J.* 2(6192):693-6 (1979).
Bakketeig, L.S., Hoffman, H.F., Titmuss-Oakley, A.R. Perinatal Mortality. In: *Perinatal Epidemiology.* M.B. Bracken (ed.), New York and London: Oxford University Press, 1984.
Balint, M. The Doctor, His Patient and the Illness. New York: International Universities Press, 1957.
Ball, K.P. Synergism of rest factors in coronary heart disease. In: A.R. Rees and H.J. Purcell (eds.), *Disease and the Environment,* Chickester and New York: Wiley, 1982.
Ballinger, C.B. Psychiatric morbidity in the menopause: journey of a gynecological outpatient clinic. *Brit. J. Psychiat.* 131:83-89 (1977).
Banden Bos, G.R. Health financing, service utilization, and national policy: a conversation with Stan Jones. *Amer. Psychologist* 8:948-955 (1983).
Bandura, A. Self-efficacy: toward a unifying theory of behavioral change. *Psychol. Rev.* 84:191-215 (1977).
Banks, M.H., et al. Factors influencing demand for primary medical care in women aged 20-44 years: a preliminary report. *Int. J. Epid.* 4:189-195 (1975).
Barbour, A.B. The meaning of care. *Stanford MD* 2-5 (Fall 1979-Winter 1980).
Barefoot, J.C., Dahlstrom, W.G. and Williams, R.B. Hostility, CHD, incidence and total mortality: a 24-year followup of 255 physicians. *Psychosom. Med.* 45:59-63 (1983).
Barnett, B.E., Hanna, B. and Parker, G. Life event scales for obstetric groups. *J. Psychosom. Res.* 27(4):313-20 (1983).
Barrera, M. and Balls, P. Assessing social support as a preventive resource: an illustrative study. *Prevention in Human Services* 2:59-74 (1983).
Barron, S.L. and Thomson, A.M. *Obstetrical Epidemiology.* New York: Academic Press, 1983.
Barsky, A.J. Patients who amplify bodily sensations. *Ann. Internal Med.* 91:63-69 (1979).
Baruffi, et al. Definition of high risk pregnancy and prediction of their predictive validity. *Am. J. Ob-Gyn.* 148:781 (1984).
Baum, A., Taylor, S.E. and Singer, J.E. *Handbook of Psychology and Health, Vol. IV: Social Aspects of Health.* Hillsdale, New Jersey: Erlbaum, 1984.
Beck, N.C. and Hall, D. Natural childbirth: a review and analysis. *Ob.Gyn.* 52:3 (1978).
Beck, N.C., Geden, E.A. and Brouder, G.T. Preparation for labor: a historical perspective. *Psychosom. Med.* 41:243-258 (1979).

Beck, N.C. and Hall, D. Natural childbirth: a review and analysis. *Ob.-Gyn.* 52:3 (1978).

Beck, N.C., Siegel, L.J., Davidson, N.P., Bormeier, S., Breitenstein, A. and Hall, D.G. The prediction of pregnancy outcome: maternal preparation, anxiety and attitudinal sets. *J. Psychosom. Res.* 24:343-51 (1980).

Beck, N.C., Siegel, L.J., Geden, E.A. and Brouder, G.T. Labor preparation and behavioral medicine. *J. Mental Health* 9:149-163 (1980).

Becker, M. and Maiman, L. Sociobehavioral determinants of compliance with medical care recommendations. *Med. Care* 13:1 (1975).

Becker, M.H., et al. Selected psychosocial models and correlates of individual health related behavior. *Med. Care* 15 (Suppl.):27-46 (1977).

Belloc, N.B. and Breslow, L. Relationship of physical health status and health practice. *Prev. Med.* 1:409ff. (1972).

Belloc, N.B. Relationship of health practices and mortality. *Prev. Med.* 2:67-81 (1973).

Belsey, E.M., et al. Predictive factors in emotional response to abortion. *Soc. Sci. & Med.* 1977:11:71-82.

Belsey, M.A. Infertility: Prevalence, Etiology, and Natural History. In: *Perinatal Epidemiology.* M.B. Bracken (ed.), New York and London: Oxford University Press, 1984.

Benedetti, J.J., Starzy, K.P. and Frost, F. Maternal deaths in Washington state. *Ob.-Gyn.* 66:99-101 (1985).

Beral, V. and Kay, C.R. Mortality among oral contraceptive users. *Lancet* 2:727-731 (1977).

Berg, P. and Snyder, D.K. Differential diagnosis of marital and sexual distress: a multidimensional approach. *J. Sex. Marital Ther.* 7(4):290-295 (Winter 1981).

Berggren, G. and Sjostedt, S. Preinvasive carcinoma of the cervix uteri and smoking. *Acta Obstet. Gynecol. Scand.* 62(6):593-598 (1983).

Berkeley, A.S., et al. The potential of digitally inserted tampons to induce vaginal lesions. *Ob.-Gyn.* 66:31-35 (1985).

Berkman, L.F. and Syme, L. Social networks, host resistance and mortality: a nine-year followup of Alameda County residents. *Am. J. Epid.* 109:186-204 (1979).

Berkman, L.F. and Breslow, L. *Health and Ways of Living: The Alameda County Study.* New York: Oxford, 1983.

Berkman, L.F. The relationship of social networks and social support to morbidity and mortality. In: S. Cohen and S.L. Syme (eds.), *Social Support and Health,* New York: Academic Press, 1985.

Berkowitz, G.S. An epidemiologic study of preterm delivery. *Am. J. Epid.* 113:81-92 (1981).

Berkowitz, G.S., Holford, T.R. and Berkowitz, R.L. Effects of cigarette smoking, alcohol, coffee and tea consumption on preterm delivery. *Early Hum. Dev.* 7(3):239-50 (1982).

Berlin, I. *Against the Current: Essays on the History of Ideas.* New York: Viking, 1955.

Bernstein, M., Zimmerman, I.L. and Eiduson, B.T. Attachment behaviors of infants reared in alternative life styles. Paper, American Psychol. Assn., 1981.

Betz, B.J. and Thomas, C.B. Individual temperament as a predictor of health or premature disease. *Johns Hopkins Med. J.* 144:81-89 (1979).

Beverage Retailers Report, Against driving drunk, Sept. 1, 1985, Washington, D.C.

Bewley, B.R., Higgs, R.H. and Jones, A. Adolescent patients in an inner London general practice: their attitudes to illness and health care. *J. Royal College Gen. Pract.* 543-546 (1984).

Bibace, R. and Walsh, M.E. Developmental stages in children's conception of illness. In: *Health Psychology*, G.C. Stone, F. Cohen, and N. Adler (eds.), San Francisco: Jossey-Bass, 1979.

Black, D., Morris, J.N. and Townsend, P. *Inequalities in Health*, HMSO (1982).

Blazer, D. Social support and mortality in an elderly community population. *Am. J. Epid.* 115:684-694 (1982).

Bloom, L.J., Shelton, J.L. and Michaels, A.C. Dysmenorrhea and personality. *J. Pers. Assess.* 42(3):272-276 (1978).

Blum, E.M. (Spitz). The uncooperative patient: the development of a test to predict uncooperativeness in medical treatment. In: *Supplementary Studies on Malpractice*, San Francisco: California Medical Assoc., 1958.

Blum, H.J. and Keranen, G.M. *Control of Chronic Diseases in Man.* Washington, D.C.: APHA, 1966.

Blum, R. Correlations and factor analysis. In: *Drugs II: Students and Drugs*, R. Blum (ed.), San Francisco: Jossey-Bass, 101-110 (1969).

Blum, R. Normal drug use. In: *Drugs I: Society and Drugs*, R. Blum (ed.), San Francisco: Jossey-Bass, 244-276 (1969).

Blum, R., Blum, E., Garfield, E. and Magista, J.G. *Drug Education Results and Recommendations.* Boston: Lexington, 1976.

Blum, R., et al. *Utopiates: a study of use and users of LSD-25.* New York: Atherton, 1964.

Blum, R.H. *Hospitals and Patient Dissatisfaction: A Study of Factors Associated with Malpractice Rates in Hospitals.* San Francisco: California Medical Assoc., 1958.

Blum, R.H. *Management of the Doctor-Patient Relationship.* New York: McGraw-Hill, 1960.

Blum, R.H. *The Psychology of Malpractice Suits.* San Francisco: California Medical Assoc., 1958.
Blum, R.H. and Ezekiel, J. *Clinical Records for Mental Health Services.* Springfield, Ill.: Charles C. Thomas, 1962.
Blum, R.H. Case identification in psychiatric epidemiology. *Milbank Memorial Fund Quarterly* 40:253-288 (1962).
Blum, R.H. *A Commonsense Guide to Doctors, Hospitals and Medical Care.* New York: Macmillan, 1964.
Blum, R.H. Social and epidemiological aspects of psychopharmacology. In C.R.B., Joyce (ed.), *Psychopharmacology*, Philadelphia: Lippincott, 1968, 243-282.
Blum, R.H. and Downing, J.J. Staff response to innovation in a mental health service. *Am. J. Pub. Health* 60:93-108 (1964).
Blum, R.H. and Blum, E.M. *Health and Healing in Rural Greece.* Stanford: Stanford University Press and Oxford: Oxford University Press, 1965.
Blum, R.H. and Blum, E.M. *Alcoholism: Modern Psychological Approaches and Treatment.* San Francisco: Jossey-Bass, 1967.
Blum, R.H., et al. *Horatio Algers Children: Role of the Family: The Origin and Prevention of Drug Use.* San Francisco: Jossey-Bass, 1972.
Blum, R.H., Herxheimer, A., Stenzl, K. and Woodcock, J. *Pharmaceuticals and Health Policy.* London: Croom Helm, 1982.
Blum, R.H., Bewley, B., Chamberlain, G., Richards, M. and Speller, M. *Improving Women's Health*, proposal submitted to the Health Promotion Research Trust, University of Cambridge Medical School, 1984.
Blum, R.H. and Haynal, A. Psychiatrie sociale aux Etats-Unis: evolution contemporaine. *Medecine et Hygiene* 43: 1893-1902 (1985).
Board on Mental Health and Behavioral Medicine, Institute of Medicine. Research on mental illness and addictive disorders: progress and prospects. Supplement to the *Am. J. of Psychiat.* 142 (1985).
Bonica, J.J. and Albe-Fessard, D.G. *Advances in Pain Research & Therapy, Vol. I.* Proceedings of the 1st World Congress on Pain, New York: Raven Press, 1976.
Boring, C.C., et. al. Patient attitude toward physician consent in epidemiological research. Am. J. Pub. Health 74:1406-1408 (1984).
Bosley, A.R., Sibert J.R. and Newcombe, R.G. Effects on maternal smoking on fetal growth and nutrition. *Arch. Dis. Child.* 56(9):727-729 (1981).
Bottoms, S.F., Rosen, M.G. and Sokol, R.J. The increase in the cesarean birth rate. *N. Engl. J. Med.* 302:559-563 (1980).
Bottom, S. Smoking. In: J.T. Queenan and J.C. Hobbins, *Protocols for High Risk Pregnancies*, Oradale, N.J.: Med. Econ. Books, 1983, 14-16.
Bourne, S. The psychological effects of stillbirths on women and their doctors. *J. Royal College Gen. Practitioners* 6:103-112 (1968).

Boyce, W.T., et al. Social and cultural factors in pregnancy complications among Navajo women. *Am. J. Epid.* 124:242-253 (1986).
Boyle, C.A., et al. Caffeine consumption and fibrocystic breast disease: a case controlled epidemiological study. *J. Natl. Cancer Inst.* 72:1015-1019 (1984).
Brackbill, Y. Obstetrical medication and infant behavior. In: J.D. Osofsky (ed.), *Handbook of Infant Development.* New York: John Wiley & Sons, 76-125 (1979).
Bracken, M.B. A causal model of psychosomatic reactions to vacuum aspiration abortion. *Soc. Psychiat.* 13:135-145 (1978).
Bradley, C., Ross, S. and Warnyca, J. A prospective study of mothers' attitudes and feelings following cesarean and vaginal births. *Birth: Issues in Perinatal Care and Education* 10:79-83 (1982).
Bradley, L.A. and van der Heider, L.H. Pain-related correlates of MMPI profile subgroups among back pain patients. *Health Psychol.* 3(2): 156-174 (1984).
Branch, L.G. and Jette, A.M. Personal health practices and mortality among the elderly. *Am. Journal of Pub. Health* 74:1126-1129 (1984).
Brandt, A.M. *No Magic Bullet: A Social History of Venereal Disease in the United States Since 1880.* New York and London: Oxford University Press, 1985.
Brazelton, T.B. and Robey, J.S. Instruments and methods: screening for the patient at risk for postpartum depression. *Am. Col. Obstet. & Gynecol.* 52:731- 736 (1978).
Brazelton, T.B. and Robey, J.S. Observations of neonatal behavior: the effect of perinatal variables, in particular that of maternal medication. *J. Amer. Acad. Child Psychiatr.* 4:613-637 (1965).
Braverman, J. and Roux, J.F. Instruments and methods: screening for the patient at risk for postpartum depression. *Am. Col. Obstet. & Gynecol.* 52:731- 736 (1978).
Brazie, J., Searls, D. and Lubchenco, L. Unpublished data, 1975. Cited in: L. Lubchenco (ed.), *The High Risk Infant.* Philadelphia: Saunders, 1976, 114 ff.
Brena, S.F., et al. Chronic pain as a learned experience. In: Ng, L.K., *New Approaches to the Treatment of Chronic Pain,* NIDA, Res.-Mngr. #36, Department of Health, Education and Welfare, 1983, 76-83.
Brenner, B.A. and McCauley, C.R. Quality of life pressures: hospital interview versus home questionnaire. *Health Psychol.* 5:171-177 (1986).
Brett, E.A. and Ostroff, R. Imagery and posttraumatic stress disorder: an overview. *Am. J. Psychiat.* 142:417-424 (1985).
Brew, T.H. *Metabolic Toxemia of Late Pregnancy and Disease of Malnutrition.* Springfield, Ill.: Charles C. Thomas, 1966.

Bridges, R.S. and Grimm, C.T. Reversal of morphine disruption of maternal behavior by concurrent treatment with the opiate antagonist naloxone. *Science* 218:166-168 (1982).

British Medical Journal, Editorial, Home or hospital, 2:6091, 845-846 (1977).

British Medical Journal, Enigmatic pelvic pain, 6144: 1041-1042 (October 1978).

Broadhead, W.E., et al. The epidemiological evidence for a relationship between social support and health. *Am. J. Epid.* 117:521-527 (1983).

Brockington, L.F. and Kumar, R. *Motherhood and Mental Health.* London: Academic Press, 1982.

Brockington, I.F. Puerperal psychosis: phenomena and diagnosis. *Archives of Gen. Psychiatr.* 38(7):829-833 (July 1981).

Brockington, L.F. and Kumar, R. *Motherhood and Mental Health.* London: Academic Press, 1982.

Brook, R.H., Williams, R.N. and Avery A.D. Quality assurance today and tomorrow. *Annals Int. Med.* 85:6 (1976).

Brooks-Gunn, J. Differentiating premenstrual symptoms and syndromes. *Psychosom. Med.* 48:385-387 (1986).

Brotman, A.W. and Stern, T.A. Osteoporosis and pathological fratures in anorexia nervosa. *Am. J. Psychiat.* 142:495-498 (1985).

Broussard, E.R. Neonatal prediction and outcome. *Child Psychiatr. & Hum. Develop.*, 7:85-93 (1976).

Brown, E., Bain, J., Lerner P. and Shaul, D. Psychological, hormonal, and weight disturbances in functional amenorrhea. *Can. J. Psychiat.* 28:624-628 (1983).

Brown, E. and Barglow, P. Pseudocyesis: a paradigm for psychophysiological interaction. *Arch. Gen. Psychiat.* 24:221 (1971).

Brown, G.W. and Harris, T. *Social Origins of Depression.* London: Tanistock, 1978.

Brown, R.A. and Lewinsohn, P.M. A psychoeducational approach to the treatment of depression: comparison of group, individual and minimal contact procedures. *J. Consult. Clin. Psychol.* 5:774-783 (1984).

Brown, S.S. Can low birth weight be prevented? *Family Planning Perspectives* 17:112-118 (1985).

Brown, Z.A., et al. Genital herpes in pregnancy: risk factors associated with recurrences and asymptomatic viral shedding. *Am. J. Ob-Gyn.* 153:24-30 (1985).

Browne, H. and Isaacs, G. Frontier nursing service. *Am. J. Ob-Gyn.* 124:14-17 (1976).

Brownell, K.D., et al. Weight loss competitions at the work site: impact on weight, morale and cost effectiveness. *Am. J. of Pub. Health* 74:1283-1288 (1984).

Bruhn, J.G., Paredes, A., Adsett, C.A. and Wolf, S. Psychological predictors of sudden death in myocardial infarction. *J. Psychosom. Res.* 18:187-191 (1974).

Buck, C., et al. The effect of single prenatal and natal complication upon the development of children with mature birthweight. A paper given at 4th European Conf. Prenatal Medicine, Prague, August, 1974.

Buckley, J.D., Doll, R., Harris, R.W.C., Vessey, M.P. and Williams P.T. Case control study of the husbands of women with dysplasia or carcinoma of the cervix of the uterus. *Lancet* 2:1010-10014 (November 1981).

Budman, S.H., Demby, A. and Feldstein, M.L. Insight into reduced use of medical services after psychotherapy. *Prof. Psychol.* 15:353-361 (1984).

Buehler, J.W., Schulz, K.F., Grimes, D.A. and Hogue, C.J.R. The risk of serious complications from induced abortion: do personal characteristics make a difference? *Am. J. Ob-Gyn.:* 153:14-20 (1985).

Bullen, B.A., Skrimar, G.S., Beitins, I.Z., Von Mering, G., Turbull, B.A. and McArthur, J.W. Induction of menstrual disorders by strenuous exercise in untrained women. *N. Eng. J. Med.* 312:1349-1353 (1985).

Burnell, G.M., Dworsky, W.A., Harrington, R.L. Post-abortion group therapy. *Am. J. Psychiat.* 129:134-137 (1972).

Bureau of the Census. Money income and poverty states of families and persons in the United States, 1984. (Advance report) #149, P-16, 1985.

Burnett, C.A., Jones, J.A., Rooks, J., Chong, H.C., Tyler, C.W., Miller, C.A. *Home Delivery and Neonatal Mortality in North Carolina, 1974-1976: A Closer Look.* Atlanta: U.S. Department of Health, Education and Welfare, Public Health Service, Center for Disease Control, Bureau of Epidemiology.

Burnett, C.A., Jones, J.A., Rooks, J., Chong, H.C., Tyler, C.W., Miller, C.A. Home delivery and neonatal mortality in North Carolina. *JAMA* 244(24):2741- 2745 (1980).

Burnham, J.D. American medicine's golden age: What happened to it? *Science* 215:1474-1479 (March 19, 1982).

Bush, J.W., Patrick, D.L., Chen, M.M. Toward an operational definintion of health. *J. Health Soc. Behav.* 14:6-23 (1973).

Bush, J.W. and Chen, M.M. Health status measures, policy and biomedical research. In: *What Is It Worth,* S. Muskin (ed.), New York: Pergamon, 1979, 15- 41.

Bush, J.W., Kaplan, R.M. and Berry, C.C. A standardizer quality of well-being scale for cost effectiveness and social decision analysis in health. *Medical Care* (1981).

Buss, D.M. Human mate selection. *Am. Scientist* 73:47-51 (1985).

Butler, N.R. and Bonham, D.G. *Perinatal mortality: the first report of the 1958 British Perinatal Mortality Survey.* Edinburgh: E. & S. Livingstone, 1963.

Butler, N.R. and Alderman, E.D. *Perinatal Problems: The Second Report of the 1958 British Perinatal Mortality Survey.* Edinburgh, E. & S. Livingstone, 1969.

Butler, W. and Brix, K. Paper presented at APHA meeting, September 30, 1986.

Butt, A.R. A method for better physician-patient communication. *Annals Int. Med.* 86:478-480 (1977).

Butterfield, L.J. Home delivery protest. *Am. Acad. Pediatrics* 8 (1978).

Butterfield, W.J.H. *Priorities in Medicine.* Nuffield Provincial Hospitals Trust, 1968.

Byrne, D.G., Rosenman, R.H., Schiller, E. and Chesney, M. Consistency and variation among instruments purporting to measure the Type A behavior pattern. *Psychosom. Med.* 47:242-261 (1985).

Byrne, D., Steinberg, M. and Schwartz, M. Relationship between repression-sensitization and physical illness. *J. Abnorm. Psychol.* 73:154-155 (1968).

Cahill, C. and Akil, H. Plasma beta-endorphin-like immunoreactivity, self reported pain perception and anxiety levels in women during pregnancy and labor. *Life Science* 31(16-17):1871-1873 (1982).

Calden, G., et al. Psychosomatic factors in the rate of recovery from tuberculosis. *Psychosomatic Medicine* 22:345-355 (1960).

Campbell, P.A. and Cohen, J.J. Effects of stress on the immune response in T.M. Field, P.M. McCabe and M. Schneiderman (eds.), *Stress and Coping,* Hillsdale, N.J.: Erlbaum, 1985, 135-145.

Campbell, J.L. and Winokur, G. Postpartum affective disorders: selected biological aspects. In: *Postpartum Psychiatric Disorders,* D.G. Inwood, Washington, D.C.: American Psychiatric Press, 1985, 20-39.

Carmody, T.P., et al. Type A behavior: attentional style and symptom reporting among adult men and women. *Health Psychology* 1:45-61 (1984).

Carnes, J.W. Psychosocial disturbances during and after pregnancy. *Postgraduate Medicine* 73(1):135-141, 144-145 (1983).

Carrie, C.M. Reproductive symptoms: interrelations and determinants. *Psychol. of Women Quart.* 6:174-186 (1981).

Cartwright, A. *Parents and Family Planning Services.* London: Routledge Kegan Paul, 1970.

Cartwright, A. Mother's experience of induction. *Br. Med. J.* 2(6039):745-749 (1977).

Cartwright, A. *Health Surveys.* King Edward's Hospital Fund for London, King's Fund Publishing Office, 1983.

Carver, C.S. and Scheier, M.F. Self consciousness, expectancies and the coping process. In: T.M. Field, P.M. McCabe, N. Schneiderman (eds.), *Stress and Coping,* Hillsdale, N.J.: Erlbaum, 1985, 305-330.

Capone, M.A., Good, R.S., Westie, K.S. and Jacobson, A.F. Psychosocial rehabilitation of gynecologic oncology patients. *Arch. Phys. Med. Rehabil.* 61(3):128-32 (1980).

Case, R.B., Heller, S.S., Case, N.B. and Moss, A.J. Type A behavior and survival after acute myocardial infarction. *N. Eng. J. Med.* 312:737-741 (1985).

Cassell, J. The contribution of the social environment to host resistance. *Am. J. Epid.* 104:107-123 (1976).

Cates, W. Legal abortion: the public and health record. *Science* 215:1586-1590 (1982).

Center for Disease Control. *Morbidity and Mortality Weekly Reports: Annual Summary, 1982.* December 1983.

Chalmers, B. Behavioral associations of pregnancy complications. *J. Psychosom. Ob-Gyn.* 3:27-39 (1984).

Chalmers, B. Psychosocial factors and obstetrical complications. *Psychol. Med.* 13:333-339 (1983).

Chalmers, D.M., Levi, A.J., Chanarin, I., North, W.R., Meader, T.W. Mean cell volume in a working population: the effects of age, smoking, alcohol and oral contraception. *Br. J. Haematol.* 43(4):631-636 (1979).

Chalmers, I., Lawson, J.G., Turnbull, A.C. Evaluation of different approaches to obstetric care. *Brit. J. Ob-Gyn.* 83:930-933 (1976).

Chalmers, I., Oakley, A., McFarlane, A. Perinatal health services: an immodest proposal. *Br. Med. J.* 280(7217):842-845 (1980).

Chalmers, I. and Richards, M.P. Intervention and causal inference in obstetrical practice. In: *Benefits and Hazards of the New Obstetrics,* T. Chard and M. Richards (eds.), London: Heinemann, 1977.

Chamberlain, G. and Garcia J. Pregnant women at work. *The Lancet* 228-230 (January 1983).

Chamberlain, G. and Dewhurst, J. *Obstetrics and Gynecology.* London: Pittman, 1984.

Chao, S. The role of risk factors in the management of pregnancy. Paper, Am. Public Health Assn., 1978.

Chapman, R.M., Sutcliffe, S.B., Malpas, J.S. Cytotoxic-induced ovarian failure in Hodgkins' disease. II. Effects on sexual dysfunction. *JAMA* 26:242(17):1882-1884 (1979).

Chard, T. and Richards, M. *Benefits and Hazards of the New Obstetrics.* London: Heinemann, 1977.

Chasnoff, I.J., Burns, W.J., Schnoll, S.H. and Burns, K.A. Cocaine use in pregnancy. *N. Eng. J. Med.* 313:666-669 (1985).

Cheek, D. Maladjustment patterns apparently related to imprinting at birth. *Am. J. Clin. Hypnosis* 18:75-82 (1975).

Chelune, G.J. and Waring, E.M. Nature and assessment of intimacy. In: McReynolds and Chelune, *Advances in Psychological Assessment, Vol. 6*, San Francisco: Jossey-Bass, 1984, 277-311.
Chesney, M. 1985, personal communication.
Chesney, M.A. Occupational setting and coronary prone behavior in men and women. In: T.J. Dembrowski, T.H. Schmidt and G. Blunchen (eds.), *Biobehavioral Bases of Coronary Heart Disease: Karger Biobehavioral Medicine Series 2*, Basel: Karger, 1983, 79-90.
Chesney, M., Black, G.W., Chadwick, J.N. and Rosenman, R.H. Physiological correlates of the Type A behavior pattern. *J. Behavior Med.* 4:217-230 (1981).
Chisholm, J.S. *Navajo Infancy: An Ethnological Study of Child Development.* New York: Aldine, 1983.
Christensen, J.F. Assessment of stress: environmental, intrapersonal and outcome issues. In: P. McReynolds, *Advances in Psychological Assessment, Vol. 5*, San Francisco: Jossey-Bass, 1981, 62-123.
Christenson, W.W. and Hinkle, L.E. Differences in illness and prognostic signs in two groups of young men. *JAMA* 177:247-253 (1961).
Chng, P.K. and Hall, M.H. Appraisal of outpatient antenatal care in a teaching hospital. In: I. Chalmers and M. Enkin (eds.), *Effectiveness and Satisfaction in Antenatal Care*, London, Heinemann, 1982.
Clark, M.M. *Health in the Mexican American Culture.* Berkeley: University of California Press, 1952.
Clark, S.D., Jr., Zabin, L.S. and Hardy, J.B. Sex, contraception and parenthood: experience and attitudes among urban black young men. *Fam. Plann. Perspect.* 16(2):77-82 (1984).
Clarke, E.A., et al. Cervical dysplasia: association with sexual behavior, smoking and oral contraceptive use. *Am. J. Ob-Gyn.* 151:612-616 (1985).
Clarke, E.A., Morgan, R.W. and Newman, A.M. Smoking as a risk factor in cancer of the cervix: additional evidence from a case-control study. *Am. J. Epidemiol.* 115(1):59-66 (1982).
Clymer, R., Baum, A. and Krantz, D.S. Preference for self care and involvement in health care. In: A. Baum, S. Taylor and J.E. Singer, *Handbook of Psychology and Health, Vol. IV*, Hillsdale, N.J.: Erlbaum, 1984, 149-166.
Cnattinguis, S., Axelsson, O., Eklund, G., and Lindmark, G. Smoking, maternal age and fetal growth. *Ob-Gyn* 66:449-452 (1985).
Cohen, D.R. and Henderson, J.B. *A Minister for Prevention.* Health Economics Research Unit, University of Aberdeen (1983).
Cohen, F. Personality, stress and the development of physical illness. In: G.C. Stone, F. Cohen and N.N. Adler (eds.), *Health Psychology*, San Francisco: Jossey-Bass Publishers, 1979, 77-111.

Cohen, F. and Lazarus, R.S. Coping with the stresses of illness. In: G.C. Stone, F. Cohen and N.N. Adler (eds.), *Health Psychology*, San Francisco: Jossey-Bass Publishers, 1979, 217-254.
Cohen S. Marijuana research; selected recent findings. Drug and Alcoholism Newsletter. Vista Hill Foundation, January 1986.
Cohen, S. and Syme, S.L. *Social Support and Health.* New York: Academic Press, 1985.
Cohen, S. and Wells, T.A. Stress, social support and the buffering hypothesis. *Psychol. Bull.* 98:310-357 (1985).
Collington, E.M., Breck, B.M., House, J.S. and Hawthorne, V.M. Psychosocial factors and blood pressure in the Michigan statewide blood pressure survey. *Am. J. Epid.* 121:515-529 (1985).
Commission on Chronic Illness. *Chronic Illness in a Large City: The Baltimore Study, 1954.* Cambridge: Harvard University Press, 1957.
Committee on Perinatal Health. *Toward Improving the Outcome of Pregnancy.* White Plains, New York: National Foundation of March of Dimes, 1976.
Committee to Study Alternative Birthing. *A Report to the 1978 Legislature.* Sacramento: State of California Health & Welfare Agency, Department of Health, December 1977.
Cooke, D.J. A Psychosocial Study of the Climacteric. In: *Psychology and Gynaecological Problems.* B.A. Broome and L. Wallace (eds.), London: Tavistock, 1984.
Cooperative Birth Center Network. *Recommendations, Rationale, and Sample Regulations for Licensure of Birth Centers.* Box 1, Route 1, Perkomenville, Pa., 18074.
Coppotella, H.C. and Orleans, C.T. Partner support and other determinants of smoking cessation maintenance among women. *J. Consult. Clin. Psychol.* 53:455-460 (1985).
Costa, P.T. and McCrae, R.R. Hypochondriasis, neuroticism and aging. *Am. Psychol.* 40:19-28 (1985).
Council on Scientific Affairs. Medical evaluations of healthy persons. *JAMA* 249:1626-1633 (1983).
Cox, C.A., Fox, J.S., Zinkin, P.S. Mathews, A.E.B. Critical appraisal of domiciliary obstetric and neonatal practice. *Brit. Med. Jr.* 1:84-86 (1976).
Cox, D. Behavior modification and diabetes, cited in *Psychol. Today* 12 (February 1985).
Cox, D.J., et al. The relationship between psychological stress and insulin dependent diabetic blood glucose control. *Health Psychol.* 3:63-75 (1984).
Craig, T.K.J. and Brown, G.W. Life events, meaning and physical illness. In: A. Steptoe and A. Mathews (eds.), *Health Care and Human Behavior*, New York and London: Academic Press, 1984, pp. 7-37.

Crandon, A.J. Maternal anxiety and obstetrical complications. *J. Psychosom. Res.* 23:109-111 (1979).

Creasey, R.K., Gummer, B. and Liggins, G.C. System for predicting spontaneous preterm birth. *Ob-Gyn.* 55:692-695 (1980).

Creasey, R.K. Threatened preterm labor. In: J.T. Queenan and J.C. Hobbins, *Protocols for High Risk Pregnancies*, Oradale, N.J.: Med. Econ. Books, 1983, pp. 206-209.

Cromwell, R.L. and Levenkron, J.C. Psychological Care of Acute Coronary Patients. In: A. Steptoe and A. Mathews, (eds.), *Health Care and Human Behavior*, New York and London: Academic Press, 1984, pp. 209-229.

Crowe, M. Some common and uncommon health and medical problems. In: *The New Our Bodies, Ourselves*. New York: Simon and Schuster, 1985, pp. 475-552.

Crowley, T.J., Wagner, J.C., Zerbe, G. and McDonald, M. Naltrexine-induced dysphoria in former opioid addicts. *Am. J. Psychiat.* 142:1081-1084 (1985).

Crue, B.L., et al. The continuing crisis in pain research. In: W.L. Smith et al., *Pain Meaning and Management*, New York: Spectrum, 1980, pp. 1-19.

Cummings, H. News report: *American Psychological Assn. Monitor*, July 1985.

Currie, B.F. and Beasley, J.W. Health promotion in the medical encounter. In: R.B. Taylor, J.R. Ureda and J.W. Denham, *Health Promotion: Principles and Clinical Applications*, Norwalk, Connecticut: Appleton-Century-Crofts, 1982, pp. 143-160.

Cushner, I.M. Maternal behavior and perinatal risk: alcohol, smoking and drugs. *Annual Rev. Public Health* 2:201-218 (1981).

Cyr, R.M., et al. Changing patterns of birth asphyxic and trauma over 20 years. *Am. J. Ob-Gyn.* 148:490-498 (1984).

Daniels, G.E. and Davidoff, E. The mental aspects of TB. *Am. Rev. of Tuberculosis* 62:532-578 (1950).

Darney, P.D. *Birthing Alternatives: Are There Differences in Outcome?* Oregon: Program for Reproductive Health, Oregon State Health Division.

Darney P.D. and Rooks, J. Unpublished working paper, 1979.

Darney, P.D. and Rooks, J. Bios: A study to answer questions about out-of-hospital birth. Paper, American Public Health Association, November 6, 1979.

Davidson, P.O. and Davidson, S.M. (eds.) *Behavioral Medicine: Changing Health Life-styles*. New York: Brunner/Mazel (1980).

Davies, A.M. and Dunlop, W. Hypertension in pregnancy. In: S.L. Barron and A.M. Thomson, *Obstetrical Epidemiology*, New York: Academic Press, 1983, pp. 167-208.

Davies, J.M, Latto, I.P., Jones, J.G., Veale, A. and Wardrop, C.A. Effects of stopping smoking for 48 hours on oxygen availability from the blood: a study on pregnant women. *Br. Med. J.* 2(6186):355-356 (1979).

Davies, M. "You've got a lovely baby, what more do you want?" *J. Pers. Assess.* 43(5):536-540 (1979).

Davis, E. *A Guide to Midwifery, Heart and Hands.* Santa Fe: N.M.: John Muir, 1981.

Davis, S.A. Maternal anxiety during pregnancy and childbirth anomalies. *Psychosom. Med.* 24:464:469 (1963).

Day, Lorber, Liu and Muller. Social and economic factors. In: S.L. Romney et al., *Gynecology and Obstetrics: The Health Care of Women,* New York: McGraw-Hill, 1975.

DeClercq, E.R. and Darney, P.D. Out-of-hospital birth in U.S.A., 1978: attendant and demographic characteristics of mothers. Unpublished, 1982.

DeGeorge, F.V., Nesbitt, R.E., Aubry, R.H. High-risk obstetrics: An evaluation of the effects of intensified care on pregnancy outcome. *Am. J. Obstet. Gyncol.* 111(5):650-657 (1971).

DeJong, R.N., Shy, K.K. and Carr, K.C. An out-of-hospital birth center using university referral. *Ob-Gyn.* 58(6):703-707 (1981).

de la Fuente, J.R. and Rosenbaum, A.H. Prolactin in psychiatry. *Am. J. Psychiatry* 138:9 (1981).

DeLeon, P.H. and Pallak, M.S. Public health and psychology. *Am. Psychol.* 37:934-935 (1982).

DeLongis, A., et al. Relationship of daily hassles and major life events to health status. *Health Psychol.* 1:119-136 (1982).

Dembrowski, T.J., Schmidt, T.H. and Blumchen, G. (eds.). *Biobehavioral Bases of Coronary Heart Disease: Karger Biobehavioral Medicine Series 2.* Basel: Karger, 1983.

Dembrowski, T.M. and MacDougall, J.M. Beyond global type A: relationships of paralinguistic attributes, hostility and anger. In: T.M. Field, P.M. McCabe and N. Schneiderman (eds.), *Stress and Coping,* Hillsdale, N.J., Erlbaum, 1985, 223- 242.

Dembrowski, T.M., MacDougall, J.M. and Musante, L. Desirability of control versus locus of control: relationship to paralinguistics in the Type A interview. *Health Psychol.* 3:14-26 (1984).

Demopoulos, R.I., Seltzer, V., Dubin, N. and Gutman, E. The association of parity and marital status with the development of ovarian carcinoma: clinical implications. *Ob.-Gyn.* 54(2):150-155 (1979).

Denney, D.R. and Gerrard, M. Behavioral treatments of primary dysmenorrhea: a review. *Behaviour Research & Therapy* 19(4):303-312 (1981).

Depue, R.A. and Monroe, S.M. Conceptualization and measurement of human disorder in life stress research: the problem of chronic disturbance. *Psychol. Bull.* 99:36-51 (1986).

Derogatus, L.R. and Kouslesis, S.M. An approach to evaluation of sexual problems in the cancer patient. *CA - Cancer J. Clin.* 31:46-50 (1981).

Detels, R. and Breslow, L. *Oxford Book of Public Health, Volume I: History Determinants, Scope and Strategies*, Holland, W.W., Detels, R. and Knox, G. (eds.), New York and London: Oxford University Press, 1984, pp. 20-32.

Dick-Read, G. *Childbirth Without Fear* (2nd rev. ed.). New York: Harper and Row, 1970.

DiMatteo, M.R. and DiNicola, D.D. *Achieving Patient Compliance*. New York: Pergamon, 1982.

Dingley, E.F. Birthplace alternatives. *Oregon Health Bulletin* 5:1-4 (October 1977).

Dingley, E.F. Birthplace and attendants: Oregon's alternative experience, 1977. *Women & Health* 4(3):239-253 (Fall 1979).

DiNichola, D.D. and DiMatteo, M.R. Practitioners, patients and compliance with medical regimens: a social psychological perspective. In: A. Baum, S.E. Taylor and J.E. Singer, *Handbook of Psychology and Health, Vol. IV, Social Psychological Aspects of Health*, Hillsdale, N.J.: Erlbaum, 1984, pp. 55-84.

Disbrow, M.S. (ed.). Meeting consumers' demands for maternity care. *Proceedings of a Conference for Nurses and Other Health Professionals, September 16, 1972.* Seattle, University of Washington Press, 1973.

Dodd, B.G. and Parsons, A.D. Psychosexual Problems. In: *Psychology and Gynaecological Problems*. B.A. Broome and L. Wallace (eds.), London: Tavistock, 1984.

Doering, P. and Steward R. The extent and character of drug consumption during pregnancy. *JAMA* 239(9):843-846 (1978).

Doering, S. and Entwisle, D.R. Preparation during pregnancy and ability to cope with labor and delivery. *Amer. J. Orthopsychiat.* 45(5):825-837 (1975).

Dohrenwend, B.P. and Shrout, P.E. "Hassles" in the conceptualization and measurement of life stress variables. *Am. Psychol.* 40:780-785 (1985).

Dohrenwend, B.S. and Dohrenwend, B.P. *Stressful Life Events: Their Nature and Effects*. New York: Wiley and Sons, 1974.

Donahoe, C.P., Lin, D.H., Kirchenbaum, D.S. and Keesey, R.E. Metabolic consequences of dieting and exercise in the treatment of obesity. *J. Consult. Clin. Psychol.* 52:827-836 (1984).

Donnelley, F.J., et al. Parental, fetal and environmental factors in perinatal mortality. *Amer. J. Ob.-Gyn.* 74:1245 (1957).

Donovan, J.W. Randomized controlled trial of anti-smoking advice in pregnancy. *Brit. J. Prev. & Social Med.* 31:6-12 (1977).

Dooher, M.E. Lamaze method of childbirth. *Nursing Research* 29(4):220-224 (1980).

Doress, P.B. Women growing older. In: *The New Our Bodies, Ourselves*. New York: Simon and Schuster, 1985, pp. 435-472.

Dow, T.G., Rooney, P.J. and Spence, M. Does anaemia increase the risks to the fetus caused by smoking in pregnancy? *Br. Med. J.* 4(5991):253-254 (1975).

Drake, T.S. and Redway, D.R. Spontaneous pregnancy during the infertility evaluation. *Fertil. Steril.* 30(1):36-38 (1978).

Drossman, D.A. Patients with psychogenic abdominal pain: six years observation in the medical setting. *Am. J. Psychiat.* 139:1549-1557 (1982).

Dryfoos, J.G. A time for new thinking about teenage pregnancy. *AJPH* 75:13-14 (1985).

Dubos, R. *Mirage of Health.* New York: Harper, 1959.

Duff, R.S. and Hollingshead, A.B. *Sickness and society.* New York: Harper and Row, 1968.

Dunbar, F. *Mind and Body: Psychosomatic Medicine.* New York: Random House, 1947.

Duncan, C.H. and Taylor, H.C. A psychosomatic study of pelvic congestion. *Am. J. Ob-Gyn.* 64:1-12 (1952).

Duncan, G.L. *Years of Poverty, Years of Plenty.* Ann Arbor: University of Michigan, Institute for Social Research, 1984.

Durant, R.H., Jay, M.S., Linder, C.W., Shoffitt, T and Litt, I. Influence of psychosocial factors on adolescent compliance with oral contraceptives. *J. Adolesc. Health Care* 5(1)1-6 (1984).

Dyk, R.B. and Sutherland, N.M. Adaptation of the spouse and other family members to the colostomy patient. *Cancer* 8:123-138 (1956).

Eddy, D.M. Probabilistic reasoning in clinical medicine. In: D. Kahneman, P. Slovie and A. Tversky (eds.), *Judgment Under Uncertainty: Heuristics and Biases,* Cambridge: Cambridge University Press, 1982.

Edwards, L.E., Barrada, M.I., Tatreau, R.W. and Hakanson, E.Y. A simplified antepartum risk-scoring system. *Ob-Gyn.* 54(2):237-240 (1979).

Effer, S.B. Management of high-risk pregnancy: Report of a combined obstetrical and neonatal intensive care unit. *Can. Med. Assoc. J.* 101:55 (1969).

Egeland, B. and Deinard, A. A prospective study of the antecedents of child abuse. Unpublished final report. University of Minnesota, 1979.

Eiduson, B.T. Comparative socialization practices in traditional and alternative families. In: M.E. Lamb (ed.), *Nontraditional Families: Parenting and Child Development,* Hillsdale, N.J.: Erlbaum, 1982, 315-346.

Eiduson, B.T. and Weisner, T. Alternative family styles: effects on young children. In: J. Stevens and M. Mathews (eds.), *Mother/Child/Father/Child Relationships,* Washington, D.C.: NAEYC, 1978.

Eisenberg, L. The ambiguities of psychosomatic medicine medicine. *J. Psychosom. Ob-Gyn.* 3:115-127 (1984).

Eisenberg, L. Health care: for patients or for profits. *Am. J. Psychiat.* 143:1015-1020 (1986).

Eisenberg, L. Is health a state of mind? *N. Eng. J. Med.* 301:1282-1283 (1979).
Eisenberg, L. Prevention: rhetoric and reality. *J. Royal Soc. Med.* 77:268-279 (1984).
Eisenberg, L. and Parron, D. Strategies for the prevention of mental disorders. In: The Surgeon General's Report on Health Promotion and Disease Prevention, 1979, 135-155.
Eisner, V., Brazie, J.V., Pratt, M.W. and Hexter, A.C. The risk of low birthweight. *Am. J. Pub. Health* 69(9):887-893 (1979).
Ellenberg, J. and Koren, Z. Infertility and depression. *Int. J. Fertil.* 27(4):219-223 (1982).
Elkin, S.A. Health care for women: a prescription for change. In: D.D. Youngs and A.A. Erhardt (eds.), *Psychosomatic Obstetrics and Gynecology*, New York: Appleton-Century-Crofts, 1980, 83-92.
Ellison, P.J. and Lager, C. Exercise induced menstrual disorder. *N. Eng. J. Med.* 313:826 (1985).
Elstein, A.S. and Bordage, G. Psychology of clinical reasoning. In: G.C. Stone et al. (eds.), *Health Psychology*, San Francisco: Jossey-Bass, 1979, pp. 333-367.
Elster, A.B. The effect of maternal age, parity and prenatal care on perinatal outcome in adolescent mothers. *Am. J. Ob. Gyn.* 149:845-847 (1984).
Engel, B.T. Stress is a noun. No, a verb. No, an adjective. In: T.M. Field, P.M. McCabe and N. Schneiderman (eds.), *Stress and Coping*, Hillsdale, N.J.: Erlbaum, 1955, 3-12.
Engel, G.L. The need for a new medical model: a challenge for biomedicine. *Science* 196:129-136 (1977).
Enkin, M. and Chalmers, I. *Effectiveness and Satisfaction in Antenatal Care.* London: Heinemann, 1982.
Epstein, L.H. The direct effects of compliance on health outcome. *Health Psychol.* 3:385-393 (1984).
Epstein, L.H., Wing, R.R. Koeske, R. and Valoski, A. Effects of diet plus exercise on weight change in parents and children. *J. Consult. Clin. Psychol.* 52:429-437 (1984).
Erb, L., Hill, G. and Houston, D. Survey of patients' attitudes toward their cesarean births in Manitoba hospitals. *Birth: Issues in Prenatal Care & Education*, 10:85-91 (1983).
Ericson, A., Kallen, B. and Westerholm, P. Cigarette smoking as an etiologic factor in cleft lip and palate. *Am. J. Obstet. Gynecol.* 135(3):348-351 (1979).
Erickson, M.T. The relationship between psychological variables and specific complications of pregnancy, labor and delivery. *J. Psychosom. Research* 20:207- 220 (1976).
Ernst, E.K.M. and Forde, M.P. Maternity care: an attempt at an alternative. *Nursing Clinics of North America* 12:241-249 (1975).

Eskenazi, B. Behavioral Teratology. In: *Perinatal Epidemiology*. M.B. Bracken, ed. New York and London: Oxford University Press, 1984.
Estes, M.N. A home obstetric service with expert consultation and back-up. *Birth and Family J.* 5(3):151-157 (1978).
Evans, D.R., Newcombe, R.G. and Campbell, H. Maternal smoking habits and congenital malformations: a population study. *Br. J. Med.* 2(6183):171-173 (1979).
Eyman, J. and Eyman, S.K. Sexual dysfunction: a review of assessment strategies. In: *Advances in Psychological Assessment, Vol. 6*, P. McReynolds and G.J. Chelune. San Francisco: Jossey-Bass, 1984, 151-193.
Fabricant, J. and Minick, R. Virus-heart link studied. (News report.) *Science* 227:735 (1985).
Fagley, N., Miller, P. and Sullivan, J. Stress, symptom proneness, and general adaptational distress during preganancy. *J. Human Stress* 8(2):15-22 (1982).
Faison, J.B., Pisani, B.J., Douglas, R.G., Cranch, G.S. and Lubic, R.W. The childbearing center: an alternative birth setting. *Ob-Gyn.* 54:527-532 (1979).
Fanelli, M.T. Promoting women's health. *Dietetic Currents* 12: 19-24 (1985).
Farer, E.A., Vaughn, B. and Egeland, B. The relationship of prenatal maternal anxiety to infant behavior and mother-infant interaction during the first six months of life. *Early Hum. Dev.* 5(3):267-277 (1981).
Farberow, N.L. Assessment of suicide. In: P. McReynolds, *Advances in Psychological Assessment, Vol. 5*, San Francisco: Jossey-Bass, 1981, pp. 124-190.
Farquhar, J.W., Maccoby, N. and Wood, P.D. Education and communication studies. In: *Oxford Textbook of Public Health*, London: Oxford Med. Pub., 1984.
Farquhar, J.W., et al. *The Stanford Five City Project.* (unpublished), 1984.
Farquhar, J.W. Changes in American lifestyle and health. In: *Marketing and Managing Health Care: Health Promotion and Disease Prevention* (Proc. Norfleet Forum, 1982), J.E. Hamner and B.J.S. Jacobs (eds.), Memphis: University of Tennessee, 1983.
Farquhar, J.W., Fortmann, S.P., Wood, P.D. and Haskell, W.L. Community studies of cardiovascular disease prevention. In: *Prevention of Coronary Heart Disease: Practical Management of the Risk Factors*, N.M. Kaplan and J. Stamler (eds.), Philadelphia: Saunders, 1983.
Farquhar, J.W. Community approaches to risk factor reduction: the Stanford project. In: J.A. Herd, *Behavior and Arteriosclerosis*, New York: Plenum, 1983, 143-148.
Fava, G.A., Fava, M., Kellner, R. Serafini, E. and Mastrogiacomo, I. Depression, hostility and anxiety in hyperprolactinemic amenorrhea. *Psychother. Psychosom.* 36(2):122-128 (1981).

Feldman, J.G., Carter, A.C., Nicasari, A.D. and Hosat, S.T. Breast self-examination, relationship to stage of disease at diagnosis. *Cancer* 47:2740-2745 (1981).
Fellman, M., Battegay, R., Raudfleisch, V. and Mall-Haefeli, M. Schweiz. *Arch. Neur., Neurochir. Psychiat.* 132:105-115 (1983).
Felton, B.J. and Revenson, T.A. Coping with chronic illness: a study of illness controllability and the influence of coping strategies on psychological adjustment. *J. Consult. Clin. Psychol.* 52:343-353 (1984).
Felton, G.S. and Segelman, F.B. Lamaze childbirth training and changes in belief about personal control. *Birth & Family J.* 5:141-150 (1978).
Ferreira, A.J. *Prenatal Environment.* Springfield: Thomas Pub., 1969.
Feverstein, M. and Kuczmierczyk, A.R. *Health Psychology.* New York: Plenum, 1985.
Field, T. Coping with separation stress by infants and young children. In: T. Field, P.M. McCabe and N. Schneiderman (eds.), *Stress and Coping*, Hillsdale, N.J.: Erlbaum, 1985, 197-219.
Field T., et al. Effects of ultra sound feedback on pregnancy anxiety, fetal activity and neonatal outcome. *Ob.-Gyn.* 66:525-528 (1985).
Fisch, I.R. and Freedman, S.H. Smoking, oral contraceptives, and obesity. Effects on white blood cell count. *JAMA* 234(5):500-506 (1975).
Fisher, B., Slack, N.H., and Bross, I. Cancer of the breast: size of neoplasm and prognosis. *Cancer* 24:1071ff. (1969).
Fitzpatrick, T.B. and Sober, A.J. Sunlight and skin cancer. *N. Eng. J. Med.* 313:818-819 (1985).
Fordney, D.S. Dyspareunia and vaginismus in counseling office practice. *Clin. Ob-Gyn.* 21:205-222 (1978).
Forester, B., Kornfield, D.S. and Fleiss, J.L. Psychotherapy during radiotherapy: effect on emotional and physical distress. *Am. J. Psychiat.* 142:22-28 (1985).
Foresti, G., Ferraro, M., Reithaar, P., Berlanda, C., Volpi, M., Drago, D., and Cerutti, R. Premenstrual syndrome and personality traits: a study on 110 pregnant patients. *Psychother. Psychosom.* 36(1):37-42 (1981).
Foster, R.S., et al. Breast self-examination practices and breast cancer stage. *N. Eng. J. Med.* 299:265ff. (1978).
Fox, B.H. Psychosocial factors and the immune system in human cancer. In: R. Ader (ed.), *Psychoneuroimmunology*, New York: Academic Press, 1981, pp. 103- 158.
Foxman, B. and Frerichs, R.R. Epidemiology of urinary tract infections I: diaphragm use and sexual intercourse. *Am. J. Pub. Health* 74:1303-1313 (1985).
Foxman, B. and Frerichs, R.R. Epidemiology of urinary tract infections II: diet, clothing and urination habits. *Am J. Pub. Health* 75:1314-1317 (1985).

France, R. and Robson, M. (News report). "Psychologists can cut GPs' drug bills," *The Times*, London, 16 January 1984.
Franceschi, S., et al. Genital warts and cervical neoplasia: an epidemiological study. *Br. J. Cancer* 48:621-628 (1983).
Frank, Jerome. *Healing: A Comparative Study of Psychotherapy.* Baltimore: Johns Hopkins, 1973.
Frederick, J. and Butler, N.R. "Intended place of delivery and perinatal outcome," *BMJ* 1:763-765 (1978).
Freedman, R. and Hermalin, A.I. Do statements about desired family size predict fertility? The case of Taiwan, 1967-1970. *Demography* 12(3):407-416 (1975).
Freeman, E.W., et al. Evaluating premenstrual symptoms in medical practice. *Ob-Gyn.* 65:500-505 (1985).
Freer, C.B. Health diaries: an efficient but under-used method for the collection of whole person health information. *J. of College of General Practice* 30:279ff. (1980).
Friederich, M.A. Psychophysiology of menstruation and the menopause. In: M.G. Romney, et al., *Gynecology and Obstetrics: The Health Care of Women*, New York: McGraw-Hill, 1975, pp. 605-617.
Friedman, D. and Jaffee, A. Influence of life style on the premenstrual syndrome. *J. Reprod. Med.* 30:715-719 (1985).
Friedman, R.C., et al. Sexual histories and premenstrual affective syndrome in psychiatric inpatients. *Am. J. Psychiat.* 139:1484-1486 (1982).
Friedrich, E.G. Vaginitis. *Am. J. Ob-Gyn.* 152:247-251 (1985).
Friedson, E. *Patients' Views of Medical Practice.* New York: Russell Sage Foundation, 1961.
Furstenberg, F.F., Jr., Herceg-Baron R., Shea, J. and Webb, D. Family communication and teenagers' contraceptive use. *Fam. Plann. Perspect.* 16(4):163-170 (1984).
Furgyk, S. and Asted, B. Gonorrheal infection followed by an increased frequency of cervical carcinoma. *Acta Ob. Gyn. Scand.* 59:521-524 (1980).
Gambrell, R.D. Proposal to decrease the risk and improve the prognosis of breast cancer. *Am. J. Ob. Gyn.* 150:119-132 (1984).
Garvey, M.J. and Tollefson, G.D. Postpartum depression. *J. Reprod. Med.* 29(2):113-116 (1984).
Gatchell, R.J., Baum, A. and Singer, J.E. *Handbook of Health Psychology, Vol. I., Psychology and Behavioral Medicine.* Hillsdale, New Jersey: Erlbaum, 1982.
Geer, J.H. and Messe, M. Sexual dysfunction. In: R.J. Gatchell et al., *Handbook of Health Psychology, Vol. I., Psychology and Behavioral Medicine*, Hillsdale, N.J.: Erlbaum, 1982.
Geller, E.S. Seat belt psychology. *Psychol. Today*, May 1985, 12-14.

Gentry, W.D. *Handbook of Behavioral Medicine.* New York: Guilford Press, 1984.

Georges, J., Giakoumaki, E., Georgoulias, N., Koumandakis, E. and Kaskarelis, D. Psychosocial stress and its relation to obstetrical complications. *Psychother. Psychosom.* 41(4):200-206 (1984).

Girard, M. Contraceptives: why all women don't use them. *Monitor,* Am. Psychol. Assn., August 11, 1986.

Gitlin, M. and Pasnair, R.O. Depression in obstetric & gynecology patients. *J. Psychiat. Treatment Evaluation* 5:421-428 (1983).

Gloingoin, E. The 'bad' patient gets better quicker. *Social Policy* 4: (November) 1973.

Golbus, M.S. Teratology for the obstetrician: Current status. *Ob-Gyn.* 55(3):269-277 (1980).

Gold, D. and Berger, C. The influence of psychological and situational factors on the contraceptive behavior of single men: a review of the literature. *Population & Environment* 6:113-127 (1983).

Gold, E.B. (ed.) *The Changing Risk of Disease in Women.* Baltimore: The Johns Hopkins University, 1983.

Gold, J.H. *The Psychiatric Aspects of Menstruation.* Washington, D.C.: American Psychiatric Press, 1985.

Goldberg, E.L. and Comstock, G.W. Life events and subsequent illness. *Am. J. Epid.* 104:146-158 (1976).

Goldberg, R.J. and Tull, R.M. *The Psychosocial Dimensions of Cancer: A Practical Guide for Health Care Providers.* New York: Macmillan, 1983.

Golden, N.L., et al. Pencyclicine use during pregnancy. *Am. J. Ob-Gyn.* 2:254-259 (1984).

Goldstein, M.S., Siegel, J.M. and Boyer, R. Predicting changes in perceived health status. *Am. J. of Pub. Health* 74:611-614 (1984).

Goldstein, S., Halbreich, U., Endicott J. and Hill, E. Premenstrual hostility, impulsivity, and impaired social functioning. *J. Psychosom. Ob. Gyn.* 5:33-38 (1986).

Goldthorp, W.O. and Richman, J. Maternal attitudes to unattended home confinement. *Practitioner* 212:1272, 845-853 (1974).

Goldzieher, J.W. The role of age, smoking habits, and oral contraceptives in the frequency of myocardial infarction in young women (author's translation). *Reproduccion* 4(1):21-27 (1980).

Golub, S. The magnitude of premenstrual anxiety and depression. *Psychosom. Med.* 38:4-12 (1976).

Good, R.S. and Capone, M.A. Emotional considerations in the care of the gynecological cancer patient. In: D.D. Youngs, and A.A. Ehrhardt (eds.), *Psychosomatic Obstetrics and Gynecology,* New York: Appleton-Century-Crofts, 1980, pp. 117-125.

Goodwin, J.W., Dunne, J.T., Thomas, B.W. Antepartum identification of the fetus at risk. *Can. Med. Assoc. J.* 101:57-67 (1969).

Gorsuch, R.L. and Key, M.I.C. Abnormalities of pregnancy as a function of anxiety and life stress. *Psychosom. Med.* 36:355-362 (1974).

Goujard, J., Rumeau, C. and Schwartz, D. Smoking during pregnancy, stillbirth and abruptio placentae. *Biomedicine* 23(1):20-22 (1975).

Graham, S., Priore, R., Graham, M., Browne, R. Burnett, W. and West, D. Genital cancer in wives of penile cancer patients. *Cancer* 44(5):1870-1874 (1979).

Grant, A. and Mohide, P. Screening and diagnostic tests in antenatal care. In: M. Enkin and I. Chalmers (eds.), *Effectiveness And Satisfaction In Antenatal Care*, London: Heinemann, 1982.

Gravell, J., Zapka, J.G. and Mamon, J. Impact of breast self examination planned educational messages in social network communications. *Health Ed. Quart.* 12:51-64 (1985).

Gray, J.D., et al. Prediction and prevention of child abuse and neglect. *Child Abuse and Neglect Intl. J.* 1:45 (1977).

Green, L.W., Dreuter, M.W., Deeds, S.G. and Partridge, K.B. *Health Education Planning.* Palo Alto: Mayfield Publishers, 1980.

Greenberg, M. The meaning of menorrhagia: an investigation into the association between the complaint of menorrhagia and depression. *J. Psychosom. Res.* 27:209-214 (1983).

Greenwood, S. *Menopause Naturally.* San Francisco: Volcano Press, 1984.

Greer, S. and Morris, T. Psychological attitudes of women who develop breast cancer: a controlled study. *J. Psychosom. Res.* 19:147-153 (1975).

Greve, W. and Schroder, S. Consultation when abortion is demanded. *Psychotherapie & Med. Psychologie* 27:58-63 (1977).

Grieco, A. and Long, C.J. Investigation of the Karnofsky performance status as a measure of quality of life. *Health Psychol* 3:129-142 (1984).

Grimes, D.A. Declining surgical case load of the obstetrician-gynecologist. *Ob-Gyn.* 67:760-762 (1986).

Grossarth-Maticek, R. Psychosocial predictors of cancer and internal disease: an overview. *Psychother. Psychosom.* 33:122ff. (1980).

Grossarth-Maticek, R., Schmidt, P., Vetter, H. and Arndt, S. Psychotherapy research in oncology. In: A. Steptoe and A. Mathews, *Health Care and Human Behavior*, New York and London: Academic Press, 1984, pp. 325-347.

Grossman, C.J. Interactions between the gonadal steroids and the immune system. *Science* 227:257ff. (1985).

Grossman, J.H. Determining origin of patient's genital herpes called clinically irrelevant. *Ob-Gyn News* 20:1 & 25 (1985).

Gruba, G.H. and Rohrbaugh, M. MMPI correlates of menstrual distress. *Psychosom. Med.* 37(3):265-273 (1975).

Gruen, R. Berkeley study finds stress is value laden. Report of a paper. *APA Monitor* 15:20 (1984).

Gwinn, M., et al. Alcohol consumption and ovarian cancer risk. *Am. J. Epid.* 123: 759-766 (1986).

Gurin, G., Veroff, J. and Feld, S. *Americans View Their Mental Health.* New York: Basic Books, 1960.

Guzinski, G. Medical gynecology: problems and patients. In: *The Woman Patient,* M.T. Notman and C.C. Nadelson (eds.), New York: Plenum, 1978, 181-202.

Haan, N.G. Psychosocial meanings of unfavorable medical forecasts. In: G.C. Stone, et al. (eds.), *Health Psychology,* San Francisco: Jossey-Bass, 1979, pp. 113-140.

Haggerty, R.J. Life stress, illness and social supports. *Dev. Med. & Child Neurology* 22:391-400 (1980).

Hall, D.C., et al. Improved detection of human breast lesion following experimental training. *Cancer* 46:408-414 (1980).

Hall, M.H., Chng, P.R. and MacGillivray, I. Is routine antenatal care worthwhile? *Lancet* 2:78-80 (1980).

Hall, R.C.W. Helping your patient deal with stress. *The Female Patient* 8:51-55 (1983).

Hall, T. What Americans eat hasn't changed much despite healthy image. *Wall St. J.,* September 12, 1985, pp. 1, 22.

Hamburg, D.A., Elliot, G.R. and Parson, D. *Health and Behavior.* Washington, D.C.: Institute of Medicine, National Academy Press, 1982.

Hamburg, D.A., et al. (eds.) *Health and Behavior: Frontiers of Research in the Biobehavioral Sciences.* Washington, D.C.: Institute of Medicine, National Academy Press, 1982.

Hamburg, D.A. Health and behavior. *Science* 30:399 (1982).

Hamburg, D.A. Frontiers of research in neurobiology. *Science,* 222 (1983), editorial.

Hamilton, J.A. *Postpartum Psychiatric Problems.* St. Louis: C.B. Mosby, 1962.

Hamilton, W.D. and Zuk, M. Heritable true fitness and bright birds: a role for parasites? *Science* 218:384-386 (1982).

Hare, M.J. Long term complications of infection of the female genital tract by intracellular sexually transmitted micro organisms: a review. *J. Royal Soc. Med.* 76:1045-1049 (1983).

Hare-Mustin, R.T. Reappraisal of the relationship between women and psychotherapy, 80 years after the case of Dora. *American Psychologist* (1983).

Harlan, W.R., et al. Weight affects blood pressure. *Ob-Gyn News* 20:24 (1985).

Harlap, S. and Shiono, P.H. Alcohol, smoking, and incidence of spontaneous abortions in the first and second trimester. *Lancet* 2(8187):173-176 (1980).

Harris, P.R. *Promoting Health-Preventing Disease: Objectives for the Nation.* Washington, D.C.: U.S. Gov't. Printing Office, 1980.

Harris, R., et al. Attitudes and perceptions of perinatal concepts during pregnancy in women from three cultures. *J. Clinical Psychol.*, 37(3):477-483 (1981).

Harrison, R.M. Women's treatment decisions for genital symptoms. *J. R. Soc. Med.* 75(1):23-26 (1982).

Hartman, R., Nielsen, J.M. and Reynolds, M. Factors affecting satisfaction with the birth experience. *NAPSAC,* 733-755 (1979).

Harvey, A.L. Risky and safe contraceptors: some personality factors. *J. Psychol.* 92(First Half):109-112 (1976).

Haskett, R. Severe premenstrual tension: delineation of the syndrome. *Biol. Psychiat.* 15:121-139 (1980).

Hatcher, R.A., et al. *Contraceptive Technology 1986-1987* (and) *Sexually Transmitted Diseases.* New York: Irvington Pub., 1986.

Hawkins, D.F. The therapeutics of normal pregnancy. In: D.F. Hawkins, *Drugs and Pregnancy,* New York: Churchill Livingston, 1983, 53-75.

Haworth, J.C., Ellestad-Sayed, J.J., King, J. and Dilling, L.A. Relation of maternal cigarette smoking, obesity, and energy consumption to infant size. *Am. J. Obstet. Gynecol.* 138(8):1185-1189 (1980).

Hayes, J. and Prokop, C.K. Sociopsychiatric characteristic of clinic patrons with repeat gonorrhea infections. *J. Am. Vener. Dis. Assoc.* 3(1):43-48 (1976).

Hayashi, K. and Bracken, M.B. Hydatidiform Mole. In: *Perinatal Epidemiology.* M.B. Bracken, ed. New York and London: Oxford University Press, 1984.

Hayes, W.J., Kilburn, K.H., Merchant, J.A. and Stokinger, H.E. Proceedings of the Workshop on Chronic Disease in the Workplace and the Environment. *Archives of Environmental Health* 1984, 39.

Haynes, S. and Feinleib, M. Women, work, and coronary heart disease: prospective findings from the Framingham heart study. *Am. J. Public Health* 70:133-141 (1980).

Hazell, D. A study of 300 elective home births. *Birth & Fam. J.* 2:11-18 (1975).

Headik, W.B., III and White, S.J. Evaluation of written reinforcement used in counseling cardiovascular patients. *Am. J. Hosp. Pharm.* 33:1277-1280 (1976).

Health Education Council. "Healthy Living: Towards a national strategy for health education and promotion." London (1983).

Department of Health & Human Services. *Preventive Health Care in Ob-Gyn Residency Training.* ACOG, 4-85.

Health Policy Analysis Program. *Midwifery Outside of the Nursing Profession: The Current Debate in Washington.* University of Washington, October, 1980.

Hebel, J.R., Nowicki, P. and Sexton, M. The effects of antismoking intervention during pregnancy: an assessment of interactions and maternal characteristics. *Am. J. Epid.* 122:135-148 (1985).

Heide, W.S. Feminism: making a difference in our health. In: M. T. Notman and C.C. Nadelson, *The Woman Patient: Medical and Psychological Interfaces*, New York: Plenum, 1978, pp. 9-19.

Heinonen, P., Slone, D. and Shapiro, S. *Birth Defects and Drugs in Pregnancy*. Littleton, Mass.: Publishing Sciences Group, 1977.

Heinrich, R.L. and Schag, C.C. Stress and activity management: group treatment for cancer patients and spouses. *J. Consult. Clin. Psychol.* 53:439-446 (1985).

Heintz, P., Haiter, W.F. and Lagasse, L.D. Epidemiology and etiology of ovarian cancer. *Ob-Gyn.* 66:127-135 (1985).

Helsing, K., Szklo, M. and Comstock, G. Factors associated with mortality after widowhood. *Am. J. Pub. Health* 71:802-809 (1981).

Hemminki, E. and Starfield, B. Prevention of low birth weight and pre-term birth. *Milbank Memorial Fund Quarterly* 56(3):339-361 (1978).

Hemminki, K., et al. Spontaneous abortions in an industrialized community in Finland. *AJPH* 73:32-37 (1983).

Hemminki, K., Mutanen, P. and Saloniemi, I. Smoking and the occurrence of congenital malformations and spontaneous abortions: multivariate analysis. *Am. J. Obstet. Gynecol.* 145(1):61-66 (1983).

Hemphill, R.E. Incidence and nature of puerperal psychiatric illness. *Br. Med. J.* 2:1232-1235 (1952).

Henderson, J.B., Hall, S.M. and Lipton, H.L. Changing self-destructive behaviors. In: G.C. Stone, et al. (eds.), *Health Psychology*. San Francisco: Jossey-Bass, 1979, pp. 141-160.

Hendler, N.H., Long, D.M. and Wise, T.N. *Diagnosis and Treatment of Chronic Pain.* New York: John Wright, 1982.

Henker, F.O. Diagnosis and treatment of nonorganic pelvic pain. *Southern Med. J.* 72:1132-1134 (1979).

Henry, J.P. and Stephens, P.M. *Stress, Health and the Social Environment: A Sociobiological Approach to Medicine.* New York: Springer Verlag, 1977.

Herd, J.A. Summary: biobehavioral perspectives: coronary arteriosclerosis. In: J.A. Herd and S.M. Weiss, *Behavior and Arteriosclerosis*, New York: Plenum Press, 1983, pp. 169-183.

Herd, J.A. and Weiss, S.M. *Behavior and Arteriosclerosis*. New York: Plenum Press, 1983.

Herd, J.A. Cardiovascular disease and hypertension. In: W.D. Gentry, *Handbook of Behavioral Medicine*, New York: Guilkford Press, 1984, pp. 222-281.

Herold, E.S., Goodwin, M.S. and Lero, D.S. Self-esteem, locus of control, and adolescent contraception. *J. Psychol.* 191(first half):83-8, 1979.

Herrenkohl, L.R. Prenatal stress reduces fertility and fecundity in female offspring. *Science* 206: 1097-1099 (1979).
Herron, M.A., Katz, R.N. and Creasey R.K. Evaluation of preterm birth prevention program. *Ob-Gyn.* 59:452-456 (1982).
Herzon, A. and Detre, T. Psychotic reactions associated with childbirth. *Disease Nerv. Syst.* 37:229-235 (1976).
Hibbard, J.H. Social ties and health status: an examination of moderating factors. *Health Ed. Quart.* 12:23-34 (1985).
Himmelberger, D.U., Brown, B.W., Jr. and Cohen, E.N. Cigarette smoking during pregnancy and the occurrence of spontaneous abortion and congenital abnormality. *Am. J. Epid.* 108(6):470-479 (1978).
Himmelfarb, S. Age and sex differences in the mental health of older persons. *J. Consult. Clin. Psychol.* 52:844-856 (1984).
Hingson, R., et al. Maternal marijuana use and neonatal outcome: uncertainty posed by self-reports. *Am. J. Pub. Health* 76:667-670 (1986).
Hinkle, L.E. and Wolff, H.G. Health and the social environment: experimental investigations. In: *Explorations and Social Psychiatry*, New York: Basic Books, 1957, 104-137.
Hinkle, L.E., Jr. The Concept of "Stress" in the Biological and Social Sciences. In: *Psychosomatic Medicine: Current Trends and Clinical Applications.* Z.J. Lipowski, D.R. Lippsitt and P.C. Whybrow (eds.), New York and London: Oxford University Press, 1977.
Hinkle, L.E. and Wolff, H.G. The nature of man's adaptation to the total environment and the relation of this to illness. *Arch. Int. Med.* 99:442-460 (1957).
Hobel, C.J., Hyvariner, M.A., Okada, D.M. and Oh, W. Prenatal and intrapartum high-risk screening. I. Prediction of the high-risk neonate. *Am. J. Ob.-Gyn.* 17:1-9 (1973).
Hobel, C.J. Recognition of the high-risk pregnant woman. In: *Management of the High Risk Pregnancy*, W.N. Spellancy (ed.), Baltimore: University Park Press, 1976, 1-28.
Hobel, C.J., Youkeles, M.A. and Forsythe, A. Prenatal and intrapartum high-risk screening. II. Risk factors reassessed. *Am. J. Ob-Gyn.* 135:1051-1056 (1979).
Holahan, C.K., Holahan, C.J. and Belk, S.S. Adjustment in aging: the roles of life stress, hassles and self efficacy. *Health Psychol.* 3:315-328 (1984).
Hollingsworth, D.R., Moser, R.J., Carlson, J.W. and Thompson, K.T. Abnormal adolescent primiparous pregnancy: association of race, human chorionic somatomammotropin production, and smoking. *Am. J. Ob-Gyn.* 126(2):230-237 (1976).
Hollis, J.F., Connor, W.E. and Matarazzo, J.D. Lifestyle, behavioral health and heart disease. In: Gatchel et al., *Handbook of Health Psychology, Vol. I., Psychology and Behavioral Medicine*, New Jersey: Erlbaum, 1982.

Hollis, J.F., et al. The nutrition attitude survey: Association with dietary habits, psychological and physical well-being and coronary risk factors. *Health Psychol.* 5:359-374 (1986).

Holmes, T.H. and Rale, R.H. The social readjustment rating scale. *J. Psychosom. Res.* 11:213-218 (1967).

Holroyd, K.A., et al. Change mechanisms in EMG biofeedback training: cognitive changes underlying improvement in tension headache. *J. Consult. Clin. Psychol.* 52:1039-1053 (1984).

Hopper, S.V., Miller, J.P., Birge, C. and Swift, J. A randomized study of the impact of home health aides on diabetic control and utilization patterns. *Am. J. of Pub. Health* 74:600-602 (1984).

Hopson, J. and Rosenfeld, A. PMS: puzzling monthly symptoms. *Psychol. Today*, August 1984, 3035.

Horder, J., et al. Medical education: an important opportunity. *Br. Med. J.* 288:1507-1511.

Horn, M.C. and Mosher, W.D. Use of services for family planning and infertility: United States, 1982. *NCHS*, Advance Data, 1984, #103.

House, J.S., Robbins, C. and Metzner, H.L. The association of social relationships and activities with mortality: prospective evidence from the Tecumseh Health Study. *Am. J. Epid.* 116:123-140 (1982).

Hovey, D.L. and Hovey, J.E. Behavioral gynecology: a new frontier. *Ob.-Gyn. World* 1:22-23.

Howard, K.I., Kopta, S.M., Krause, M.S. and Orlinsky, D.E. The dose-effect relationship in psychotherapy. *Am. Psychol.* 41:159-164 (1986).

Howe, H.L. Age specific hysterectomy and ophorectomy prevalence rates and the risks for cancer of the reproductive system. *Am. J. Pub. Health* 74:560-563 (1984).

Hughes, G.H., et al. The multiple risk factor intervention trial (MRFIT) V. Intervention on smoking. *Prev. Med.* 10:476-500 (1981).

Huguley, C.M. and Brown, R.L. The value of breast self examination. *Cancer* 47:989 ff.

Humphrey, M. Infertility and Alternative Parenting. In: *Psychology and Gynaecological Problems.* A. Broome and L. Wallace, eds. London: Tavistock, 1984.

Hunt, E.B. and MacLeod, C.M. Cognition and information processing in patient and physician. In: G.C. Stone, F. Cohen and F. Adler (eds.), *Health Psychology*, San Francisco: Jossey-Bass, 1979, 303-332.

Hunt, W.A. and Bespalec, D.A. The evaluation of current methods of modifying smoking behavior. *J. Clin. Psychol.* 30:431-438 (1974).

Hurney, C. and Holland, J. Psychosocial sequelae of ostomies in cancer patients. *CA - Cancer Jr. Clinicians* 35:170-183 (1985).

Huston, K. Ethical decisions in treating battered women. *Prof. Psychol.* 15:822-832 (1984).

Huttunen, M.O. and Niskanen, P. Prenatal loss of father and psychiatric disorders. *Arch. Gen. Psychiatry* 35(4):429-431 (1978).
Illich, I. *Medical Nemesis: the Expropriation of Health.* New York: Bantam, 1976.
Illsley, R. Social aspects of pregnancy outcome. In: S.L. Barron and A.M. Thomson (eds.), *Obstetrical Epidemiology,* New York: Academic Press, 1983, 449-476.
Institute for Health Policy Studies. *Smoking During Pregnancy: What Can Be Done?* III, San Francisco: University of California, 1985, 1-4.
Institute of Medicine. Committee to Study Prevention of Low Birthweight. *Preventing Low Birthweight.* Washington, National Academy Press, 1985. Also reported in *The Nation's Health, APHA,* March, 1985.
Institute of Medicine. National Research Council. Research Issues in the Assessment of Birth Settings. Washington, D.C., 1982.
Inwood, D.G. *Recent Advances in Postpartum Psychiatric Disorders.* Washington, D.C.: American Psychiatric Press, 1985.
Jain, A.K. Cigarette smoking, use of oral contraceptives, and myocardial infarction. *Am. J. Obstet. Gynecol.* 126(3):301-307 (1976).
James, W.H. Birth ranks of spontaneous abortions in sibships of children affected by anencephaly or spina bifida. *Br. Med. J.* 1(6105):72-73 (1978).
James, S.A. and Kleidbaum. Socioecologic stress and hypertension-related mortality rates in North Carolina. *Am. J. Pub. Health* 66:354-358 (1976).
Jamison, K., et al. Correlation of personality profile with pain syndrome. In: J.J. Bonica and D.G. Albe-Fessard, *Advances in Pain Research and Therapy, Vol. I.,* Proceedings of the 1st World Congress on Pain, New York: Raven Press, 1976, pp. 317-325.
Janis, I. *Psychological Stress.* New York: Wiley, 1958.
Janis, I.L. and Rodin, J. Attribution, control and decision making: social psychology and health care. In: G.C. Stone, F. Cohen and F. Adler (eds.), *Health Psychology,* San Francisco: Jossey-Bass, 1982, 487-521.
Janis, I., Defares, P. and Grossman, P. Hyper-vigilant reactions to threat. In: *Guide to Stress Research, Vol. III,* H. Selye, et al. (eds.), 1983.
Janis, I.L. The patient as decision maker. In: W.D. Gentry, *Handbook of Behavioral Medicine,* New York: Guilford Press, 1984, pp. 326-368.
Janis, I.L. The role of social support in adherence to stressful decisions. *Am. Psychologist,* 38:143-160 (1983).
Janis, I.L. Stress innoculation in health care: theory and research. In: D. Meichenbaum and M.E. Jaremko, *Stress Prevention and Management,* New York and London: Plenum Press, 1983.
Jemmott, J.B. and Locke, S.T. Psychosocial factors, immunological mediation and human susceptibility to infectious disease. *Psychol. Bull.* 95:78-108 (1984).

Jenkins, C.D. Recent evidence supporting psychological and social risk factors for coronary disease. *N. Eng. J. Med.* 294:987-994, 1033-1038 (1976).
Jensen, J. Advertising plays a key role in making women aware of special services. *Modern Healthcare* (August 1986), 68-70.
Joffe, J.M. *Prenatal Determinants of Behavior*. London: Pergamon, 1962.
Johansson, D.B. The sterile menstrual cycle. *Acta Ob. Gyn. Scand.* Supp. 123:147-150 (1984).
Johnson, J.E. Psychological interventions and coping with surgery. In: *Handbook of Psychology and Health, Vol. IV*, Baum, Taylor and Singer (eds.), 1982, 167-187.
Johnstone, C. Cigarette smoking and the outcome of human pregnancies. *Clin. Toxicology* 18:189-209 (1981).
Joklik, W.K. *Virology*. Norwalk, Connecticut: Appleton-Century-Crofts, 1985.
Jones, A.C. Life changes and psychological distress in predictors of pregnancy outcome. *Psychosom. Med.* 40:402-412 (1978).
Jordan, J. and Meckler, J.R. The relationship between life change events, social supports, and dysmenorrhea. *Res. Nurs. Health* 5(2):73-79 (1982).
Jorgensen, C., Uddenberg, N. and Ursing, I. Ultrasound diagnosis of fetal malformation in the second trimester: the psychological reactions of women. *J. Psychosom. Ob-Gyn.* 4:31-40 (1985).
Jorgensen, S.R. and Sonstegard, J.J. Predicting adolescent sexual and contraceptive behavior: an application of the Fishbein model. *J. Marriage & Fam.* 43-55 (February 1984).
Jospe, M., Nieberding, J. and Cohen, B.D. (eds.), *Psychological Factors in Health Care*. Boston: Lexington Books, 1980.
Julius, M., et al. Anger-coping types, blood pressure and all cause mortality: a follow up in Tecumseh, Michigan, 1971-1983. *Am. J. of Epid.* 124:220-233 (1986).
Meichenbaum, D. and Jaremko, M.E. Theory and research. In: *Stress Reduction and Prevention*, D. Meichenbaum and M.E. Jaremko, New York and London: Plenum Press, 1983.
Kandel, D.B., et al. The stressfulness of daily social roles for women: marital occupational and household roles. *J. Health Soc. Behav.* 26:64-78 (1986).
Kaplan, B.H., Cassel, J.C. and Gore, S. Social support and health. *Med. Care* 15th Supp. #5, 47-58 (1977).
Kaplan, H. *The Evaluation of Sexual Disorder: Psychological and Medical Aspects*. New York: Brunner Mazel, 1983.
Kaplan, R.M. and Bush, J.W. Health-related quality of life measurement for evaluation research and policy analysis. *Health Psychol.* 1:61-80 (1982).

Kaplan, R.M. The connection between clinical health promotion and health status: a critical overview. *Am. Psychol.* 39:755-765 (1984).
Kaplan, R.M., Atkins, C.J. and Reinsch, S. Specific efficacy expectations mediate exercise compliance in patients with COPD. *Health Psychol.* 3:223-242 (1984).
Kagan, A.R. and Levi, L. Health and environment—psychosocial stimuli. A review. *Soc. Sci. Med.* 8:225-241 (1974).
Kashiwagi, T., McClure, J.N. and Wetzel, R.D. Premenstrual affective syndrome and psychiatric disorder. *Disease Nerv. Sys.* 37:116-119 (1976).
Kasl, S.V., Ostfelt, A.M., Brody, G.M., Snell, L. and Price, D.A. Effects of 'Involuntary' Relocation on the Health and Behavior of the Elderly. In: *Second Conference on the Epidemiology of Aging.* S.G. Haynes and M. Feinleib, eds. NIH Pub. 80-969, USDHHS, 211-236 (1980).
Katon, W., Egan, K. and Miller, D. Chronic pain: lifetime psychiatric diagnosis and family history. *Am. J. Psychiat.* 142:1156-1160 (1985).
Katon, W.J., Ries, R.K., Bokan, J.A. and Kleinman, A. Hyperemesis gravidarum: a biopsychosocial perspective. *Int. J. Psychiatry Med.* 10(2):151-162 (1980).
Kaunitz, A.M., et al. Causes of maternal mortality in the U.S. *Ob-Gyn.* 65:605-612 (1985).
Keehn, R.J., Goldberg, I.D. and Beebe, G.W. Twenty-four year follow-up of army veterans with disability separations for psychoneurosis. *Psychosom. Med.* 36:27-46 (1944).
Kellner, R., Buckman, M.T., Fana, G.A. and Pathak, D. Hyperprolactinemia, distress and hostility. *Am. J. Psychiat* 141:759-767 (1984).
Kennell, J.H. and Klaus, M.H. Early mother-infant contact: effects on the mother and the infant. *Bulletin Menninger Clinic* 43:69-78 (1979).
Keown, C., Solvic, P. and Lichthenstein, S. Attitudes of physicians, pharmacists, and laypersons toward seriousness and need for disclosure of prescription drug side effects. *Health Psychol.* 3:1-11 (1984).
Kessner, D.M., et al. Infant death: An analysis by maternal risk and health care. *Contrasts in Health Status, Vol. 1*, Published by OSBN.
Ketai, R.M. and Brandwin, M.A. Childbirth-related psychosis and familiar symbiotic conflict. *Am. J. Psychiatry* 136(2): 190-193 (1979).
Keye, W.R. Psychological testing can clarify PMS (report of paper presented to Am. Fertility Soc.). *Ob-Gyn News* 20:8 (1985).
Kiecolt-Glaser, J.K., et al. Psychosocial enhancement of immuno-competence in a geriatric population. *Health Psychol.* 4:25-41 (1985).
Kiernen, B.V. The development, direction and evaluation of the child development and parenting project. Unpublished review, 1979.
Kiesler, C. A 'top down' look at public policy. Paper delivered to Vermont Conference on the Primary Prevention of Psychopathology. *Am. Psychol. Monitor* 24, September 1983, p. 5.

Kilmartin, A. *Cystitis: The Complete Self-Help Guide*. New York: Warner, 1980.
Kinch, R.A.H. and Steinberg, S. Psychosocial problems. In: S.L. Romney et al., *Gynecology and Obstetrics: The Health Care of Women*, New York: McGraw-Hill, 1975, pp. 513-525.
King, S. and Cobb, S. Psychosocial factors in the epidemiology of rheumatoid arthritis. *J. Chronic Dis.* 7:466-475 (1958).
Kirscht, J.P. and Rosenstock, I.M. Patients' problems in following recommendations of health experts. In: *Health Psychology*, G.C. Stone, F. Cohen and N.I. Adler (eds.), San Francisco: Jossey-Bass, 1979, 189-215.
Kirscht, J.P. Preventive health behavior: a review of research and issues. *Health Psychology* 2(3):277-301 (1983).
Kirz, D.S., Dirchester, W. and Freeman, R.K. Advanced maternal age: the mature gravida. *Am. J. Ob-Gyn.* 152:7-11 (1985).
Kissen, D.M., Brown, R.I.F. and Kissen, M. A further report on personality and psychosocial factors in lung cancer. *Ann. N.Y. Acad. Sci.* 164:535-544 (1969).
Kitzinger, S. Anxiety in pregnancy. *J. Maternal & Child Health.* September 1977, 358-360.
Kitzinger, S. and Davies, J.A. *The Place of Birth.* Oxford: Oxford University Press, 1978.
Klaus, M.H., et al. *Maternal Attachment and Mothering Disorders: A Round Table.* New Brunswick, New Jersey: Johnson & Johnson Baby Products, 1976.
Klaus, M.H., Trause, M.A., Kennell, J.H. Does human maternal behaviour after delivery show a characteristic pattern? *Parent-Infant Interaction.* New York: Elsevier, 69-85.
Klaus, M.H. and Kennell, J.H. *Maternal and Infant Bonding.* St. Louis: C.V. Mosby, 1976.
Klein, M. Papegeorgiou, A.N., Westreich, R., Spector-Dunsky, L., Elkins, V., Kramer, M. and Gelfand, M. A randomized controlled trial of medical/psychological outcomes in a birth room versus conventional labor and delivery. Paper. American Public Health Assn., Montreal, 1982.
Klein, R. *The Politics of the National Health Service.* London: Longman, 1983.
Klerman, G.L. and Izen, J.F. The effects of bereavement and grief on physical health and general well-being. *Adv. Psychosom. Med.* 6:63-104 (1977).
Kliegman, R.M. and Gross, T. Perinatal problems of the obese mother and her infant. *Ob.-Gyn.* 66:299-306 (1985).
Kline, J. and Stein, Z. Spontaneous Abortion (Miscarriage). In: *Perinatal Epidemiology.* M.B. Bracken, ed. New York and London: Oxford University Press, 1984.
Kline, J., Stein, Z.A., Susser, M. and Warburton, D. Smoking: a risk factor for spontaneous abortion. *N. Eng. J. Med.* 297(15):793-796 (1977).

Kline, J., Stein, Z., Strabinow, B., Susser, M. and Warburton, D. Surveillance of spontaneous abortions: power in environmental monitoring. *Am. J. Epid.* 106:345-350 (1977).

Kline, J., Levin, B., Shrout, P., Stein, Z., Susser, M. and Warburton, D. Maternal smoking and trisomy among spontaneously aborted conceptions. *Am. J. Hum. Genet.* 35(3):421-431 (1983).

Kloosterman, G.J. In S. Kitzinger and J.A. Davis (eds.), *The Place of Birth.* Oxford: Oxford University Press, 1978, 85-92.

Knapp, F.T., et al. Some psychologic factors in prolonged labor due to insufficient uterine action. *Comprehensive Psychiat.* 4:9-17 (1963).

Knesper, D.J., Pagnucco, J.D. and Wheeler, J.R.S. Similarities and differences across mental health services providers and practice settings in the United States. *Am. Psychol.* 40: 1352-1369 (1985).

Knodel, J. and Hermalin, A.J. Effects of birth rank, maternal age, birth interval and sibship size on infant and child mortality: evidence from the 18th and 19th century reproductive histories. *Am. J. Pub. Health*, 1098-1106 (1984)

Knorr, K. The effect of tobacco and alcohol on pregnancy course and child development. *Bull. Schweiz. Akad. Med. Wiss.* 35(1-3):137-146 (1979).

Knowles, J.H. The responsibility of the individual. *Daedalus* 106:57-80 (1977).

Knox, E.G. A suitable case for treatment. *Times Literary Supplement* 17:169 (1984). (A critical review of Klein, R., *The Politics of the National Health Service*, and Iliffe, S., *The NHS: A Picture of Health?*)

Kok, F.J., et al., Dietary sodium, calcium and potassium and blood pressure. *Am. J. Epid.* 123:1043-1048 (1986).

Kolata, G. Lowered cholesterol decreases heart disease. *Science* 223:381-382 (1984).

Kolata, G. Obesity declared a disease. News report. *Science* 227:226-227.

Kolata, G. Heart panel's conclusions questioned. News report. *Science* 227:40-41 (1985).

Kolata, G. Why do people get fat? News report. *Science* 227:1327-1328 (1985).

Kolodny, R.C. and Masters, W.H. *Textbook of Sexual Medicine.* Boston: Little, Brown, 1979.

Koop, C.E. Physician's attitude called one of biggest obstacles to improving patient compliance. News report. *Ob-Gyn News*, February 1985, 24.

Koos, T.L. *The Health of Regionville.* New York: Columbia University Press, 1954.

Korenbrot, C.C. *Cost Effectiveness of Improving Prenatal Care to Low Income Women.* Research Highlights, San Francisco: University of San Francisco, Center for Population and Reproductive Health Policy, 1984, 2.

Korte, D. and Scaer, R. A survey of maternal preferences: what mothers want—not what they have. In: *Compulsory Hospitalization or Freedom of choice in Childbirth*, Vol. 3, Stewart and Stewart (eds.), Marble Hill, Mo.: NAPSAC Reproductions, 1979, 725-731.

Kotelchuck, M., Schwartz, J.B., Anderka, M.T. and Finison, K.S. WIC participation and pregnancy outcomes: Massachusetts statewide evaluation project. *Am. J. Pub. Health* 74:1086-1092 (1984).

Krant, M.J. Psychosocial impact of gynecologic cancer. *Cancer* 48(2 Suppl.):608-612 (1981).

Krantz, D.S., Baum, A. and Singer, J.E. *Handbook of Psychology and Health, Vol. 3, Cardiovascular Disorders and Behavior.* Hillsdale, New Jersey: Erlbaum, 1983.

Krantz, D.S. and Glass, D.C. Personality, behavior patterns and physical illness: conceptual and methodological issues. In: W.D. Gentry, *Handbook of Behavioral Medicine*, New York: Guilford Press, 1984, pp. 38-86.

Krantz, D.S. and Manuck, S.B. Acute psychophysiological reactivity and risk of cardiovascular disease: a review and methodological critique. *Psychol. Bull.* 96- 435-464 (1984).

Krouse, H.J. and Krouse, J.H. Psychological factors in postmastectomy adjustment. *Psychol. Reports* 48:275-278 (1981).

Kucera, H., Pavelka, R., Rudelstorfer, B. and Reinold, E. The influence of socioeconomic factors on the results of a premature-Dysmaturity prevention programme (author's translation). *Wien. Lin. Wochenschr.* 89(9):307-311 (1977).

Kuhn, T.S. *The Structure of Scientific Revolution.* Chicago: University of Chicago Press, 1970.

Kumar, K. Previous induced abortion and ante-natal depression in primiparae. *Psychol. Med.* 8:711-715 (1978).

Kung, H., et al. Patterns of site-specific displacement: cancer mortality among migrants: the Chinese in the U.S. *Am. J. Pub. Health* 75:237-424 (1985).

Kurata, J.H., Elashoff, J.D., Nogawa, A.N. and Haile B.M. Sex and smoking differences in duodenal ulcer mortality. *Am. J. Pub. Health* 76: 700-702 (1986).

Kushner, R. Psychosocial aspects of breast cancer. In: D.D. Youngs and A.A. Ehrhardt, *Psychosomatic Obstetrics and Gynecology*, New York: Appleton-Century-Crofts, 1980, pp. 165-274.

Labarba, R.C. Prenatal and neonatal influences on behavioral health development. In: J.D. Matarazzo et al., *Behavioral Health: A Handbook of Health Enhancement and Disease Prevention*, New York: Wiley, 1984, pp. 41-55.

Labrum, A.H. Psychological antecedents in gynecological cancer. In: D.D. Youngs and A.A. Ehrhardt, *Psychosomatic Obstetrics and Gynecology*, New York: Appleton-Century-Crofts, 1980, pp. 275-287.

Lalonde, M. Beyond a new perspective. APH Association, October 1976.
Lalos, A., Lalos, O., Jacobsson, L. and Von Schoultz, B. A psychosocial characterization of infertile couples before surgical treatment of the female. *J. Psychosom. Ob-Gyn.* 4:83-93 (1984).
Lammer, E.J., et al. Retinoic acid embryopathy. *N. Eng. J. Med* 313:837-841 (1985).
Lancet, Incontinent women. 1:521-522 (1977).
Langer, E.J. and Rodin, J. The effects of choice and enhanced personal responsibility for the aged: a field experiment in an institutional setting. *J. Personality Soc. Psychol.* 34:191-198 (1976).
Lark, S. *Premenstrual Syndrome Self Help Book.* Los Angeles: Forman, 1984.
Laukaran, V.H. and Van den Berg, B.J. The relationship of maternal attitude to pregnancy outcomes and obstetric complications. A cohort study of unwanted pregnancy. *Am. J. Ob.-Gyn.* 136(3):374-379 (1980).
LaVecchia, C. Benign breast disease, oral contraceptive use and the risk of breast cancer. *J. Chron. Dis.* 37:869 (1984).
Lawlor, C.L. and Davis, A.M. Primary dysmenorrhea. Relationship to personality and attitudes in adolescent females. *J. Adolesc. Health Care* 1(3):208-212 (1981).
Lazarus, R.S. The trivialization of distress. In: B.L. Hammonds and C.J. Scheirer (eds.), *Psychology and Health: The Master Lecture Series,* Washington, D.C.: Am. Psychol. Assn., 1983, pp. 125-144.
Lazarus, R.S., Kanner, A.D. and Folkman, S. Emotions: a cognitive- phenomenological analysis. In: R. Plutchik and H. Kellerman (eds.), *Emotion: Theory, Research and Experience,* New York: Academic Press, 1980, 189-218.
Leck, I. Fetal malformations. In: S.L. Barron and A.M. Thompson, *Obstetrical Epidemiology,* London and New York: Academic Press, 1983, 263-318.
Lawlor, C.L. and Davis, A.M. Primary dysmenorrhea. Relationship to personality and attitudes in adolescent females. *J. Adolesc. Health Care.* 1(3):208-212 (1981).
Lazarus, R.S., DeLongis, A., Folkman, S. and Gruen, R. Stress and adaptational outcome: the problem of confounded measures. *Am. Psychol.* 40:770-779 (1985).
Leck, I. Fetal malformation. In: S.L. Barron and A.M. Thomson, *Obstetrical Epidemiology,* New York: Academic Press, 1983, 265-318.
Lederman, R.P., Lederman, E., Work, B.A. and McCann, D.S. The relationship of maternal anxiety, plasma catecholamines, and plasma cortisol to progress in labor. *Am. J. Ob. Gyn.* 132:495-500 (1978).
Lederman, E., Lederman, R.P., Work, B.A., Jr. and McCann, D.C. Maternal psychological and physiologic correlates of fetal-newborn health status. *Am. J. Ob. Gyn.* 139:956 (1981).

Lederman, R.P., Lederman, E., Work, B.A., Jr. and McCann, D.S. Relationship to psychological factors in pregnancy to progress in labor. *Nursing Research*, p. 84.

Lehtovirta, P., Forss, M., Rauramo, I. and Kariniemi, V. Acute effects of nicotine on fetal heart rate variability. *B. J. Obs. and Gyn.* 90:710-715 (1983).

Lerner, M. *Occupational Stress Groups and the Psychodynamics of the World of Work.* Berkeley: Institute for Labor and Mental Health, 1985.

Leiva, J.L., et al. Microorganisms in semen used for artificial insemination. *Ob.-Gyn.* 65:669-672 (1985).

Lenfant, C. and Schweizer, M. Contributions of health relating biobehavioral research to the prevention of cardiovascular diseases. *Am. Psychol.* 40:217-220 (1985).

LeRoy, P.L. *Current Concepts in the Management of Chronic Pain,* Pro DoLore Symposium. New York: Stratton Medical Book Corporation, 1977.

LeShan, L. An emotional life history pattern associated with neoplastic disease. *Annal. N.Y. Acad. Sci.* 125:780-793 (1966).

Lesinsky, J. High risk pregnancy. *Ob.-Gyn.* 46:599-603 (1975).

Leventhal, H. Rewards and adolescent health behavior: promise or promise missed. *Health Psychol.* 3:347-349 (1984).

Leventhal, H., Zimmerman, R. and Gutman, M. In: W.D. Gentry, *Handbook of Behavioral Medicine,* New York: Guilford Press, 1984, pp. 369-436.

Levi, L. Psychosocial factors in preventive medicine. In: Surgeon General's Report, *Healthy People,* 1979, 207-252.

Levine, S. and Coe, C.L. The use and abuse of cortisol as a measure of stress. In: T.M. Field, P.M. McCabe and N. Schneiderman (eds.), *Stress and Coping,* Hillsdale, N.J.: Erlbaum, 1985, 149-160.

Levy, B., et al. Reducing neonatal mortality rate with nurse midwives. *Am. J. Ob.-Gyn.* 109:509 (1971)

Levy, S.M. *Behavior and Cancer.* San Francisco: Jossey-Bass, 1985.

Lewis, C.M., et al. Relationships between birth with selected social, environmental and medical care factors. *Am. J. Pub. Health* 63:973-981 (1973).

Lewis, F. Mourning by the family after a still birth or neonatal death. In: *Coping With Physical Illness,* R.H. Moos (ed.), New York: Plenum, 1984, 43-50.

Liddell, H.S. *Emotional Hazards in Animals and Man.* Springfield, Illinois: Thomas, 1956.

Liddell, H.S. Sheep and goats: the psychological effects of laboratory experience of deprivation and stress upon certain experimental animals. In *Beyond the Germ Theory,* I. Galdston (ed.), New York: Health Education Council, 1954, 106-119.

Lilienfeld, A.M. and Pasamanick, B. The associations of maternal and fetal factors with the development of cerebral palsy and epilepsy. *Am. J. Ob.-Gyn.* 70:93-101 (1955).

Lilienfeld, A.M. and Parkhurst, E. A study of the association of factors of pregnancy and parturition with the development of cerebral palsy. *Amer. J. Hygiene* 53:262 (1951).

Lin, H.B., Carter, W.B. and Kleinman, A.M. An exploration somatization among Asian refugees and immigrants in primary care. *Am. J. Pub. Health* 75:1080-1084 (1985).

Lindbohm, M.L., Hemminki, K. and Kyyronen, P. Parental occupational exposure and spontaneous abortions in Finland. *Am. J. Epidemiol.* 120(3):370-378 (1984).

Lindemann, E. *Beyond Grief: Studies in Crisis Intervention.* New York: Aronson, 1979.

Lindheimer, M.D. and Katz, A.I. Hypertension in pregnancy. *N. Eng. J. Med.* 313:674-676 (1985).

Link, B. and Dohrenwend, B.P. Formulation of Hypotheses About the True Prevalence of Demoralization in the United States. In: *Mental Illness in the United States: Epidemiological Estimates.* B.P. Dohrenwend et al., eds. New York: Praeger, 1980.

Linn, S., et al. The association of marijuana use with outcome of pregnancy. *AJPH* 73:1161-1164 (1983).

Lipid Research Clinic Program. The lipid clinic coronary primary prevention brief results: The relationship of reduction in incidence of coronary heart disease to cholesterol lowering. *JAMA* 251:365-374 (1984).

Lipkin, M. and Kupka, K. *Psychosocial Factors Affecting Health.* New York: Praeger, 1982.

Littman, B. and Parmalee, A. Medical correlates of infant development. *Pediatrics* 61:470-474 (1978).

Little, B.C., Hayworth, J., Benson, P., Bridge, L.R., Dewhurst, J. and Priest, R.G. Psychophysiological ante-natal predictors of post-natal depressed mood. *J. Psychosom. Res.* 26(4):419-428 (1982).

Little, R.E. and Hook, E.B. Maternal alcohol and tobacco consumption and their association with nausea and vomiting during pregnancy. *Acta Obstet. Gynecol. Scand.* 58(1):15-17 (1979).

Locke, S.E. Stress, adaptation and immunity. *Gen. Hosp. Psychiat.* 4:49-58 (1982).

Longo, L. Prenatal care and its evolution in America. Unpublished manuscript (1983). Cited with author's permission.

Lovchik, J.C. and Alger, L. Chlamydia infection causes risks to pregnancy. *Nation's Health* 4 (May-June 1986).

Lubic, R.W. Effect of cost on patterns of maternity care. *Nursing Clinics of No. Amer.* 10:229-239 (1975).

Lubic, R.W. Evaluation of an out-of-hospital maternity center for low risk patients. In: *Health Policy and Nursing Practice,* L. Aiken (ed.), New York: McGraw-Hill, 1980.

Lubic, R.W. Alternative childbirth practices. In: *Pregnancy, Childbirth and Parenthood: Coping with Medical Issues*, P. Ahmed (ed.), 1981, 274-286.

Lubin, B., Gardener, S.H. and Roth, A. Mood and somatic symptoms during pregnancy. *Psychosom. Med.* 37(2):136-146 (1975).

Lumley, J. and Astbury, J. Advice in pregnancy: perfect remedies and imperfect science. In: *Effectiveness and Satisfaction in Internatal Care*, Enkin, M. and Chalmers, I. (eds.), London: Heinemann, 1982, pp. 132-150.

Lund, A.K. and Kegeles, S.S. Psychology, serendipity and public health: a reply to Suls and O'Leary. *Health Psychol.* 3:381-383 (1984).

Lunenfeld, E., Rosenthal, J., Larholt, K.K. and Insler, V. Childbirth experience – psychological, cultural and medical associations. *J. Psychosom. Ob.-Gyn.* 3:165-171 (1984).

Lutz, D.J. and Holmes, D.S. Instructions to change blood pressure and diastolic blood pressure biofeedback: their effects on diastolic blood pressure, systolic blood pressure and anxiety. *J. Psychosomatic Res.* 25:479-485 (1981).

Lux, E., Pa'al, M. and Solymos, A. Psychological and gynecological characteristics of rejection of the maternal role and its significance for sterility. *Wiad Led.* 36(8):687-690 (1983).

Lyon, J.L., Gardner, J.W., West, D.W., Stanish, W.M., Hebertson, R.M. Smoking and carcinoma in situ of the uterine cervix. *Am. J. Public Health* 73(5):558-562 (1983).

Lynch, M.A. and Roberts, J. Ill-health and child abuse. *Lancet* 317-319 (August 1975).

Lynch, M.A. and Roberts, J. Predicting child abuse: signs of bonding failure in the maternity hospital. *Br. Med. J.* I(6061):624-626 (1977).

Magni, A., et al. Ti fattore psicosociali e complicazze della gravedenza e del parto. *Medicina Psychosomatica* 28:129-137 (1983).

Mahlstedt, P.O. The psychological component of infertility. *Fertility and Sterility* 43:335-346 (1985).

Maimon, J.A. and Zapka, J.G. Improving frequency and proficiency of breast self-examination: effectiveness of an education program. *Am. J. Public Health* 75:618-624 (1985).

Mann, E.C. Habitual abortion: a report, in two parts, on 160 patients. *Am. J. of Ob-Gyn.* 77:706-718 (1959).

Mann, E.C. Psychiatric investigation of habitual abortion. *Ob-Gyn.* 7:589-601 (1956).

Marbury, M.C. The association of alcohol consumption with outcome of pregnancy. *Am. J. Pub. Health* 73:1165-168 (1983).

Marmot, M.G. and Morris, J.N. Social Factors Have a Powerful Influence on Health Status. In: *Oxford Book of Public Health*, Vol. I. New York and London: 1986.

Marshall, J.R., Graham, S., Byers, T., Swanson, M. and Brasure, J. Diet and smoking in the epidemiology of cancer of the cervix. *JNCI* 70(5):847-851 (1983).
Martin, H. *The Abused Child: A Multi-disciplinary Approach to Developmental Issues and Treatment.* Cambridge, Mass.: Ballinger Press, 1976.
Martin, J.E., et al. Behavioral control of exercise in sedentary adults: studies 1 through 6. *J. Consult. Clin. Psychol.* 52:795-811 (1984).
Martin, P.M. and Hill, G.B. Cervical cancer in relation to tobacco and alcohol consumption in Lesotho, southern Africa. *Cancer Det. Prev.* 7:109-115 (1984).
Martin, R.A. and Lefcourt, H.B. Sense of humor as a moderator of the relation between stress and moods. *J. Pers. Soc. Psychol.* 45:1313-1321 (1983).
Maruta, T., Swanson, D.W. and Swenson, W.M. Chronic pain: which patients may a pain management program help? *Pain* 7:321-329 (1979).
Masters, W.H. and Johnson, V.E. *Human Sexual Inadequacy.* Boston: Little, Brown, 1970.
Matarazzo, J.D. Behavioral health's challenge to academic, scientific and professional psychology. *Am. Psychologist* 37:1, 1-14 (1982).
Matarazzo, J.D. Behavioral immunogens and pathogens in health and illness. In: *Psychology and Health*, Vol. 3, Master Lectures. Washington, D.C.: APA, 1983, 5-44.
Matarazzo, J.D. Behavioral immunogens and pathogens: psychology's newest challenge. *Prof. Psychol.* 14:414-416 (1983).
Matarazzo, J.D. Behavioral health: a 1990 challenge for the health sciences professions. In: J.D. Matarazzo et al. (eds.), *Behavioral Health: A Handbook of Health Enhancement and Disease Prevention,* New York: Wiley, 1984, 3-40.
Matarazzo, J.D. *The Changing Patterns of Disease, Disability and Death: Pagan Gods, Harsh Environment and Microbial Pathogens,* 1984 (unpublished).
Matarazzo, J.D., Weiss, S.M., Herd, J.A. and Miller, N.E. *Behavioral Health: A Handbook of Health Enhancement and Disease Prevention.* New York: Wiley, 1984.
Matarazzo, J.D. Behavioral health and behavioral medicine: frontiers for a new health psychology. *Am. Psychol.* 35:9, 807-817.
Maternity Alliance Reports 1984-85, London, 1985.
Mathews, A. and Ridgeway, V. Psychological preparation for surgery. In: A. Steptoe and A. Mathews, *Health Care and Human Behavior,* New York and London: Academic Press, 1984, 231-259.
Mathews, K.A., Glass, D.C., Rosenman, R.N. and Bortner, R.H. Competitive drive, pattern A, and coronary heart disease. *J. Chron. Diseases* 30:489-498 (1977).
Mayberry, R.M. Cigarette smoking, herpes simplex virus type 2 infection and cervical abnormalities. *Am. J. Pub. Health* 75:676-678 (1985).

Mayo, R. Psychological morbidity in a clinic for sexually transmitted disease. *Br. J. Vener. Dis.* 51(1):57-60 (1975).

McCarthy, M. *Epidemiology and Policies for Health Planning*, King Edward's Hospital Fund for London (1983).

McCleod, B. Rx for health: a dose of self-confidence. *Psychol. Today* 46-50 (October 1986).

McDonald, R.L. The role of emotional factors in obstetrical complications. *Psychosom. Med.* 30:222-237 (1968).

McGinnis, J.M. Recent history of federal initiatives in prevention policy. *Am. Psychol.* 40:205-212 (1985).

McKeown, T. and Lowe, C.R. *An Introduction to Social Medicine.* Oxford: Blackwell Scientific Publications, 1966.

McKeown, T. *The Role of Medicine: Dream, Mirage or Nemesis.* London: Nuffield Provincial Hospitals Trust, 1976.

McKuldy, S.M. Menopause and mental health. Cited in *Psychol. Today* 12 (February 1985).

McKinley, J.B. The new latecomers to antenatal care. *Brit. J. Prev. Soc. Med.* 24:52-57 (1970).

McNeil, T.F., Kaij, L. and Malmquist-Larsson, A. Pregnant women with nonorganic psychosis: life situation and experience of pregnancy. *Acta Psychiatr. Scand.* 68:445-457 (1983).

McQuilty, L.L. Opportunities for cluster analysis: a review of Corr, *Cluster Analysis for Social Scientists.* In: *Contemporary Psychol.* 29:977 (1984).

McReynolds, P. *Advances in Psychological Assessment, Vol. 5.* San Francisco: Jossey-Bass, 1981.

McReynolds, P. and Chelune, G.J. *Advances in Psychological Assessment, Vol. 6.* San Francisco: Jossey-Bass, 1984.

Meade, T.W. Oral contraceptives, clotting factors, and thrombosis. *Am. J. Ob.Gyn.* 6 (2):768-761 (142).

Mechanic, D.C. *The Growth of Bureaucratic Medicine.* New York: Wiley, 1976.

Mechanic, D.C. The stability of health and illness behavior: results from a 16-year follow-up. *Am. J. Pub. Health* 69:1142-1145 (1977).

Mednick, S.A. Birth defects and schizophrenia. *Psychol. Today* 4:48-50 (1971).

Mehl, L.E., Peterson, G.H., Whitt, M.C. and Hawes, W.H. Outcomes of 1,146 elective home deliveries. *J. Reprod. Med.*, 1977

Mehl, L.E. Screening for risk. In: G.H. Peterson (ed.), *Birthing Normally: A Personal Growth Approach to Childbirth,* Berkeley: Mind-Body Press, 1981.

Mehl, L.E. and Peterson, G.H. An existential approach to risk screening and childbirth preparation. In: P. Ahmed (ed.), *Pregnancy, Childbirth and Parenthood: Coping with Medical Issues,* New York: Elsevier, 1981, 225-260.

Mehl, L.E. and Peterson, G.H. Matched comparison study of home vs. hospital birth. In: P. Ahmed (ed.), *Psychosocial Aspects of Pregnancy*, New York: Elsevier, 1981.

Mehl, L.E. The outcome of home delivery research in the United States. In: S. Kitzinger and J.A. Davis (eds.), *The Place of Birth*, Oxford: Oxford University Press, 1978, 93-117.

Mehlman, M.A., Shapiro, R.E., Cranmer, M.F. and Norvell, M.J. Hazards from toxic chemicals. National Center for Toxicological Research and the National Institutes of Health, Conference Proceedings. *J. Environmental Path. and Tox.*, 1978.

Melamed, B.G. *Health Intervention: Psychology and Health.* Master Lectures, Vol. 3. Washington, D.C.: APA, 1983, 78-119.

Melamed, B. Personal communication, 1983.

Melzak, R. and Wall, P.D. Pain mechanisms: a new theory. *Science* 150:971-979.

Melzak, R., Taenzer, P., Feldman, P. and Kinch, R. Labour is still painful after prepared childbirth training. *Can. Med. Assn. Jr.* 125:357-363 (1981).

Mendenhall, R.C. *Obstetrics - Gynecology Practice Study Report*, Los Angeles, USC School of Medicine, unpublished contract report, 1977.

Mergler D. and Vezina, D. Dysmenorrhea and cold exposure. *J. Repro. Med.* 30:106-111 (1985).

Merrick, T. The effect of piped water on early childhood mortality in urban Brazil, 1970-1970, Paper #594. Washington, D.C.: World Bank, 1983.

Merskey, H. Psychological and psychiatric aspects of pain control. In: W.L. Smith et al. (eds.), *Pain: Meaning and Management*, New York: Spectrum, 1980, 105-117.

Meyer, A. *The Commonsense Psychiatry of Adolph Meyer.* New York: McGraw Hill (1948).

Meyer, M.B., Tonascia, J.A. and Buck, C. The interrelationship of maternal smoking and increased perinatal mortality with other risk factors. Further analysis of the Ontario Perinatal Mortality Study, 1960-1961. *Am. J. Epidemiol.* 100(6):443-452 (1974).

Meyer, M.B., Jonas B.S. and Tonascia, J.A. Perinatal events associated with maternal smoking during pregnancy. *Am. J. Epidemiol.* 103(5):464-476 (1976).

Meyer, M.B. and Tonascia, J.A. Maternal smoking, pregnancy complications, and perinatal mortality. *Am. J. Obstet. Gynecol.* 128(5):494-502.

Meyer, M.B. How does maternal smoking affect birth weight and maternal weight gain? Evidence from the Ontario Perinatal Mortality Study. *Am. J. Obstet.- Gynecol.* 131(8):888-893 (1978).

Meyerowitz, B.E. Postmastectomy coping strategies and quality of life. *Health Psychology* 2(2):117-132 (1983).

Michael, J.M. The second revolution in health: health promotion and its environmental base. *Am. Psychol.* 37:936-941 (1982).

Miller, H.C., Hassanein, K. and Hensleigh, P.A. Fetal growth retardation in relation to maternal smoking and weight gain in pregnancy. *Am. J. Obstet. Gynecol.* 125(1):55-60 (1976).

Miller, H.C. and Jekel, J.F. Associations between unfavorable outcomes in successive pregnancies. *Am. J. Ob. Gyn.* 153:20-24 (1985).

Miller, H.L., Fowler, R.D. and Bridgers, W.T. The public health psychologist: an ounce of prevention is not enough. *Am. Psychol.* 37:9459 (1982).

Miller, M.W. Effects of alcohol on the generation and migration of cerebral cortical neurons. *Science* 233:1308-1321 (1986).

Miller, W.B. Sexual and contraceptive behavior in young unmarried women. In: D.D. Youngs and A.A. Ehrhardt, *Psychosomatic Obstetrics and Gynecology*, New York: Appleton-Century-Crofts, 1980, 211-238.

Miller, W.R. Motivation for treatment: a review with special emphasis on alcoholism. *Psychol. Bull.* 98:84-107 (1985).

Mindick, B., Oskamp, S. and Berger, D.E. Prediction of success or failure in birth planning: an approach to prevention of individual and family stress. *Am. J. Community Psychol.*, 5(4):447-459 (1977).

Mindick, B., Oskamp, S. and Snortnum, J. Personality characteristics as trans-situational predictors of contraceptive behavior. *Personality Soc. Psychol. Bull.* 4:362 (1978).

Moldofsky, H., et al. The relationship of interleukin-1 and immune functions to sleep in humans. *Psychosom. Med.* 48:309-318 (1986).

Moldofsky, H., Lue, F.A. and Smythe, H.A. Alpha EEG sleep and morning symptoms in rheumatoid arthritis. *J. Rheumatol.* 10:373-379 (1983).

Molfese, V.J., Thomson, B.K. and Bennett, A.G. Perinatal outcome: similarity and predictive value of antepartum assessment scales. *J. Repro. Med.* 30:30-38 (1985).

Monroe, S.M. Bromet, E.J., Connell, M.M. and Steiner, S.C. Social support, life events, and depressive symptoms: a 1-year prospective study. *J. Consult. Clin. Psychol.* 54:424-431 (1986).

Moore, J.E. and Chaney, E.F. Outpatient group treatment of chronic pain: effects of spouse involvement. *J. Consult. Clin. Psychol.* 53:326-334 (1985).

Moos, R.H. *Coping With Physical Illness.* New York: Plenum, 1984.

Mor, V., McHorney, C. and Sherwood, S. Secondary morbidity among the recently bereaved. *Am. J. Psychiat.* 143:158-168 (1986).

Morisky, D.E., et al. Evaluation of family health education to build social support for long term control of high blood pressure. *Health Ed. Quart.* 12:35-50 (1985).

Morrison, D.M. Adolescent contraceptive behavior: a review. *Psychol. Bull.* 98:538-568 (1985).

Mozley, P.D. Emotional parameters of infertility. In: D.D. Youngs and A.A. Ehrhardt (eds.), *Psychosomatic Obstetrics and Gynecology*, New York: Appleton-Century-Crofts, 1980, 241-253.

Nadelson, CC. The emotional impact of abortion. In: M.T. Notman and C.C. Nadelson, *The Woman Patient: Medical and Psychological Interfaces*, New York: Plenum, 1978, 173-179.

Naeye, R.L. Abruptio placentae and placenta previa: frequency, perinatal mortality, and cigarette smoking. *Ob.-Gyn.* 55(6):701-704 (1980).

Naeye, R.L. Causes of perinatal mortality in the U.S. collaborative perinatal project. *JAMA* 238(3):228-229 (1977).

Naeye, R.L. The duration of maternal cigarette smoking, fetal and placental disorders. *Early Hum. Dev.* 3(3):229-237 (1979).

Naeye, R.L. Relationship of cigarette smoking to congenital anomalies and perinatal dealth. A prospective study. *Am. J. Pathol.* 90(2):289-293 (1978).

Nathanson, C.A. and Becker, M.H. The influence of client-provider relationships on teenage women's subsequent use of contraception. *Am. J. Pub. Health* 75:33-38 (1985).

National Center for Health Statistics. Series 13, #45. National Ambulatory Medical Care Survey, 1977.

National Center for Health Statistics. Series 13, #63. National Health Survey: Use of health services for disorders of the female reproductive system, 1977-1978.

National Center for Health Statistics. Advanced Data #30, July 1978.

National Center for Health Statistics. Vital Statistics of the U.S., Vol. II, Mortality, Part 1, 1979.

National Center for Health Statistics. Advanced Data #45, February 1979. Use of family planning services by currently married women 15-44.

National Center for Health Statistics. Advanced Data #54, February 1981. Fats, cholesterol and sodium intake in the diet of persons 1-74 years.

National Center for Health Statistics. National Ambulatory Medical Care Survey, 1980-1981.

National Center for Health Statistics. Health Promotion and Disease Prevention, #119 (1986).

National Center for Health Statistics. Vital and Health Statistics. Maternal Weight Gain and the Outcome of Pregnancy. Series 21, #44, PHS #86-1922.

National Center for Health Statistics. Vital and Health Statistics. Morbidity and Mortality Weekly Reports: Annual Summary, 1982. Behavioral risk factors, December 1983.

National Center for Health Statistics. Vital and Health Statistics. Advanced Data. Health care of adolescents by office based physicians, 1984.

National Center for Health Statistics, 1985. News release of July 10, for 1984. *Peninsula Times Tribune*, October 11, 1985.

National Center for Health Statistics. Advanced Data, Diagnosis related groups using data from the National Hospital Discharge Survey: U.S. 1982, #105, 1985.

National Institute of Medicine. *Health and Behavior: Frontiers of Research in the Biobehavioral Sciences.* Washington, D.C.: National Academy Press, 1982.

National Institutes of Health. Consensus Development Conference Osteoporosis, 5:#3 (1984).

Nation's Health. Little known on safety of birth settings. (February 1983).

Nation's Health. Call for increase of hepatitis vaccination. (January 1985), 1, 9.

Nation's Health. News article reporting: a national agenda to address women's mental health needs. (April 1985), 8.

Nation's Health. Doctors can double number of smokers who quit. (January 1986), 11.

Nelson, E.C., et al. Medical self care education for elders: a controlled trial to evaluate impact. *Am. J. Pub. Health* 74:1357-1362 (1984).

Nesbitt, R. and Aubrey, R. High risk obstetrics II: Value of semiobjective grading system in identifying the vulnerable group. *Am. J. Ob.-Gyn.* 103:972-985 (1969).

Newton, W. and Keith, L.G. Role of sexual behavior in the development of pelvic inflammatory disease. *J. Repro. Med.* 30:77-81 (1985).

Nisbett, R.E. and Wilson, T.D. Telling more than we know: verbal reports on mental health processes. *Psychol. Review* 84:231-259 (1977).

Niemiec, M.A. and Chen, S.P. Seeking clinic care for veneral disease: a study of teenagers. *J. Sch. Health* 48(1):681-686 (1978).

Ng, L.I. *New Approaches to the Treatment of Chronic Pain*, NIDA Research Monograph 36, Washington, D.C.: Department of Health, Education and Welfare, 1983.

Norbeck, J. and Tilden, V. Lifestress, social support and emotional disequilibrium in complications of pregnancy: a prospective multivariate study. *J Health Soc. Behav.* 24:30-46 (1983).

Norris, R.V. *PMS/Premenstrual Syndrome.* New York: Rawson, 1983.

Notman, M.T. and Nadelson, C.C. *The Woman Patient: Medical and Psychological Interfaces.* New York: Plenum, 1978.

Nuckolls, K.B., Cassel, J. and Kaplan, B. Psychosocial assets, life crisis and the prognosis of pregnancy. *Am. J. of Epid.* 95(5):531-441 (1972).

Nunes, M.C., Sobrinho, L.G., Calhaz-Jorge, C., Santos, M.A., Mauricio, J.C. and Sousa, M.F. Psychosomatic factors in patients with hyperprolactinemia and/or galactorrhea. *Ob-Gyn.* 55:591-595 (1980).

Nyswander, K.R. and Gordon, M. *The Women and Their Pregnancies: Collaborative Perinatal Study of the National Institute of Neurological Disease and Stroke.* Washington, D.C.: U.S., Department of Health, Education and Welfare, 1972.

Oakley, A., MacFarlane, H. and Chalmers, I. Social class, stress, and reproduction. In: A.R. Rees and H.J. Purcell, *Disease and the Environment*, Chichester and New York: Wiley, 1982, 11-50.

Obayuwana, A.O., Carter, A.C. and Barnett, R.M. Psychosocial distress and pregnancy outcome: a 3-year prospective study. *J. Psycho. Ob.-Gyn.* 3:173-183 (1984).

O'Brien. P.M.S.: The premenstrual syndrome: a review. *J. Repro. Med.* 30:113-126 (1985).

O'Brient, M. and Smith, C. Women's views and experiences of ante natal care. *The Practitioner* 225:123-126 (1981).

O'Hara, M.W., Rehm, L.P. and Campbell, S.B. Postpartum depression: a role for social network and life stress variables. *J. Nerv. Ment. Dis.* 171(6):336-341 (1983).

O'Hoy, K.M. and Tang, G.W.K. Sexual function following treatment for carcinoma of cervix. *J. Psychosom. Ob-Gyn.* 4:41-48 (1985).

Okada, F. Depression after treatment with thiazide diuretics for hypertension. *Am. J. Psychiat.* 142:1101-1102 (1985).

Olasov, B. and Jackson, J. Effects of expectancies on women's reports of moods during the menstrual cycle. *Psychosomatic Medicine*, 1986, in press.

Oleskier, E. and Walsh, L.V. Childbearing among lesbians. *J. Nurse Midwifery* 29:322-327 (1984).

Oliver, J.M. and Simmons, M.E. Depression as measured by the DSM II and the Beck Depression Inventory in an unselected adult population. *J. Consult. Clin. Psychol.* 52:892-898 (1984).

Olsen, J., Rachootin, P., Schiodt, A.V. and Damsbo, N. Tobacco use, alcohol consumption and infertility. *Int. J. Epid.* 12:179-184 (1983).

O'Neill, C.P. and Zeichner, A. Working women: a study of relationships between stress, coping and health. *J. Psychosom. Ob.-Gyn.* 4:105-116 (1985).

Osborne, D. The MMPI in medical practice. *Psychiat. Annals* 15:534-541 (1985).

Osofsky, H.J. and Blumenthal, S.J. *Premenstrual Syndrome: Current Findings and Future Directions.* Washington, D.C.: Am. Psychiat. Press, 1985.

Osofsky, H.J. and Keppel, W. Psychiatric and gynecological evaluation and management of premenstrual symptoms. In: *Premenstrual Syndrome: Current Findings and Future Directions*, H.J. Osofsky and S.J. Blumenthal (eds.), Washington, D.C.: American Psychiatric Press, 1985, 39-54.

Osofsky, H.J. and Osofsky, J.D. Transition to parenthood—risk factors for mothers and infants. *American Society of Psychosomatic Ob-Gyn,* April 1985.

Osofsky, J.D. *Handbook of Infant Development.* New York: Wiley, 1979.

Oster, G. and Epstein, A.M. Primary prevention and coronary heart disease: the economic benefits of lowering serum cholesterol. *Am. J. Pub. Health* 76:647-656 (1986).

Othner, E. and DeSouza, C. A screening test for somatization disorder (hysteria). *Am. J. Psychiat.* 142:1146-1149 (1985).

Paavonen, J., et al. Etiology of cervical inflammation. *Am. J. Ob. Gyn.* 154:556-564 (1986).

Page, I.H. and McCubbin, J.W. The physiology of arterial hypertension. *Handbook Physiol., Sect. 2, Circ. 3* 3:3163-2208 (1965).

Pakter, J. Births at home create debate on safety. *The Nation's Health,* February 1977, 12.

Parazzini, F., et al. Risk factors for pathologically confirmed benign breast disease. *Am. J. Epid.* 12:115-122 (1984).

Parboosingh, J. and Kerr, J. Innovations in the role of obstetrical hospitals in prenatal care. In: M. Enkin and I. Chalmers, *Effectiveness and Satisfaction in Antenatal Care,* London: Heinemann, 1982, 254-264.

Parson, D. *Health and Behavior.* Washington, D.C.: Institute of Medicine, National Academy Press.

Patel, C. A new dimension in the prevention of coronary heart disease. In: T.J. Dembrowski, T.H. Schmidt and G. Blumchen (eds.), *Biobehavioral Bases of Coronary Heart Disease: Karger Biobehavioral Medicine Series 2,* Basel: Karger, 1983, 416-438.

Paxton, N.F. and Franklin, J.G. The first 1,000 deliveries at the booth maternity center in Philadelphia. *Transactions of the American Assoc. of Obstet. & Gynecol.,* 85:152 (1974).

Paykel, E.S. Contribution of life events to causation of psychiatric illness. *Psychol. Med.* 8:245-253 (1978).

Paykel, E.S., Emms, E.M., Fletcher, J. and Rassaby, E.S. Life events and social support in puerperal depression. *Br. J. Psychiatry* 136:339-346 (1980).

Pearce, S. and Beard, R.W. Chronic Pelvic Pain. In: *Psychology and Gynaecological Problems.* A. Broome and L. Wallace (eds.), London: Tavistock, 1986.

Pearse, W.H. Home birth. *J. Am. Med. Assoc.,* 241:95-110 (1979).

Peckham, C.S. and Marshall, W.C. Infections in pregnancy. In: S.L. Barron and A.M. Thomson. *Obstetrical Epidemiology,* New York: Academic Press, 1983, 210-256.

Peele, S. The cultural context of psychological approaches to alcoholism. *Am. Psychol.* 39:1137-1351 (1984).

Pennebaker, J.W. Accuracy of symptom perception. In: *Social Psychological Aspects of Health, Handbook of Health Psychology, Vol. IV*, S.E. Taylor and J. E. Singer (eds.), Hillsdale, New Jersey: Erlbaum, 1984, 189-217.

Pennebaker, J.W. *The Psychology of Physical Symptoms*. New York: Springer Verlag, 1982.

Peoples, M.D., Grimson, R.C. and Daughtry, G.L. Evaluation of the effects of the North Carolina improved pregnancy outcome project: implications for state-level decision-making. *Am. J. Pub. Health* 74:549-554 (1984).

Perez, R. Effects of stress, social support and coping style in adjustment to pregnancy among Hispanic women. *Hispanic J. Behav. Sci.* 5:141-161 (1983).

Peterson, D.R. Sudden Infant Death Syndrome. In: *Perinatal Epidemiology*. M.B. Bracken (ed.), New York and London: Oxford University Press, 1984.

Peterson, G.H., Mehl, L.E. and Leiderman, P.H. The relation of prenatal attitude and birth experience to father attachment. *Am. J. Orthopsychiat.*, April 1979.

Peterson, G.H. and Mehl, L.E. Some determinants of maternal attachment. *Amer. J. Psychiat.*, October, 1978.

Peterson, L.G., Peterson, McK., O'Shanick, G.J. and Swann, A. Selfinflicted gunshot wounds. *Am. J. Psychiat.* 142:228-232.

Peterson, O.L., et al. An analytical study of North Carolina medical practice. *J. Med. Educ.* 31(II), December 1956.

Petitti, D.B. and Klatsky, A.L. Malignant hypertension in women aged 15 to 44 years and its relation to cigarette smoking and oral contraceptives. *Am. J. Cardiol.* 52(3):297-298 (1983).

Petitti, D.B., Wingerd, J., Pellegrin, F. and Ramcharan, S. Oral contraceptives, smoking, and other factors in relation to risk of venous thromboembolic disease. *Am. J. Epidemiol.* 108(6):480-485 (1978).

Petitti, D.B. and Wingerd, J. Use of oral contraceptives, cigarette smoking, and risk of subarachnoid haemorrhage. *Lancet* 2(8083):234-235 (1978).

Petitti, D.B., Wingerd, J., Pellegrin, F. and Ramcharan, S. Risk of vascular disease in women. Smoking, oral contraceptives, noncontraceptive estrogens, and other factors. *JAMA* 242(11):1150-1154 (1979).

Petterson, K. *Psychophysiological Correlates of Premenstrual Tension*. Reports Dept. Psychology, University of Stockholm, 1975, 446, p. 16.

Pharaoh, P.O.D. Obstetrical and neonatal care related to outcome: a comparison of two maternity hospitals. *Brit. J. Prev. Soc. Med.* 3,4:256, 261 (1976).

Pierog, S., Chandavasu, O. and Wexler, I. The fetal alcohol syndrome: some maternal characteristics. *Int. J. Gynaecol. Obstet.* 16(5):412-415 (1979).

Pierson, E.C. Gynecological approach to counseling the sexually active young woman. *Clin. Ob.-Gyn.* 21:235-248 (1978).

Piper, J.M., Matonoski, G.M. and Tonascic, J. Bladder cancer in young women. *Am. J. Epid.* 123:1033-1045 (1986).

Plant, S.M. and Friedman, S.B. Psychosocial factors in infectious disease. In: R. Ader (ed.), *Psychoneuroimmunology*, New York: Academic Press, 1981, 3-30.
Polit, D.F. and LaRocco, S.A. Social and psychological correlates of menopausal symptom. *Psychosom. Med.* 42:335-345 (1980).
Polivy, J. and Herman, P.C. Dieting and binging. *Am. Psychol.* 40:193-201 (1985).
Porreco, R.P. High cesarian section rate: a new perspective. *Ob.-Gyn.* 65:307-311 (1985).
Porter, J.B., Hunter, J.R., Jick, H. and Stergachis, A. Oral contraceptives and nonfatal vascular disease. *Ob.-Gyn.* 66:1-4 (1985).
Porter, W.P., et al. Toxicant-disease-environment interactions associated with suppressing of immune system, growth and reproduction. *Science* 224:1014ff. (1984).
Powers, W.T. *Behavior: The Control of Perception.* Chicago: Aldine, 1973.
Pratt, L. *Family Structure and Effective Health Behavior.* Boston: Houghton, Mifflin, 1976.
Prechtl, H.F.R. Neurological sequela of prenatal and perinatal complications. *Brit. Med. J.* 34:763 (1967).
Prevention Index '86, Prevention Research Center. Emmaus, Pennsylvania: 1986.
Pritchard, J.A., MacDonald, P.C. and Grant, N.F. *Williams Obstetrics.* Norwalk, Conn.: Appleton-Century-Crofts, 1985.
Proctor, N.H. and Hughes, J.P. *Chemical Hazards of the Workplace.* Philadelphia: Lippincott, 1978.
Prokop, C.K. and Bradley, L.A. (eds.), *Medical Psychology: Contributions to Behavioral Medicine.* New York: Academic Press, 1981.
Prutting, J. Autopsies-benefits for clinicians. *Am. J. Clin. Path* 69 (Supp. 1):223-225 (1978).
Psychosomatic determinants in hyperprolactinemic women. *Ob.-Gyn. Lit. News* 1984, 4.
Public Health Service, *Women's Health: Report of The Task Force on Women's Health Issues.* Washington, D.C. (1985).
Queenan, J.T. and Hobbins, J.C. *Protocols for High Risk Pregnancies.* Oradele, N.J.: Med. Econ. Books (1983).
Rabin, A.I. Are the mentally abnormal dangerous? (book review). *Cont. Psychol.* 30:38-39 (1985).
Rabkin, J.G. and Struening, E.L. Life events, stress and illness. *Science* 194:1013-1020 (1976).
Rahe, R.H. The pathway between subjects' recent life changes and their nearfailure illness report. In: B.S Dohrenwend and B.P. Dohrenwend, *Stressful Life Events: Their Nature and Effects*, New York: Wiley and Sons, 1974.

Rainwater, L. and Weinstein, J. *And the Poor Get Children.* Chicago: Quadrangle Books, 1960.

Rannevik, G., Starup, J. and Doberi, A. Current concepts on fibrocystic breast disease. *Acta Ob. Gyn. Scand.* Supp. 123:147-196 (1984).

Rayburn, W.F. and McKean, H.E. Maternal perception of fetal movement and perinatal outcome. *Ob.-Gyn.* 38(3):504-512 (1982).

Reading, A.E. The influence of maternal anxiety on the course and outcome of pregnancy: a review. *Health Psychology* 2(2):187-202 (1983).

Reading, A.E., Cox, D.N., Sledmere, C.M. and Campbell, S. Psychological changes over the course of pregnancy: a study of attitudes toward the fetus/neonate. *Health Psychol.* 3:211-221 (1984).

Realini, J.P. and Goldheizer, J.W. Oral contraceptives and cardiovascular disease: a critique of the epidemiological studies. *Am. J. Ob. Gyn.* 152(2):729- 795 (1985).

Reddy, D.M. Breast self examination, correlates and research needs. *The Health Psychologist*, 1984, winter.

Rees, A.R. and Purcell, H.J. *Disease and the Environment.* Chichester and New York: Wiley, 1982.

Rehu, M. The effect of education, marital status and sexual behaviour on the incidence of puerperal endometritis and bacteriuria. *Ann. Clin. Res.* 19(6):315- 319 (1980).

Reich, J., Tupin, J.P. and Abramowitz, S.I. Psychiatric diagnosis of chronic pain patients. *Am. J. of Psychiatry.* 141:11 (1983).

Reich, T. and Winokur, G. Postpartum psychoses in patients with manic depressive disease. *J. Nerv. & Ment. Dis.* 151(1):60-68 (1970).

Renaer, M., Vertonimer, I.H., Nijs, P., Wageman, L. and Van Hemelrijck, T. Psychological aspects of chronic pelvic pain in women. *Am. J. Ob. Gyn.* 134:75- 78 (1979).

Revicki, D.A. and May, H.J. Occupational stress, social support and depression. *Health Psychol.* 4:61-77 (1985).

Riegle, D.W. The psychological and social effects of unemployment. *Am. Psychol.* 37:1124-1127 (1982).

Riley, V., Fitzmaurice, M.A. and Spackman, D.H. Psychoneuroimmunological Factors in Neoplasia: Studies in Animals. In: R. Ader (ed.), *Psychoneuroimmunology*, New York: Academic Press, 1981, 31-102.

Ringler, M. and Krizmanits, A. Psychosomatic aspects of emesis gravidarum: somatic and psychosocial status of females in early pregnancy. *Z. Geburtshilfe Perinatol.* 188(5):234-238 (1984).

Rizzardo, R., et al. Psychosocial aspect during pregnancy and obstetrical complications. *J. Psychosom. Ob. Gyn.* 4:11-22 (1985).

Roback, H.B. *Helping Patients and Their Families Cope with Medical Problems.* San Francisco: Jossey-Bass, 1985.

Robbins, L.C. and Blankenbaker, R. Prospective medicine and the health hazard appraisal. In: R.B. Taylor, J.R. Vreda and J.W. Denham (eds.), *Health Promotion: Principles and Clinical Applications*, Norwalk, Ct.: Appleton-Century-Crofts, 1982, 67-121.

Roberts, M. Nationwide screening for breast cancer plea. *London Times*, July 5, 1985.

Robitaille, Y. and Kraner, M.S. Does participation in prenatal courses lead to heavier babies? *Am. J. Pub. Health* 75:1187-1189 (1985).

Rodin, G. Aging and health: effects of the sense of control. *Science* 233: 1271-1276 (1986).

Rodin, G. and Voshard K. Depression in the medically ill: an overview. *Am. J. Psychiat.* 143:696-705 (1986).

Rodin, J. A sense of control. *Psychology Today*, 38-42 (December 1984).

Roeske, N.C.A. Hysterectomy and other gynecological surgeries. In: M.T. Notman and C.C. Nadelson, *The Woman Patient: Medical and Psychological Interfaces*, New York: Plenum, 1978.

Roethlisberger, F.J. and Dickson, W.T. *Management and the Worker*. Cambridge, Massachusetts: Harvard University Press, 1946.

Rofe, Y. and Goldberg, J. Prolonged exposure to a war environment and its effects on the blood pressure of pregnant women. *Br. J. Med. Psychol.* 56 (Pt. 4):3-5-311 (1983).

Rogel, M.J. and Zuehlke, M.E. Adolescent contraceptive behavior. In: I.R. Stuart and C.F. Wells (eds.), *Pregnancy in Adolescence: Needs, Problems and Management*, New York: Van Nostrand, 1982.

Rogers, D.F. Adjusting to a no-growth future: Imperatives for academic medicine in the 1980s. *Cornell U. Med. College Alum. Quart.* 43:3-9 (1980).

Roman, E., Doyle, P., Beral, V., Alberman, E. and Pharoah, P. Fetal loss, gravidity, and pregnancy order. *Early Hum. Dev.* 2(2):131-138 (1978).

Roman, E. and Stevenson, A.C. Spontaneous abortion. In: S.L. Barron and A.M. Thomson, *Obstetrical Epidemiology*, New York: Academic Press, 1983, 61-87.

Romano, J.M. and Turner, J.A. Chronic pain and depression: does the evidence support a relationship? *Psychol. Bull.*, 97:18-34 (1985).

Romero, R. First trimester vaginal bleeding. In: J.T. Queenan and J.C. Hobbins, *Protocols for High Risk Pregnancies*, Oradele, N.J.: Med. Econ. Books, 1983, 196- 200.

Romney, S.L., Gray, M.J., Little, A.B., Merrill, J.A., Wuilligan, E.J. and Stander, R. *Gynecology and Obstetrics: The Health Care of Women*. New York: McGraw-Hill, 1975.

Rosen, M. Pain and its relief. In Chard and Richards (eds.), *Benefits And Hazards Of The New Obstetrics*, Ondon, Heinemann 1977.

Rosen, M.G. and members of the task force on cesarean childbirth. *Consensus Development Conference on Cesarean Childbirth.* U.S. Department of Health and Human Services, Public Health Services, National Institutes of Health, July 1980.

Rosenfield, A. and Maine, D. Maternal mortality: a neglected tragedy. *Lancet* 2(8446):83-85 (July 13, 1985).

Rosenman, R.H., Brand, R.J., Jenkins, C.D., Friedman, M., Straus, R. and Wurm, M. Coronary heart disease and the Western Collaborative Study Group: Find follow up experience after 8 years. *JAMA* 233:872-877 (1975).

Rosenstock, I.M. and Kirscht, J.R. Why people seek health care. In: G.C. Stone, F. Cohen and N.N. Adler (eds.), *Health Psychology*, San Francisco: Jossey-Bass Publishers, 1979, 161-188.

Rosenthal, D. and Frank, J.D. Psychotherapy and the placebo effect. *Psychol. Bull.* 53:294-302 (1956).

Roth, S. and Cohen, L.J. Approach, avoidance and coping with stress. *Am. Psychol.* 41:813-819 (1986).

Rubin, R. Bonding-in in the postpartum period. *Maternal & Child Nursing J.* 6(2):67-75 (1977).

Rubinow, D.R. and Roy-Byrne, P. Premenstrual syndromes: overview from a methodologic perspective. *Am. J. Psychiat.* 141:163-172 (1984).

Rubinow, D.R., et al. Menstrually related mood disorders. In: H.J. Osofsky and S.J. Blumenthal, *Premenstrual Syndrome: Current Findings and Future Directions*, Washington, D.C.: Am. Psychiatric Press, 1985, 27-36.

Rubinow, D.R., et al. Prospective assessment of menstrually related mood disorders. *Am. J. Psychiat.* 141:684-686 (1984).

Ruble, D.N. and Brooks-Gunn, J. Menstrual symptoms: a social cognition analysis. *J. Behav. Med.* 2(2):171-194 (1979).

Ruddell, H., et al. Coronary-prone behavior and blood pressure reactivity in laboratory and life stress. In: T.J. Dembrowski, T.H. Schmidt and G. Blumchen (eds.), *Biobehavioral Bases of Coronary Heart Disease: Karger Biobehavioral Medicine series 2*, Basel: Karger, 1982, 185-196.

Ruff, M.R., Pert, C.B., Weber, R.J., Wahl, L.M., Wahl, S.M. and Paul, S.M. Benzodiazepam receptor-mediated chemotaxis of human monocytes. *Science* 229:1281-1283 (1985).

Russell, J.R. Maternal Mortality. In: S.L. Barron and A.M. Thomson (eds.), *Obstetrical Epidemiology*, New York: Academic Press, 1983, 399-416.

Russell, M.A.H., Wilson, C., Taylor, C. and Baker, C.D. Effect of general practitioners' advice against smoking. *Br. Med. J.* 2:231-235 (1979).

Russell-Briefel, R., Ezzati, T. and Perlman, J. Prevalence and trends in oral contraceptive use in premenopausal females ages 12-54 years, U.S., 1971-80. *Am. J. Pub. Health* 75:1173-1176 (1985).

Ryan, G., Sweeney, P. and Sorola, A. Pregnancy care and pregnancy outcome. *Ob.-Gyn.* 137:876-888 (1980).

Sadet, D.L. and Haynes, R.R. *Compliance with Therapeutic Regimes.* Baltimore: Johns Hopkins Press, 1976.

Sadeghi, S.B., et al. Prevalence of cervical intraepithelial neoplasia in sexually active teenagers and young adults. *Am. J. Ob-Gyn.* 148:726-729 (1984).

Sakiyama, R. and Quan, M. Galactorrhea and hyperprolactinemia. *Ob.-Gyn. Survey* 38:689-700 (1983).

Saks, B.R., et al. Depressed mood during pregnancy and the puerperium: clinical recognition and implications for clinical practice. *Am. J. Psychiat.* 142:728-732 (1985).

Salonen, J.T. Oral contraceptives, smoking and risk of myocardial infarction in young women. A longitudinal population study in eastern Finland. *Acta Med. Scand.* 212(3):141-144 (1982).

Sameroff, A.J. and Chandler, M.J. Reproductive risk and the continuum of caretaking causality. In: F.D. Horowitz (ed.), *Review of Child Development Research,* Vol. 4, Chicago, University of Chicago Press, 1975.

Sandberg, D., Field, T.M., Quetel, T.A., Garcia, R. and Rosario, M. Prenatal stress and fetal activity in humans. In: T.M. Field, P.M. McCabe and N. Schneiderman (eds.), *Stress and Coping,* Hillsdale, N.J.: Erlbaum, 1985, 161-178.

Sandler, D.P., Everson, R.B., Wilcox, A.J. and Browder, J.P. Cancer risk in adulthood from early life exposure to parents smoking. *Am. J. Pub. Health* 75:487-492 (1985).

Sansom, C.D., MacInery, J., Oliver, J. and Wakefield, J. Differential response to recall in a cervical cancer screening program. *Brit. J. Prev. Soc. Med.* 29:4047 (1975).

Sarason, I.G. and Sarason, B.R. Life change, moderators of stress, and health. In: A. Baum, S.E. Taylor and J.E. Singer (eds.), *Handbook of Psychology and Health,* Vol. IV, *Social Psychological Aspects of Health.* Hillsdale, N.J.: Erlbaum, 1984, 279-299.

Schafer, R. The pursuit of failure and the idealization of unhappiness. *Am. Psychol.* 39:398-405 (1984).

Schecter, M.T., Miller, A. and Howe, G.R. Cigarette smoking and breast cancer. *Am. J. Epid.* 121:479-487 (1985).

Schmale, A.H. and Iker, H.P. The affect of hopelessness and the development of cancer. *Psychosom. Med.* 28:714-721 (1966).

Schmale, A.H. and Iker, H. Hopelessness as a predictor of cervical cancer. *Soc. Sci. and Med.* 5:95-100 (1971).

Schmale, H. and Iker, H. The psychological setting of uterine cervical cancer. *Annals N.Y. Acad. Sci.* 125:794-780 (1965).

Schneiderman, N. and McCabe, P.M. Biobehavioral responses to stressors. In: T.M. Field, P.M. McCabe, and N. Schneiderman (eds.), *Stress and Coping*, Hillsdale, N.J.: Erlbaum, 1985, 43-61.

Schnider, S.M., et al. Uterine blood flow and plasma norepinephrine changes during maternal stress in the pregnant ewe. *Anesthesiology* 50:524-527 (1979).

Schofield, B.S. *Sexually Transmitted Diseases*. Edinburgh: Churchill Livingstone, 1979.

Schramm, W.F. WIC Prenatal participation and its relationship to newborn Medicaid costs in Missouri: a cost/benefit analysis. *Am. J. Pub. Health* 75:851- 857 (1985).

Schreiber, C., Florin, I. and Rost, W. Psychological correlates of functional secondary amenorrhea. *Psychother. Psychosom.* 39(2):106-111 (1983).

Schuckit, M.A., Daly, V., Herrman, G. and Hineman, S. Premenstrual symptoms and depression in a university population. *Dis. Nerv. Syst.* 36(9):516-517 (1975).

Schwartz, G. The brain as a health care system. In: G.C. Stone, F. Cohen and N.N. Adler (eds.), *Health Psychology*, San Francisco: Jossey-Bass, 1979, 549-572.

Schwartz, G. Psychological patterning and emotion: implications for the self-regulation of emotion. In: K.R. Blankstein and J. Policy. *Self-control and Self-modification of Emotional Behavior*, Plenum Publishing Corp., 1982.

Schwartz, G. Testing the biopsychosocial model: the ultimate challenge facing behavioral medicine? *J. Consulting and Clinical Psychol.* 50:6, 1040-1053 (1982).

Schwartz, G.E. Disregulation theory and disease: applications to the repression/cerebral disconnection/cardiovascular disorder hypothesis. *Int. Rev. Applied Psychol.* 32:95-118 (1983).

Schwartz, M.A. and Wiggins, O.P. Systems and the structuring of meaning: contributions to a biopsychosocial medicine. *Am. J. Psychiat.* 143: 1213-1221 (1986).

Schwartz, M.F. and Masters, W.H. The Masters and Johnson treatment program for dissatisfied homosexual men. *Am. of Psychiatry* 141:2 (1984).

Science, Depression research advances, treatment lags. 233:723-725 (1986).

Science, ADAMHA Funding 227:147-149 (1985).

Science, How important is dietary calcium in preventing osteoporosis? 233:519-520 (1986).

Science, Is the war on cancer being won? 229:543-544 (1985).

Seibel, M.M., Freeman, M.G. and Graves, W.L. Carcinoma of the cervix and sexual function. *Obstet. Gynecol.* 55(4):484-487.

Seligman, M.E.P. *Helplessness or Depression, Development and Death*. San Francisco: Freeman, 1975.

Selye, H.A. *The Stress of Life*. New York: McGraw Hill, 1976, 2nd edition.
Selye, H.A. A syndrome produced by diverse nocuous agents. *Nature*: 138:32 (1936).
Sexton, M. and Hebel, J.R. A clinical trial of change in maternal smoking and its effect on birth weight. *JAMA* 251(7):911-915 (1984).
Shanok, S.S. and Lewis, D.O. Medical histories of abused delinquents. *Child Psychiatry & Human Dev.* 11(4):222-231 (Spring, 1981).
Shapiro, S., Schlesinger, E.R. and Nesbitt, R.E.L. *Infant Perinatal, Maternal and Childhood Mortality in the United States*. Boston: Harvard University Press, 1968.
Shavit, Y., et al. Opioid peptides mediate the suppressive effect of stress on natural killer cell cytotoxicity. *Science* 223:188-190 (1984).
Shekelle, R.B. et al. Dietary vitamin A and risk of cancer in the Western Electric Study. *Lancet* 2: 1185-1190 (November, 1981).
Shekelle, R.B., et al. Psychological depression and 17 year risk of death from cancer. *Psychosom. Med.* 43:117-125 (1981).
Sheridan, M.D. Infants at risk of handicapping conditions. *Mon. Bul. Health & PHLS* 21:238 (1962).
Shetulle, R.B., Gale, M., Ostfeld, A.M. and Paul, O. Hostility, risk of coronary heart disease and mortality. *Psychom. Med.* 45:109-114 (1983).
Showstack, J.A., Budetti, P.P. and Minkler, D. Factors associated with birthweight: an exploration of the roles of prenatal care and length of gestation. *Am. J. Pub. Health* 74:1003-1008 (1984).
Shy, K.K., Frost, F. and Ullom, J. Out-of-hospital delivery in Washington State, 1975 to 1977. *Am. J. Ob.-Gyn.* 137:547-552 (1980).
Siebold, D. and Roper, R. Psychosocial determinants of health care intention: test of the Triandis and Fishbein models. In: D. Nimmo (ed.), *Communication Yearbook 3*, New Brunswick: Transaction Books, 1979.
Siegel, E., Gillings, D., Campbell S. and Guild, P. A controlled evaluation of rural regional perinatal care: impact on mortality and morbidity. *Am. J. Pub. Health* 75:246-254 (1985).
Siegel, J.M., Johnson, J.H. and Sarason, I.G. Life changes and menstrual discomfort. *J. Hum. Stress* 5:41-46 (1979).
Siever, L.J. and Davis, K.L. Overview: toward a dysregulation hypothesis of depression. *Am. J. Psychiat.* 142:1017-1031 (1985).
Sifneos, P.E. *Short Term Psychotherapy and Emotional Crisis*. Cambridge, Massachusetts: Harvard University Press, 1972.
Silverman, W. A. *Retrolentil Fibroplasia: A Modern Parable*. New York: Grune and Stratton, 1980.
Simons, R.C. and Pardes, H. *Understanding Human Behavior in Health and Illness*. Baltimore: Williams and Wilkins, 1981.
Singer, A., Walker, P.G. and McCance, D.J. Genital wart infestations: nuisance or potentially lethal? *Br. Med. Jr.* 288:735-736 (1984).

Singer, E., Garfinkle, R. and Cohen, S.M. Mortality and mental health evidence from the Midtown Manhattan Restudy. *Soc. Sci. and Med.* 10:517-525 (1976).
Sklar, L.S. and Anisman, H. Stress and cancer. *Psychol. Bull.* 89:369-406 (1981).
Sloan, D. In Vicki Walton (ed.), *Have It Your Way.* New York: Bantam, 1976.
Slome, C., Wetherbee, H., Daly, M., Christensen, K., Meglen, M. and Thiede, H. Effectiveness of certified nurse-midwives. *Am. J. Ob.-Gyn.* 124:177-182 (1976).
Sloss, E.M. and Frerichs, R.R. Smoking and menstrual disorders. *Int. J. Epidemiol.* 12(1):107-109 (1983).
Smith, C.V.M. *The Problem of Life: An Essay on the Origins of Biological Thought.* New York: Wiley, 1976.
Smith, D.K. Psychological aspects of gynecology and obstetrics. *Ob. Gyn. Annual* 8:457-473 (1979).
Smith, E.M., Johnson, S.R. and Guenther, S.M. Health care attitudes and experiences during gynecologic care among lesbians and bisexuals. *Am. J. Pub. Health* 75:1085-1087 (1985).
Smith, P.G., Kinlen, L.J., White, G.C., Adelstein, A.M. and Fox, A.J. Mortality of wives of men dying with cancer of the penis. *Br. J. Cancer* 41(3):422-428 (1980).
Smith, W.L. and Duerksen, D.L. Personality and the relief of chronic pain. In: W.L. Smith, H. Merskey and S.C. Gross (eds.), *Pain: Meaning And Management*, New York, Spectrum 1980.
Smith, W.L., Merskey, H. and Gross, S.C. *Pain: Meaning and Management.* New York: Spectrum, 1980.
Smith, T.W. and Frohm, K.D. What's so unhealthy about hostility? Construct validity and psychosocial correlates of the Cook and Medley Ho scale. *Health Psychol.* 4:503-520 (1985).
Smithells, R.W. The demonstration of teratogenic effects of drugs in humans. In: D.F. Hawkins (ed.), *Drugs and Pregnancy: Human Teratogens and Related Problems*, New York: Churchill and Livingston, 1983, 22-30.
Snowdon, D.A. and Phillips, R.L. Does a vegetarian diet reduce the occurrence of diabetes? *Am. J. Pub. Health* 75:507-512 (1985).
Sobrenho, L.G., et al. Hyperprolactinemia in women with paternal deprivation during childhood. *Ob.-Gyn.* 64:465-468 (1984).
Sokol, R.J., Rosen, M.G., Stojkov, J. and Chjik, L. Clinical application of high-risk scoring on an obstetrical service. *Am. J. Ob.-Gyn.* 128:652-661 (1977).
Solomon, G.F. Emotional and personality factors in the onset and course of autoimmune disease, particularly rheumatoid arthritis. In: R. Ader (ed.), *Psychoneuroimmunology*, 1981, 159-182.

Solomon, G.F. and Amkraut, A. Emotions, immunity and disease. In: C. Van Dyke and L.S. Zegans (eds.), *Emotions in Health and Illness*. New York: Grune and Stratton, 1982, 167-186.

Sontag, S. *Illness as Metaphor*. New York: Random House, 1979.

Sorensen, S.S. Infertility factors: their relative importance and share in an unselected material of infertility patients. *Acta Ob. Gyn. Scand.* 59:513-552 (1980).

Sosa, R., Kennel, J. and Klaus, M. The effect of a supportive companion on perinatal problems: length of labor, and mother-infant interactions. *N. Eng. J. Med.* 305:597-600 (1980).

Spencer, S.W. and Snyder, M.L. The menstrual cycle and punitiveness. *Health Psychol.* 3:143-155 (1984).

Speroff, L. Exercise induced amenorrhea and anorexia, news report. *Ob.-Gyn. News* 20:2,23 (1985).

Spicer, G. Home births. *The Practicing Midwife* 1(15):8-11 (April 1982).

Stallones, R.A. Ischemic heart disease and lipids in blood and diet. *Annual Rev. Nutrition* 3:155-185 (1983).

Statistical Abstracts of the United States, 1982-1983, Bureau of the Census.

Statistical Abstracts of the United States, 1985, Bureau of the Census.

Steege, J.F., Stout, A.L. and Rupp, S.L. Relationships among premenstrual symptoms and menstrual cycle characteristics. *Ob.-Gyn.* 65:398-402 (1985).

Steiner, H. and Neligan, G.A. Perinatal mortality and the quality of the survivors. In: S.L. Barron and A.M. Thomson (eds.), *Obstetrical Epidemiology*, New York: Academic Press, 1983, 417-448.

Steinhorn, S.C., Myers, M.H., Hankey, B.F. and Pelham, V.F. Factors associated with survival differences between black women and white women with cancer of the uterine corpus. *Am. J. Epid.* 124:85-93.

Steinlauf, B. Problem-solving skills, locus of control, and the contraceptive effectiveness of young women. *Child Dev.* 50(1):268-271.

Stellman, S.D., Austin, H. and Wynder, E.L. Cervix cancer and cigarette smoking: a case-control study. *Am. J. Epidemiol.* 111(4):383-388 (1980).

Stembera, Z.K., et al. Identification and quantification of high-risk factors affecting fetus and newborn. *Proceedings of the 4th European Congress of Perinatal Medicine*, Prague, August 1974.

Steptoe, A. Psychophysiological processes in disease. In: A. Steptoe and A. Mathews (eds.), *Health Care and Human Behavior*, New York and London: Academic Press, 1984, 77-112.

Steptoe, A. and Mathews, A. *Health Care and Human Behavior*. New York and London: Academic Press, 1984.

Steward, D. and Steward L. *Safe Alternatives in Childbirth*. Chapel Hill, N.C.: NAPSAC, 1977, second edition.

Stewart, A.J. and Salt, P. Life stress, life styles, depression and illness in adult women. *J. Person. Soc. Psychol.* 40: 1063-1069 (1981).
Stewart, P. Patients' attitudes to induction and labour. *Br. Med. J.* 2(6089):749- 752 (1977).
Stewart, P.J. Most mothers quit, cut smoking during pregnancy. *Ob.-Gyn. News* 19:3 (1984).
Steward, T.D. Introduction to *A Guide to Midwifery.* Sante Fe: John Muir Press, 1981.
Sternbach, R.A. Psychological factors in pain. In: J.J. Bonica and D.G. Hibe-Fessard (eds.), *Advances in Pain Research & Therapy, Vol. I.*, Proceedings of the 1st World Congress on Pain, New York: Raven Press, 1976, 293-300.
Stillman, M. Women's health beliefs about breast cancer and breast self examination. *Nursing Research* 26:121-127 (1977).
Stone, G.C., Cohen, F. and Adler F. (eds.). *Health Psychology.* San Francisco: Jossey-Bass, 1979.
Strain, J.J. *Psychological Interventions in Medical Practice.* New York: Appleton-Century-Crofts, 1978.
Straub, L.R., Ripley, H.S. and Wolf, S. Disturbances in bladder function in women and men. *JAMA* 141:1139-1143 (1949).
Straub, L.R., Ripley, H.S. and Wolf S. An experimental approach to psychosomatic bladder disorders. *New York State J. of Medicine* 49:635-638 (1949).
Strauss, J.S., Halfez, H., Lieberman, M.D. and Harding, C.M. The course of psychiatric disorder, III: longitudinal principles. *Am. J. Psychiat.* 142:289-296 (1985).
Streissguth, A.P., Darby, B.L., Barr, H.M., Smith, J.F. and Martin, D.C. Comparison of drinking and smoking patterns during pregnancy over a six-year interval. *Am. J. Ob. Gyn.* 145:716-724 (1983).
Strickland, B.R. Internal-external expectancies and health-related behavior. *J. Consult. Clin. Psychol.* 46:1192-1211 (1978).
Stverre-Pedersen, B. and Stverre-Pedersen, S. Etiological factors and subsequent reproductive performance in 195 couples with a prior history of habitual abortion. *Am. J. Ob. Gyn.* 148:140-146 (1984).
Suarstad, B. Physician-patient communication and patient conformity with medical advice. In: *The Growth of Bureaucratic Medicine,* D. Mechanic (ed.), New York: Wiley, 1976.
Suchman, E.A. Stages of illness and medical care. *J. Health Hum. Behav.* 6:114-128 (1965).
Summary of the ten thousand confinement records of the Frontier Nursing Service. *Quart. Bull. Frontier Nursing Service* 33:45-55 (1958).
Surgeon General's Report on Health Promotion and Disease Prevention. *Healthy People.* Two volumes, report and background papers. Washington, D.C.: U.S., Department of Health, Education and Welfare, 1979.

Suruutt, R. Behavior modification and diabetes. Cited in *Psychology Today* (February 12, 1985).
Swanson, D.W. Chronic pain as a third pathologic emotion. *Am. J. of Psychiatry* 141:2 (1984).
Syme, S. and Torfs, C.P. Epidemiological research in hypertension: a critical appraisal. *J. of Health and Human Stress* 4:43-48 (1978).
Syme, S.L. Sociocultural factors and disease etiology. In: W.D. Gentry (ed.), *Handbook of Behavioral Medicine*, New York: Guilford Press, 1984, 13-37.
Syme, S.L. Remarks cited in: Reducing risk: a change of heart? *Science* 231,669-670 (1986).
Syrfanen, K.J. Current concepts of human papilomavirus infections in the genital tract and their relationship to intraepithelial neoplasia and squamous cell carcinoma. *Ob-Gyn. Survey* 39:252-264 (1984).
Szasz, T. *The Myth of Mental Illness*. New York: Hoeber Harper, 1963.
Tapp, J.T. Multisystems: holistic model of health, stress and coping. In: T.M. Field, P.M. McCabe and N. Schneiderman (eds.), *Stress and Coping*, Hillsdale, N.J.: Erlbaum, 1985, 285-304.
Taylor, H.C., Jr. Vascular congestion and hyperemia: their effect on structure and function in the female reproductive system. *Am. J. of Ob.-Gyn.* 57:211-230 (1949).
Taylor, C.W. Promoting health strengthening and wellness through environmental variables. In: J.D. Matarazzo et al. (eds.), *Behavioral Health: A Handbook of Health Enhancement and Disease Prevention*, New York: Wiley, 1984, 130-149.
Taylor, G.J. Alexithymia: concept, measurement and implications for treatment. *Am. J. Psychiat.* 141:725-732 (1984).
Taylor, R.B., Ureda, J.R. and Denham, J.W. *Health Promotion: Principles and Clinical Applications*. Norwalk, Connecticut: Appleton-Century-Crofts, 1982.
Taylor, S.E. Adjustment to threatening events: a theory of cognitive adaptation. *Am. Psychol.* 38:1161-1173 (1983).
Taylor, S.E. The changing patterns of disease, disability and death. In: J.D. Matarazzo (ed.), *Behavioral Immunogens*, draft ms., UCLA, 1983.
Taylor, S.E., Lichtman, R.R. and Wood, J.V. Compliance with chemotherapy among breast cancer patients. *Health Psychol.* 3:553-562 (1984).
Temostiok, L. Emotional adaptation and disease. In: C. VanDyke and L.S. Zegans (eds.), *Emotions in Health and Illness: Theoretical and Research Foundations*, New York: Grune and Stratton, 1982, 207-233.
Terman, G.W., et al. Intrinsic mechanisms of pain inhibition: activation by stress. *Science* 226:1270-1277 (1984).
Tew, M. The case against hospital deliveries. In: S. Kitzinger and J. Davies (eds.), *The Place of Birth*, Oxford: Oxford University Press, 1978.

Thomas, C.B., Duszynski, K.R. and Shaffer, J.W. Family attitudes reported in youth as potential predictors of cancer. *Psychosom. Med.* 41:287-301 (1979).

Thomas, C.B. and Greenstreet, R.L. Psychological characteristics in youth as predictors of five disease states: suicide, mental illness, hypertension, coronary heart disease and tumors. *Johns Hopkins Med. J.* 132:16-43 (1973).

Thomsen, S.G., Isagers, S.L., Lange, A.P., Saurbrey, N. and Schiolier, V. Smoking habits and maternal serum alpha-fetoprotein levels during the second trimester of pregnancy. *Br. J. Obstet. and Gyn.* 90:716-717 (1983).

Thomson, A.L. Fetal growth and size at birth. In: S.L. Barron and A.M. Thomson, *Obstetrical Epidemiology*, New York: Academic Press, 1983, 89-142.

Thomson, A.M. and Barron, S.L. In: S.L. Barron and A.M. Thomson (eds.), *Obstetrical Epidemiology*, New York: Academic Press, 1983, 347-398.

Thoresen, C., Friedman, M. and Gill, J. News Report. *Science 84*, p. 14.

Thurlow, H.J. General susceptibility to illness. *Can. Med. Assn. J.* 97:1397-1404 (1967).

Tietze, C. Induced abortion. In: S.L. Barron and A.M. Thomson (eds.), *Obstetrical Epidemiology*, New York: Academic Press, 1983, 319-346.

Tilden, V.P. The relation of life stress and social support to emotional disequilibrium during pregnancy. *Res. Nurs. Health* 6(4):167-174 (1983).

Tilson, H.H. Governmental and Legislative Policies to Control and Direct the Promotion of Health. In: *Oxford Book of Public Health*. New York and London: Oxford University Press, 1984, 161-169.

Timmermans, M. and Sternbach, R.A. Human chronic pain and personality. In: J.J. Bonica and D.G. Albe-Fessard (eds.), *Advances in Pain Research & Therapy, Vol. I.*, Proceedings of 1st World Congress on Pain, New York: Raven Press, 1976, 307-310.

Timmins, N. "Psychologists can cut GPs' drug bills," survey shows. *The Times*, London, January 16, 1984.

Topliss, E.P. Selection procedures for hospital and domiciliary confinements. In G. McLachan and R. Skegog (eds.), *In the Beginning: Studies of Maternity Services*. Oxford: Oxford University Press, 1970.

Trevathan, E., Layde, P., Webster, L.A., Adams, J.B., Benigno, B.B. and Ory, H. Cigarette smoking and dysplasia and carcinoma in situ of the uterine cervix. *JAMA* 250(4):49-502 (1983).

Trichinosis. *Science* 227:621-624 (1985).

Trussell, R.E. and Elinson, J. *Chronic Illness in a Rural Area*. Cambridge, Harvard University Press, 1959.

Tsuzng, M.T., Boor, M. and Fleming, M.S. Psychiatric aspects of traffic accidents. *Am. J. Psychiat.* 142:538-546 (1985).

Tuchman-Duplessis, H. *Drug Effects on the Fetus: A Survey of the Mechanisms and Effects of Drugs on Embryogenesis and Fetogenesis*. Sydney: Adis Press, 1975.

Tudiver, F. Dysfunctional uterine bleeding and prior life stress. *J. Fam. Pract.* 17(6):999-1003 (1983).

Tulandi, T. and Lal, S. Menopausal hot flash. *Ob.-Gyn. Survey* 40:553-563 (1985).

Twining, T.C. Some interrelationships between personality variables, obstetrical outcome and perinatal mood. *J. Repro. and Infant Psychol.* 11-17 (1983).

U.S., Department of Health, Education and Welfare. Collaborative Perinatal Study of the National Institute of Neureological Diseases. Storke, Nyswander and Gordon (eds.), *The Women and Their Pregnancies*, 1972.

Utian, W.H. *Menopause in Modern Perspective: A Guide to Clinical Practice*, Norwalk, Ct.: Appleton-Century-Crofts, 1981.

Utian, W.H. *Guide for Today's Women.* Norwalk, Ct.: Appleton-Century-Crofts, 1981.

Vaillant, G.E. Natural history of male psychological health: effects of mental health on physical health. *N. Eng. J. Med.* 301: 1249-1254 (1979).

van Alten, D., et al. A place to be born. *Brit. Med. J.*, 1:771 (1976).

van den Berg, B.J. and Oeschsli, F.W. Prematurity. In: *Perinatal Epidemiology*. M.B. Bracken (ed.), New York and London: Oxford University Press, 1984, 69-85.

van Dyke, C. and Zegans, L.S. *Emotions in Health and Illness.* New York: Grune and Stratton, 1982.

Verbrugge, L.M. and Steiner, R.P. Prescribing drugs to men and women. *Health Psychol.* 4:79-98 (1985).

Verney, T. *The Secret Life of the Unborn Child.* New York: Summit, 1981.

Vital and Health Statistics, Public Health Service. Current Estimates from National Health Interview Survey Questionnaire, 1979.

Vital and Health Statistics, Public Health Service. Drug Utilization in Office Based Practice, 1980.

Vital and Health Statistics, Public Health Service. Health Characteristics According to Family and Personal Income, Series 10, #147, DHHS, 1985.

Vital Statistics of the U.S. Life Tables, Public Health Service, NCHS, 1980.

Vital and Health Statistics, Public Health Services, National Health Survey: Personal Health Practices and Consequences. Series 15, 1979.

Vouk, V.B. and Sheehan, P.J. *Methods for Assessing the Effects of Chemicals on Reproductive Function.* SGOMSEC 1, New York: Wiley, 1983.

Wadde, T.A., Stunkard, A.J., Brownell, K.D. and Day, S.D. Treatment of obesity by behavior therapy and a very low calorie diet: a pilot investigation. *J. Consult. Clin. Psychol.* 52:692-696 (1984).

Wadsworth, M.E.J. Health and sickness: the choice of treatment. *J. Psychosom. Res.* 18:271-276 (1974).
The Wall Street Journal, August 31, 1985, p. 12.
Wanger, P.J. and Curran, P. Health beliefs and physician identified "worried well." *Health Psychol.* 3:459-474 (1984).
Ware, J.E., Manning, W.G., Duan, N., Wells, K.B. and Newhouse, J.P. Health status and the use of outpatient mental health services. *Am. Psychol.* 39:1090-1100 (1984).
Warner, K.E. Cigarette smoking in the 1970s: the impact of the antismoking campaign. *Science* 211:729-730 (1983).
Watson, D. and Clark, L.A. Negative affectivity: the disposition to experience aversive emotional states. *Psychol. Bull.* 96:465-490 (1984).
Watson, J.P. and Bamber, R.W. Some relationships between sex, marriage and mood. *J. Int. Med. Res.* 8 Suppl. 3:14-19 (1980).
Watts, R.J. Sexual functioning, health beliefs, and compliance with high blood pressure medications. *Nurs. Res.* 31(5):278-283 (1982).
Weber, J.C.P. Limitation of a Voluntary Reporting System. In: D.F. Hawkins, *Drugs and Pregnancy*, New York: Churchill Livingston, 1983, 31-40.
Webber, L.S., Hunter, S.M., Baugh, J.G., Srinivasan, S.R., Sklov, M.C. and Berenson, G.S. The interaction of cigarette smoking, oral contraceptive use, and cardiovascular risk factor variables in children: the Bogalusa Heart Study. *Am. J. Pub. Health* 72(3):266-274 (1982).
Weinstein, N.D. Why it won't happen to me: perceptions of risk factors and susceptibility. *Health Psychol.* 3:431-457 (1984).
Weisman, A.D. A model for psychosocial phasing in cancer. In: *Coping With Physical Illness. Two New Perspectives*, R.H. Moos (ed.), New York: Plenum, 1984, 107-122.
Weisman, A.D. Understanding the cancer patient: the syndrome of the caregiver's plight. In: *Coping With Physical Illness, Two New Perspectives*, R.H. Moose (ed.), New York: Plenum, 1984, 345-358.
Weiss, J.M. Behavioral and psychological influences in gastrointestinal pathology: experimental techniques and findings. In: W.D. Gentry, *Handbook of Behavioral Medicine*, New York: Guilford Press, 1984, 174-221.
Weiss, N.S., Young, J.L. Jr. and Roth, G.L. Marital status and incidence of ovarian cancer: the U.S. Third National Cancer Survey, 1969-71.
Weiss, W. and Jackson, F.C. *Maternal Factors Affecting Birth Weight, Perinatal Factors Affecting Human Development*. Washington, D.C.: Pan American Health Organization, 1969.
Weissman, M.Y., et al. Depression and perception of health in an urban community. In: C. Van Dyke and L.S. Zegans (eds.), *Emotions in Health and Illness*, New York: Grune and Stratton, 1982.

Welisch, D., Landsverk, J. Giudera, K., Pasnau, R.O. and Fawzy, F. Evaluation of psychosocial problems of the homebound cancer patient. I: Methodology and problem frequencies. *Psychosom. Med.* 45:11-21 (1983).

Wells, H.B., et al. North Carolina fetal and neonatal death study: 1. Study design and some preliminary results. *Am. J. Obstet. & Gynecol.* 48:1583 (1968).

Wells, P. Calcium deficiency. *Special Delivery* (Maternal Center Association) 2:3 (1984).

Wenderlein, J.M. The IQ in gynaecology. *Geburtshilfe Frauenheilkd* 38(8):619-28 (1978).

Wenderlein, J.M. Hormonal contraceptives cause depression? *Med. Clin.* 76(10):288-290 (1981).

Wenderlein, J.M. The psychosomatic aspects of complaints of varicose veins during pregnancy. A psychosometric investigation in 345 antenatal patients. *Geburtshilfe Frauenheilkd* 36(11):997-1003 (1976).

Wengraf, F. *Psychosomatic Approach to Gynecology and Obstetrics.* Springfield: Thomas Publishers, 1953.

Wentz, W.B., Heggie, A.D., Anthony, D.D. and Reagan, J.W. Effect of prior immunization on induction of cervical cancer in mice by Herpes Simplex Virus Type 2. *Science* 222:1128-1129 (1983).

Wertz, R.W. and Wertz, D.C. *Lying-In: A History of Childbirth in America.* New York: Free Press, 1977.

White, K.L., William, T. and Greenberg, B.G. The ecology of medical care. *N. Eng. J. Med.* 265:885-892 (1961).

Whitehead, W.E., Busch, C.M., Heller, B.R., and Costa, P.T. Social learning influences on menstrual symptoms and illness behavior. *Health Psychol.* 5:13-24 (1986).

Wicker, A.W. Nature and assessment of behavior settings: recent contributions from the ecological perspective. In: P. McReynolds (ed.), *Advances in Psychological Assessment,* San Francisco: Jossey-Bass, 1981, Volume 5, 22-61.

Wiebe, D.J. and McCallum, D.M. Health practices and hardiness as mediators in the stress illness relationship. *Health Psychol.* 5:425-438 (1986).

Wijma, K. Psychological functioning after noncancer hysterectomy: a review of methods and results. *J. Psychom. Ob-Gyn.* 3:133-154 (1984).

Wiley, J.A. and Camacho, T.C. Life styles and future health: evidence from the Alameda County Study. *Prev. Med* 9:1-21 (1980).

Williams, C.A., et al. The Edgecombe County high blood pressure control program: III, social support, social stressors, and treatment dropout. *Am. J. Pub. Health* 75:483-486 (1985).

Williams, J.B.W. and Spitzer, R.L. (eds.), *Psychotherapy Research.* New York: Fuilford Press, 1984.

Williams, N.A. and Deffenbacher, J.L. Life stress and chronic yeast infections. *J. Human Stress* 9(1):26-31 (1983).
Williams, R.L., Binkin, N.J., and Clingman, E.J. Pregnancy outcomes among Spanish-surname women in California. *Am. J. Pub. Health* 76:387-391 (1986).
Williams R.L. and Chen, P.M. Identifying the sources of the recent decline in perinatal mortality rates in California. *N. Eng. J. Med.* 306(4):207-214 (1982).
Williams, R.L. and the Staff of the California Department of Health Services. *Out-of-Hospital births in California: 1970-1977.* Santa Barbara: Community & Organization Research Institute, University of Santa Barbara, 1979. (Cited with permission of the author.)
Williams, R.L. Measuring the effectiveness of perinatal care. *Medical Care* 17:95-110 (1979).
Williams, R.L. *Measuring the Effectiveness of Perinatal Care.* Santa Barbara: Community & Organization Research Institute, University of Santa Barbara, 1980. Final report to the Maternal & Child Health & Crippled Children's Services Research Grants Program.
Williams, R.R. Breast & thyroid cancer and malignant melanoma promoted by alcohol-induced pituitary secretion of prolactin, TSH and MSH. *Lancet* 1:996- 999 (1976).
Wilsnack, R.W., Wilsnack, S.C. and Klassen, A.D. Women's drinking and drinking problems: patterns from a 1981 national survey. *Am. J. Pub. Health* 74:1231-1237 (1984).
Wilson, R. and Schifrin, B. Is any pregnancy low risk? *Ob.-Gyn.* 55:653-656 (1980).
Wingard, D. and Berkman, L.F. A multivariate analysis of health practices and social networks. In: L.F. Berkman and L. Breslow, *Health and Ways of Living: The Alameda County Study,* New York: Oxford, 1983.
Windard, D., Suarez, L. and Barrett-Conner, L. The sex differential in mortality from all causes and ischemic heart disease. *Am. J. Epid.* 117:165-172 (1983).
Winters, R.W. Arousal, sleep and stress. In: T.M. Field, P.M. McCabe and N. Schneiderman. *Stress and Coping.* Hillsdale, N.J.: Erlbaum, 1985, 63-92.
Wolff, B.B. Psychosocial aspects of the patient with chronic pain. In: P.L. LeRoy, *Current Concepts in the Management of Chronic Pain,* Pro Dolore Symposium. New York: Stratton Medical Book Corporation, 1977, 45-52.
Wolff, B.R., Cohen, P. and Green, C.T. Behavioral mechanisms of human pain: effects of expectancy, magnitude and type of cross-modal stimulation. In: J.J. Bonica and D.G. Albe-Fessard (eds.), *Advances in Pain Research & Therapy, Vol. I.,* Proceedings of the 1st World Congress on Pain, New York: Raven Press, 1976,327-333.

Wolff, H.G. and Wolf, S. *Pain.* Springfield, Thomas Publishers, 1958.
Wolff, H.G. (Wolf, S.G. and Goodell, H.G., eds.) *Stress and Disease.* Springfield: Thomas Publishers, 1960.
Wolf, S.G. *Life Stress and Essential Hypertension: A Study of Circulatory Adjustments in Man.* Baltimore: William and Wilkins, 1955.
Wolf, S.G. and Wolff, H.G. *Headaches: Their Nature and Treatment.* Boston: Little, Brown, 1953.
Wolf, S.G. and Wolff, H.G. *Human Gastric Function. An Experimental study of a Man and His Stomach.* London: Oxford University Press, 1943.
Wood, Y.R. Social support and social networks: nature and measurement. In: P. McReynolds and G.J. Chelune (eds.), *Advances in Psychological Assessment, Vol. 6,* San Francisco: Jossey-Bass, 1984, 312-353.
Woods, N.F., Dery, G.K. and Most, A. Stressful life events and perimenstrual symptoms. *J. Human Stress* 8(2):23-31 (1982).
World Health Statistics, WHO, Geneva, 1983.
Worthington, E.L., Jr. Labor room and laboratory: clinical validation of the cold pressor as a means of testing preparation for childbirth strategies. *J. Psychosomatic Res.* 26(2):223-230 (1982).
Wrede, G., Mednick, S.A., Huttunen, M.O. and Nilsson, C.G. Pregnancy and delivery complications in the births of an unselected series of Finnish children with schizophrenic mothers. *Acta Psychiatr. Scand.* 62(4):369-381 (1980).
Wright, V.C., et al. Age at beginning of coitus versus chronological age as basis for Papanioleaou smear screening: an analysis of 747 cases of preinvasive disease. *Am. J. Ob. Gyn.* 149:824-830 (1984).
Wynn, M. and Wynn, A. *The Prevention of Handicap of Early Pregnancy Origin.* London: Foundation for Education and Research in childbearing, 1981.
Yalom, I.D., Lunde, D.T., Moos, R.H. and Hamburg, D.A. "Postpartum blues" syndrome: a description and related variables. *Arch. Gen. Psychiat.* 18:16-27 (1968).
Yanover, M.J., Jones, D. and Miller, M.D. Perinatal care of low-risk mothers and infants: Early discharge with home care. *N. Eng. J. Med.* 294:702-705 (1976).
Youngs, D.D. and Ehrhardt, A.A. *Psychosomatic Obstetrics and Gynecology.* New York: Appleton-Century-Crofts. 1980.
Youngs, D.D. and Works-Lind, M. Practical strategies for managing PMS. *Contemporary Ob/Gyn* 111-122 (October 1985).
Youngs, D.T. and Wise, T.N. Psychological sequelae of elective gynecologic surgery. In: D.D. Youngs and A.A. Ehrhardt (eds.), *Psychosomatic Obstetrics and Gynecology,* New York: Appleton-Century-Crofts, 1980, 256-274.
Zackler, J., et al. The young adolescent as an obstetrical risk. *Am. J. Obstet. & Gynecol.* 103:305-312 (1969).

Zacur, H.A., Chapanis, N.P., Lake, C.R., Ziegler, M. and Tyson, J.E. Galactorrhea-amenorrhea: psychological interaction with neuroendocrine function. *Am. J. Obstet. & Gynecol.* 125(6):859-862 (1976).

Zappert, L.T. and Weinstein, H.M. Sex differences in impact of work on physical and psychological health. *Am. J. Psychiat.* 142:1174-1178 (1985).

Zarski, J. Hassles and health: a replication. *Health Psychol.* 3:243-251 (1984).

Zax, M., Sameroff, A. and Babigian, H. Birth outcomes in the offspring of mentally disordered women. *Am. J. Orthopsychiat.* 47:218-230 (1977).

Zbella, E.A., Depper, G. and Elrad, H. Gonococcal arthritis in pregnancy. *Ob.-Gyn. Survey* 39:8-12 (1984).

Zborowski, M. Cultural components in response to pain. *J. Soc. Issues* 8:16-30 (1952).

Zegans, L.S. Emotions in health and illness: an attempt at integration. In: Van Dyke, C. and Zegans, L.S. (eds.), *Emotions, Health and Illness: Theoretical and Research Foundations*, New York: Grune and Stratton, 1982, 235-256.

Zeichner, A. and Dickson, B.E. Cardiovascular risk factors: a multisystem assessment approach. In: P. McReynolds and G.J. Chelune (eds.), *Advances in Psychological Assessment, Vol. 6*, San Francisco: Jossey-Bass, 1984, 194-235.

Zimmerman, M., O'Hara, M.W. and Corenthal, C.P. Symptom contamination of life event scales. *Health Psychol.* 3:77-81 (1984).

Zola, I. Pathways to the doctor— from person to patient. *Soc. Sci. & Med.* 7:677-689 (1973).

Zola, I. Studying the decision to see the doctor. *Social Issues* 8:16-30 (1972).

Author Index

Abelson, 94
ACOG, 11, 12, 169
Adamson, 168
Ader, 122, 129, 167
Adler, xv, 15, 107, 146, 149, 319
Ahmed, 135, 151
Akhtan, 156
Alagna, 196
Alameda study, 118
Albe-Fessard, 194
Alberman, 156
Alcoholics Anonymous, 5
Alderman, 156
Aldrich, 221
Alexander, 60
Algert, 260
Allan, 243
Almy, 201
Alter, 143
American Academy of General Practice, 27
American Cancer Society, 3, 107, 182, 288
American College of Obstetricians and Gynecologists, 233
American College of Obstetrics and Gynecologists, 87
American College of Obstetrics and Gynecology, 347
Amkraut, 182, 185
Anderman, 141

Andersen, 198, 235
Anderson, 179, 181, 185, 235, 311, 313
Andreasen, 337
Angel, 22
Anisman, 18, 59, 122
Anisman, 129, 182, 196, 198, 211
Antley, 243
Antonovsky, 34, 54, 98, 354
Appel, 301
Appels, 179, 310
Aral, 184, 194
Arms, xv, 37, 131, 152
Aro, 143
Ashbury, 173
Ashford, 152, 170
Assaf, 196
Assal, 253
Astbury, 135, 141, 230
Asted, 198
Aubrey, 135, 136, 156, 163, 166, 170
Avery, 314
Axelrod, 122, 130, 167

Babigian, 137, 139
Backstrom, 189
Bagigian, 163
Baird, 10, 19, 131, 157, 170
Baker, 149, 179, 181
Bakketeig, 137

Balint, 301
Ball, 179, 210
Ballantyne, 132
Ballentyne, 10, 11
Ballinger, 195
Ballon, 270
Balls, 135
Banber, 95
Band, 201
Bandura, 68, 244
Banks, 54
Barefoot, 110
Barfglow, 221
Barlar, 196
Barracla, 156
Barrera, 135
Barron, 10, 128, 131, 132, 137, 147, 153, 170, 171
Barskey, 300
Barsky, 66, 69, 77
Baruffi, 166
Baum, 54, 181
Beard, 194
Beasley, 298
Beck, 152, 156, 172
Becker, 42, 147, 229, 236, 237
Beer, 156
Beeson, 229
Bellack, 262
Belloc, 109, 122
Belsey, 149, 201
Benedetti, 103
Bennett, 162
Beral and Kay, 179
Berger, 146
Bergren, 198
Berkeley, 200
Berkman, 22, 109, 111, 112, 205
Berkowitz, 139
Berlin, 22, 125
Bernard, 60, 122, 167

Bernstein, 151
Betz, 67, 110
Bewley, xv, 53, 58
Blaney, 54, 61, 114, 149
Blankenbaker, 23, 27, 181, 183, 275, 279
Blankerbaker, 17
Blazer, 115, 118
Blondel, 10, 11
Bloom, 191
Blum, xxiii, 3, 4, 35, 37, 40, 43, 52, 53, 71, 74, 77, 93, 95, 128, 152, 227, 233, 236, 240, 252, 263, 294, 315, 332, 347, 352, 353
Blumberg, 243
Blumer, 194
Boker, 211
Bone, 235
Bonica, 194
Bordage, 125
Boring, 240
Bottom, 152
Bottoms, 153
Bourne, 320
Boyce, 135
Boyle, 202
Bracken, 146, 202
Bradley, 152, 194
Brahn, 179
Branch, 110
Brandt, 31, 32, 208
Brandwin, 149
Braverman, 149
Brazie, 156, 163
Brem, 156
Brena, 194
Breslau, 109, 122, 205
Breslow, 3, 22
Brix, 140
Broadhead, 114
Broods-Gunn, 189

Author Index

Brook, 93
Brooks-Gunn, 76
Brotman, 187
Broussard, 156
Browder, 172
Brown, 6, 61, 63, 97, 122, 63, 139, 170, 180, 181, 194, 196, 221, 301
Brownell, 251
Brozne, 156
Bruckington, 149
Buck, 167
Buckley, 198
Budman, 6
Budmen, 304
Buehler, 135
Bullen, 190
Bureau of Census, 297
Bureau of Labor Statistics, 79
Burnap, 235
Burnell, 267
Burnett, 137, 156, 170
Burnham, 35, 36
Bush, xv, 207, 209
Buss, 64, 170
Butler, 135, 140, 156
Butt, 233, 234
Butterfield, 54, 56, 159
Butts, 149
Byrne, 66, 72, 171, 194
Byrnes, 119

Calder, 42
Camacho, 122
Campbell, 59, 149, 168, 231
Candide, 351
Cannon, 18, 60, 122, 173
Capone, 313, 314
Carnegie Foundation Subcommittee on Modification of Patient Behavior for Health Maintenance and Disease Control, 2

Carnes, 149
Carregal, 194
Carrie, 80, 135
Carter, 36, 242
Cartwright, 53, 93, 95, 107, 146, 156, 235
Carver, 68
Case, 119, 179, 207
Cassel, 129
Cassell, 15
Cates, 23, 196
Chalmers, 125, 132, 135, 139, 143, 152, 155, 156, 158, 165, 169, 170, 230, 231
Chamberlain, xv, 139, 155, 235
Chandler, 121
Chapman, 313
Chard, 25, 131, 132, 159
Charles, 186
Chase, 243
Chasmoff, 153
Chasnoff, 140
Cheek, 313
Chellune, 68
Chelune, 180
Chen, 156, 180
Chesney, 180, 206, 210
Chihal, 189
Chik, 156
Chilah, 211
Childs, 243
Chisholm, 144
Choe, 158
Christensen, 68, 122, 123, 333
Clark, 77, 146, 170
Clarke, 198
Clayton, 112
Cloosterman, 170
Clumer, 54
Clymer, 55, 114, 233, 305
Cnattinguis, 139
Cobb, 186

Coe, 129, 168
Cohen, 15, 56, 59, 60, 95, 114, 122, 143, 168, 180, 182, 185, 194, 205, 236, 305, 306
Collington, 181
Comstock, 112
Cooper, 190
Coppotelli, 260
Cormon, 337
Costa, 68, 302
Council on Resident Education in Obstetrics and Gynegology, 87
Cox, 112, 170, 186
Craig, 61, 63, 122, 180, 181, 194, 301
Craighead, 251
Cranden, 152
Crandon, 144
Creacy, 156
Creasey, 153, 158
Creasy, 139
Cromwell, 119
Crowley, 229
Crue, 194
Cullen, 313
Cummings, 305
Currie, 298
Cushner, 156
Cyr, 25

Dahlstrom, 110
Daniels, 42
Darney, xv, 170
Darvey, 156
Darvish, 112
Davidoff, 42
Davies, 144
Davis, 42, 59, 156, 191
Day, 146, 184
De Longis, 63

de Georges, 135
de la Fuente, 196
de Tocqueville, 352
Declerq, 170
Define, 60
Dembroski, 206, 210
Dembrowski, 67
Dembrowsky, 119
Demopoulis, 198
Denham, 14
Dennerstein, 269
Depue, 64
Depuis, 63
Derogates, 235
Derogitise, 196
DeSouza, 71, 335
Detels, 3
Deutsch, 60
Dewhurst, 155, 235
DHHS, 3
Dickson, 180, 259
DiMatteo, 230, 231
Dingley, 170
DiNicola, 230, 231
Dodd, 235
Dodson, 199
Doering, 143, 152, 156
Dohrenwend, 60, 63, 73, 122
Doll, 27
Dombrowski, 180
Donnelly, 156
Donnison, 18
Drake, 201
Drantz, 122
Drause, 205
Drossman, 194
Duekson, 194
Duff, 93
Duke, 312
Dunbar, 42, 60
Duncan, 29, 194, 318
Dunlop, 144
Dunner, 156

Dupue, 72, 73
Durant, 146
Dyk, 259

Eakins, xv
Eddy, 125, 274
Edwards, 135, 156
Ehrlich, 32
Eiduson, 151
Eisenberg, 7, 15, 26, 28, 34, 72, 98, 122, 171, 180, 194, 257, 300, 301
Eisner, 139, 156
Elkin, 39
Elleberg, 201
Elliot, 14, 180
Ellison, 190
Elster, 156
Elstien, 125
Empedocles, 32
Engel, 60, 75, 306, 67
Enkin, 125, 132, 139, 152, 155, 169, 230, 231
Entwisle, 152
Entwistle, 156
Epstein, 65, 265
Erb, 152
Erhardt, 22, 182, 189, 196
Ericson, 143
Eriken, 143
Erikson, 156
Escalona, 337
Eskenazi, 151
Estes, 170
Euland, 170
Evans, 143, 205
Exman, 71
Ezekiel, 52

Fagley, 135
Fanelli, 187
Faratian, 189

Farber, 135
Farquhar, 3, 237, 355
Fava, 190
Fedrick, 170
Feinleib, 79, 119, 180
Fellman, 199
Felton, 156
Fentz, 65
Feuerstein, 20, 60
Field, 129, 135, 139
Filner, 156
Fink, 239
Finney, 239
Fisher, 196
Fitzpatrick, 183
Fleg, 302
Flemmings, 32
Folkman, 60
Ford, 112
Forester, 313
Foresti, 189
Forohm, 180
Forreit, 146
Fortney, 158
Foster, 196
Fox, 18, 182, 313
Foxman, 201
Framingham Heart Study, 118
Framingham, 79
France, 304
Franceschi, 198
Frank, 73, 303
Frankenhaeusen, 180
Frederiksen, 237, 206
Freeman, 211
Freiderich, 201
Frerichs, 201
Freud, 60, 125, 173
Fried, 156
Friederich, 191, 199
Friedman, 185, 189, 211, 242
Friedrichs, 189

Friedson, 43
Fries, 305
Frontier Nursing Service, 170
Frost, 103
Funch, 114
Furgyik, 198

Galen, 9, 18, 277
Galler, 45
Gambrell, 196
Gant, 10, 141, 155
Garcia, 139, 152, 234
Garvry, 149
Gath, 243, 300, 301
Geden, 172
Geere, 235
Gelman, 196
Gentry, 7, 15
Gerber, 112
Gesell, 110
Girard, 146
Gittin, 199
Glasgow, 42
Glass, 112, 180, 181, 182, 206
Glick, 112
Globus, 143
Golbus, 156, 243
Gold, 146, 149, 190, 191, 195, 269
Goldberg, 112, 144, 182, 199, 235, 259
Golden, 235
Goldheizer, 180
Goldstein, 57, 189
Goldziher, 180
Golub, 189
Good, 313, 314
Goodell, 19
Goodwin, 135, 137, 156
Gordon, 9
Gorusch, 135
Goujard, 153

Graham, xx, 10, 27, 198
Grant, 158, 206
Grantz, 206
Gravell, 261
Green, 8, 60, 233
Greenberg, 191
Greenblatt, 112
Greene, 194
Greenfield, 185
Greenstreet, 110
Greenwood, 187, 195
Greer, 18, 196, 311
Greve, 139, 149
Grimes, 90
Gross, 137, 144, 194
Grossarth, 118
Grossarth-Maticek, 114, 182, 259
Grossman, 107, 122
Gruba, 189
Gummer, 156
Gurin, 64
Guten, 263
Gutman, 231
Gutmann, 95, 254
Guy, 18
Guzinski, 39, 40
Gwinn, 198

Haan, 42, 229, 241, 243, 244, 301
Hacker, 235, 311, 313
Hafner, 211
Hagerty, 185
Hakanson, 156
Hall, 169, 256, 303
Halliday's, 18
Hamburg, 5, 14, 23, 180
Hamilton, 9
Hammond, 27
Hann, 43
Hare, 201

Author Index

Harlage, 243
Harlan, 181
Harlap, 140
Harris, 23, 97, 263
Hartmann, 152, 156
Harvey, 146
Haskett, 189, 211
Hatcher, 23, 93, 180, 181, 190, 198, 201, 202
Haukins, 155
Hayashi, 202
Hayes, 28, 184
Haynes, 79, 119, 180, 227
Hazel, 170
Health Education Council's, 3
Hebel, 139
Hector, 156
Heide, 39
Heilbronn, 194
Heinonen, 143
Heinrich, xxiii, 260
Helsing, 112
Heminki, 139
Hemman, 156
Hemminki, 140, 143, 144, 156, 205, 294
Hemphill, 149
Henderson, 278
Hendler, 194
Henker, 194, 318
Henry and Stephens, 18
Henry, 14, 18, 19, 181, 201, 354
Herd, 4, 180, 181
Herman, 278
Herold, 146
Herrenkohl, 201
Herzlich, 301
Herzog, 149
Hesse, 235, 311
Hesselius, 200
Higgs, 53
Hill, 27

Himmelberger, 140
Hingson, 143
Hinkle, 19, 62, 63, 73, 122, 123
Hirsch, 204
Hladik, 234
Hobbins, 136
Hobel, xv, 135, 139, 156, 158, 163, 165, 166
Hoffman, 137
Holland, 311, 312, 313
Hollingshead, 93, 297
Hollingsworth, 135, 144
Holmes, 9, 122, 135, 170
Holroyd, 256, 257
Hook, 135, 155
Hopper, 186
Hopson, 189
Horn, 27
Horstmann, 141
House, 111, 115
Hovey, 189
Howard, 234
Hughes, 155, 211
Hughs, 258
Huguley, 196
Hull, 198
Humphrey, 201
Hung, 125
Hunt, 252
Hurney, 311, 312, 313
Hyvarinen, 163
Hyvarmer, 156

Iacone, 191
Iker, 198
Illich, 36
Illsley, 29, 151, 170
Ilm, 199
Imboden, 185
Innui, 237
Institute for Health Policy Studies, 97

Institute for Health Policy, 255
Institute of Medicine, 3, 159
Inui, 305
Inwood, 149
Isaacs, 170
Isen, 313
Izen, 182, 191, 198

Jackson, 156, 189
Jaffe, 189
Jain, 180
James, 140, 181
Jamis, 253
Jamison, 194
Janis, 43
Janis, 185, 227, 232, 250, 262, 301
Jemmott, 185
Jenkins, 180
Jensen, 41
Jette, 110
Jochimsen, 235
Jochinsen, 235, 311
Joe, 146
Joffe, 121, 156
Johansson, 202
John Hopkins, 112, 237
Johnson, 185
Johnstone, 156
Joklik, 141, 184
Jones, 53, 135, 156
Jordan, 191
Jorensen, 319
Jorgensen, 146
Jospe, 95
Julius, 111
Jung's, 18

Kagen, 183
Kandel, 80
Kannel, 180
Kaplan, 129, 203, 207, 209, 236, 253, 313

Kappel, 321
Kashiwagi, 189, 211
Kasl, 115
Katon, 194
Katz, 190
Kaunitz, 147
Kauntiz, 103
Keehn, 111
Keeler, 304
Kegals, 205
Keith, 194
Kelly, xviv
Kennel, 151
Kenton, 194
Keppel, 189, 269
Kernanen, 53
Kerr, 8, 10
Kessner, 137
Keye, 189
Keys, 135
Kilata, 196
Killilea, 5
Kilmartin, 201, 212
Kinch, 200
King, 186, 196
Kintz, 135
Kirsch, 53, 228, 237, 239, 242
Kirscht, 95, 263
Kissen, 182
Kitai, 149
Klatsky, 181
Klaus, 151
Kleidbaum, 181
Kleigman, 137
Klein, 34, 152, 156
Klerman, 66, 182, 191, 198
Kliegman, 144
Kline, 140
Knapp, 254
Knesper, 95
Knodel, 156
Knorr, 139

Knowles, 15, 25
Kobassa, 44
Kok, 181
Kolata, 198, 204
Koop, 230
Koos, 65
Koren, 201
Korenbrot, 156
Kourlesis, 235
Kramer, 172
Krant, 313
Krantz, 54, 112, 180, 181, 182, 206
Krishmer, 196
Kroger, 140
Krouse, 313
Kruckman, 149
Kuczmierczyk, 20, 60
Kuera, 139
Kuhn, 346
Kumar, 149
Kunin, 201
Kupka, 98
Kuptia, 104
Kurtsin, 18

Labarba, 8, 135
Labbe, 20, 60
Labrum, 196, 198
Lacey, 19, 122
Lachman, 123
Lager, 190
Lakatta, 302
Lal, 195
Lalos, 201, 317
Lamaze, 171, 173
Lammen, 141
Lamong, 313
Langer, 42, 112, 241
Lanson, 180
Lark, 269
LaRocca, 195

Laukaran, 135, 137, 141, 143, 153
Lawl, 191
Lazarus, 60, 63, 68, 122, 194, 236, 305, 306, 314, 348
Leake, 9
Leck, 143, 171
Lederman, 152, 156, 168
Leibel, 204
Leiva, 184
Lelonde, 3
Lenenthal, 95
Lenfant, 118, 258, 264
Leonard, 243
Lerner, 79, 255
LeRoy, 194
LeShan, 182
Lesinski, 156
Lesinsky, 163
Levankron, 119
Leventhal, 231, 251, 254, 255
Levi, 98, 181, 183
Levine, 118, 129, 168
Leviz, 137
Levy, 44, 113, 114, 122, 182, 198, 211
Lewinsohn, 6
Lewis, 320
Ley, 228
Lidell, 129
Lieber, 311
Liggel, 172
Liggin, 156
Lilienfeld, 151, 132
Lillienfeld, 121
Lin, 64, 77
Lindbohm, 144
Lindemann, 112
Lindheimer, 144
Linenthal, 205
Link, 73
Linn, 156, 240

Lipkin, 98, 104
Lister, 10
Little, 10, 135, 149, 155, 156
Littman, 163
Lock, 185
Locke, 66
LoGerfo, 305
Long, 194
Longo, 132, 170
Lotgoring, 135, 139, 156
Love, 196
Lowe, 53
Lubchenco, 163
Lubin, 135
Lumley, 135, 141, 173
Lumly, 230
Lund, 204
Lundin, 184
Lunenfeld, 152
Lutkinds, 112
Luttman, 156
Lux, 201
Lwies, 240
Lynch, xx, 151
Lyon, 198

MacDonald, 10, 141, 155
MacDougal, 67
MacDougall, 119, 206
Macentyre, 152
Macintyre, 171
Maddison, 112
Magmi, 135
Maguire, 235
Mahlstedt, 317
Maiman, 229, 236, 237, 261
Maine, 82
Malamud, 261
Malmo, 67
Mamlin, 233
Mandler, 66
Mann, 140, 250, 318

Manuck, 122, 180, 181
Marbury, 97, 156
Marine Hospital Service, 17
Marmot, 180, 181
Marshall, 114, 141, 198
Martin, 198, 259, 300
Maruta, 318
Marx, 353
Masuda, 135
Matarazzo, 14, 24, 25, 27, 45, 129, 263
Matarrazo, 7, 156
Mathew, 60
Mathews, 66, 68, 180, 185, 230
Maticek, 118
Mattson, 189
May, 43, 44
Mayberry, 198
Mayer, 153
Mayo Clinic, 69
Mayou, 135, 146, 184
McCabe, 60, 63, 66, 69, 180, 181
McCallum, 61
McCormack, 93
McCormick, 201
McCrae, 68, 243, 302
McDonald, 135, 140, 152, 155
McDougall, 180, 210
McDowell, xviv
McGinnis, 17
McHorney, 113
McHugh, 304
McKean, 136
McKenney, 239
McKeown, 34
McKewon, 53
McKinley, 156
McKuldy, 195
McLeod, 125, 244
McNeill, 149
McReynolds, 68, 333

Meade, 180
Mechanic, 93, 263
Mehl, 135, 170
Mehlman, 28
Melamed, 196, 251, 252, 253, 318
Melzak, 194
Mendenhall, 11, 91
Menzer, 319
Merrick, 9
Merskey, 194
Metal, 198
Mettlin, 114
Metzer, 111
Meyer, 121, 137, 139, 153, 167, 185, 306
Miller, 135, 143, 146, 241, 261
Mindick, 146
Mochizuke, 121
Mohide, 158, 206
Molfese, 159, 162, 163, 165, 166
Molinski, 135
Monroe, 60, 63, 64, 72, 73, 116
Montgomery, 137
Moore, 305
Moos, 182, 314
Moose, 244
Mor, 113
Morgan, 144
Morisky, 238
Morison, 156
Morris, 18, 19, 57, 169, 180, 181, 196, 228, 235
Morrison, 137, 146, 180
Morton, 184
Moskowitz, 44
Mosley, 201
Mossey, 57
Mozley, 190, 310, 317
Mulder, 179, 310
Mumford, 6, 303, 304, 306

Nadelson, 37, 38, 149, 311, 319
Naeye, 135, 153
Najman, 73
Nathanson, 42, 147
National Center for Health Statistics, 74
National Collaborative Study, 97
National Health Service, 34
National Institute of Medicine, 14, 23, 132, 170
National Institutes for Health, 17
Nayeye, 143
Neligan, 121, 132, 151
Nelson, 228, 240
Nesbitt, 135, 156, 163
Newcombe, 158
Newton, 194
Ng, 194
Nieberding, 95
Nielsen, 156
Niemiec, 184
Nilsen, 121
Nisbet, 302
Nisbett, 125
Norbeck, 129, 136, 151
Norris, 79, 80, 189, 257, 268, 318, 321
Notman, 37, 38
Nuckolls, 129, 136
Nunes, 190

O'Brien, 156, 189, 257, 321
O'Hara, 149
O'Hoy, 235
O'Neill, 78
Oakley, 10, 136, 139, 152, 156, 190, 234
Obayama, 136
Obayuwana, 156

Ochsner, 27
Oeschsli, 158
Okada, 156, 163, 229
Olasov, 189
Olesker, 38
Olsen, 137, 156, 201
Operation Lifestyle, 3
Orleans, 260
Osborne, 69
Oschsner, xx
Oshner, 10
Osofsky, 189, 269, 321, 333
Ostfeld, 302
Othermer, 71
Othner, 335

Paavonen, 202
Page, 18
Paklulainen, 205
Panchieri, 63
Papiernik-Berhauer, 158
Parazzini, 202
Parboosing, 8
Parks, 112
Parmalee, 156, 163
Parron, 98, 180
Parson, 14
Parsons, 235
Pasamanick, 121, 132, 151
Pasnau, 38, 199
Patel, 180
Paykel, 23, 124, 149
Pearse, xv, 156, 194
Peckinham, 141
Peele, 97
Pehl, 181
Peirson, 199
Pennebaker, 53, 54, 64, 65, 66, 67, 74
Pennington, 135, 156, 163
Perez, 152
Peterson, 135, 143, 211
Petterson, 189
Pettite, 180

Pettiti, 181
Phelan, 243
Phillips, 186
Pied Piper, 263
Pierson, 194
Pinsky, 194
Piper, 183
Pitts, 79
Plast, 185
Plato, 351
Pokhilko, 199
Pokorny, 15
Polivy, 278
Pollinger, 170
Porreco, 90
Porter, 129, 156
Powers, 67
Pratt, 41
Pratt, 156
President's Commission on Mental Health, 98
Pritchard, 10, 137, 141, 155, 194
Proctor, 211
Prue, 259
Prutting, 93
Public Health Service, 89

Quan, 190
Queenan, 136

Rabin, 211
Rabkin, 180, 186
Raener, 194
Rahe, 122
Rainwater, 147
Rannevik, 202
Rasputin, 263
Rayburn, 136, 181
Read, 171, 173
Reading, 136, 139, 152, 156, 231

Realini, 180
Reamy, 200
Reddy, 196
Redman, 144
Redway, 201
Rees, 112
Rehu, 154
Reich, 149
Reid, 198
Reisine, 130, 167
Reseine, 122
Revicki, 43, 44
Reynolds, 156, 243
Rice, 98
Richards, xv, 25, 125, 131, 132, 136, 156, 159, 165
Richmond, 156
Ridgeway, 185
Riegle, 156
Riley, 18
Ripley, 201
Risenbery, 255
Rizzardo, 136
Roback, 310
Robbins, 17, 23, 27, 111, 181, 183, 275, 279
Robert Wood Johnson Foundation, 24
Roberts, 151, 191, 208
Robitaille, 172
Robson, 304
Roden, 42, 112
Rodin, 69, 112, 227, 232, 241, 301
Roeske, 318
Roethlisberger, 259
Rofe, 144
Rogel, 147
Rogers, 24
Rohrbaugh, 189
Roman, 137, 140
Romano, 194

Romney, 105, 191, 194
Rooks, xv, 156, 170
Roper, 198
Rosen, 152, 156, 194, 205
Rosenbaum, 196
Rosenfeld, 189
Rosenfield, 82
Rosenman, 207
Rosenmann, 180
Rosenstock, 53, 95, 228, 237, 239, 242
Rosenthal, 255, 262, 303
Roth, 56
Rousseau, 351
Roux, 149
Roy-Byrne, 189
Rozensky, 262
Rubinow, 189
Ruble, 189
Ruff, 338
Russell, 8, 103, 147, 157, 248, 259
Russell-Briefel, 180
Ryan, 156

Sacket, 227
Sacks, 149
Sadeghi, 198
Sakiyama, 190
Salonen, 180
Salt, 80
Sameroff, 121, 139, 162
Sandberg, 136, 143, 151, 152, 231
Sandbert, 139
Sanders, 36
Sandler, 182, 317
Sansom, 198
Sarason, 63, 180
Schacter, 255
Schafer, 70
Schag, 260

Schecter, 196
Scheier, 68
Schifrin, 156, 166
Schlesinger, 156
Schmale, 198
Schneiderman, 60, 63, 66, 69, 180, 181
Schnider, 168
Schofield, 93
Schramm, 139
Schreiber, 190
Schroder, 139, 149
Schwartz, 20, 66, 67, 75, 181, 251
Schweizen, 264
Schweizer, 118, 258
Scientific Council of the American Medical Association, 13
Searls, 163
SEC, 170
Segelman, 156
Sehgal, 156
Sely, 122
Selye, 20, 60, 122
Semmelweis, 10
Seyle, 18
Shagass, 67
Shanock, 151
Shapiro, 156, 201
Shavit, 129
Sheehan, 143, 171
Shekelle, 111, 113, 119, 182
Sherwood, 113
Shiono, 140
Showstack, 156
Shrout, 60, 63
Shukit, 189
Sibinga, 242
Siebel, 313
Siebold, 198
Siegel, 156, 189
Siever, 59

Silen, 196
Silverman, 151, 158, 169
Sims, xxiv
Singer, 57, 107, 156, 172, 173, 198
Sjostee, 198
Sklar, 18, 59, 122, 129, 182, 196, 198, 211
Sloane, 156
Sloss, 189
Smith, 32, 96, 156, 180, 194, 198
Smithells, 140, 143
Smizer, 181
Snowden, 186
Sober, 183
Sobrihno, 195
Sokel, 136, 139
Sokol, 156, 158
Solomon, 182, 185, 186
Someroff, 137
Sonstegard, 146
Sontag, 30, 31, 32
Sorenson, 201
Sosa, 152, 172
Speller, xv
Speroff, 190
Spitz, 129
Spitzer, 332, 335
Stallones, 204
Starfield, 139, 156, 294
Starzyk, 103
Steege, 189
Stein, 140, 156, 186
Steinberg, 66, 200
Steiner, 94, 121, 132, 151
Steinhorn, 198
Steinlau, 147
Stellman, 198
Stembera, 156, 166
Stephans, 14
Stephen, 181

Author Index

Stephens, 18, 19, 201, 354
Steptoe, 60, 66, 68, 183
Sterbach, 194
Stern, 149, 187
Sternbach, 194
Steward, 97, 156
Stewart, 80
Stolkov, 156
Stone, 15, 53, 72
Storms, 302
Storthlz, 107
Strabinow, 156
Strickland, 114
Struab, 201
Struening, 180
Stuening, 186
Stunkard, 251, 252
Suchman, 53, 228
Surgeon General, 11, 23
Surwitt, 186
Susser, 156
Sutherland, 259, 311
Svengali, 263
Sverre-Pederson, 201
Syme, 111, 114, 205, 264
Syrjanen, 198
Szasz, 36
Szklo, 112

Tang, 235
Tapp, 67
Tatreau, 156
Taylor, 14, 71, 170, 194, 257, 318
Tazaras, 185
Telden, 129
Temoshok, 196
Terman, 194
Tew, 170
The Institute of Health Policy, 230
Thiessen, 170

Thomas, xx, 67, 110, 112, 115, 153, 156
Thomson, 10, 128, 131, 132, 137, 139, 147, 162, 170, 171
Thurlow, 62, 73
Tietze, 147
Tiger, 18
Tilden, 136, 149, 151
Tilson, 13
Timmermans, 194
Tollefson, 149
Tonascia, 167
Topless, 152, 156
Townly, 243
Tranethan, 198
Trussell, 74
Tsuang, 186
Tuchman-Duplessis, 143
Tudiver, 191
Tulandi, 195
Tull, 112, 182, 199, 235, 259
Turner, 194
Twinning, 156
Tyler, 123

U.S. Public Health Service, 17
Ueland, 103
Ureda, 14

Vaillant, 110
Van Alten, 170
Van der Heide, 194
Van Dyke, 60, 66
van den Berg, 135, 137, 141, 143, 158
Vecchia, 202
Verbrugge, 94
Verney, 131, 156
Vickery, 305
Vico, 125
Viola, 112

Voshart, 69
Vouk, 143, 171

Wadsworth, 54, 56
Waldo, 24
Wall, 194
Walsh, 38
Waring, 180
Warner, 8
Washington, 17, 156
Watson, 95, 170
Watt, 315
Weber, 210
Weinberg, xv
Weinberger, 233
Weiner, 18
Weinstein, 79, 147, 254
Weisman, 259, 313
Weisner, 151
Weiss, 156, 180, 183, 198
Weissman, 69
Welisch, 314
Wells, 156
Wenderlein, 154, 200, 315
Wengrad, 191
White, 54, 234
Whitehead, 191
Whitehorne, 158
Who, 82
Wideman, 156, 172, 173
Wiebe, 61
Wiggins, 75
Wilcox, 201
Wiley, 122
William, 156
Williams, v, xx, 110, 139, 156, 196, 238, 332
Wilsmick, 96
Wilsneck, 97
Wilson, 125, 156, 166, 248, 255
Winokur, 149
Winters, 340

Wise, 194, 199, 318, 319
Wolf, xxi, 19, 60, 201, 300
Wolff, 19, 60, 62, 63, 122, 194
Wolfson College, v
Woods, 189
Worden, 259
Works-Lind, 321
World Health Organization, 82
Wortis, 139
Wrede, 136
Wright, 198
Wynn, 139, 156, 190

Youkeles, 156
Young, 182, 189, 196
Youngs, 199, 318, 319, 321
Yudkin, 170

Zackler, 137, 156
Zacur, 190
Zapka, 261
Zappert, 79
Zax, 139, 162
Zbella, 202
Zborowski, 77
Zegans, 60, 66
Zeicher, 78
Zeichner, 180
Zimmerman, 95, 231
Zimmermann, 251
Zola, 54, 55, 77
Zuihlke, 147
Zuspan, xviii, 181

Subject Index

(MMPI) 113
(SEC) 9, 28

abdominal pain 61, 92, 104, 191, 212, 300
abnormal bleeding 91
abortion 6, 24, 37, 56, 90, 91, 103, 104, 105, 107, 128, 135, 138, 131, 136, 144, 146, 147, 148, 184, 196, 202, 222, 243, 267, 274, 314, 318, 319, 320, 328, 341
abruptio placenta 153
Absenteeism 79
abstinence 252, 260, 262, 356
accident 275, 282, 284, 286, 292
accidents 29, 44, 102, 111, 112, 147, 153, 181, 261, 278, 279
acquired immune deficiency syndrome 22, 30, 94, 140
act 17
adaptive Potential for Pregnancy Scale 336
addiction 254
addictions 279
additives 256
adherence 8, 237, 238, 249, 250, 253, 259, 263, 265, 266, 267, 270, 274, 276, 296, 304, 309, 310, 316, 352

adolescence 105
adrenal insufficiency 219
adrenalectomy 96
adultery 315
affective disorder 69, 188
aftercare 91
age 134, 136, 137, 139, 140, 141, 143, 146, 147, 156, 183, 186, 189, 236, 278, 303, 319
AIDS 31, 140, 184, 289, 325, 350
Aitken Visual Analog 335
alcoholism 1, 4, 5, 15, 25, 29, 33, 43, 55, 77, 88, 96, 104, 106
Alameda study 109, 122, 340
albumin 222
alcohol 3, 13, 22, 55, 100, 109, 110, 112, 113, 121, 124, 128, 130, 135, 142, 150, 176, 182, 183, 186, 193, 195, 196, 197, 198, 211, 247, 252, 254, 261, 266, 268, 269, 278, 279, 280, 285, 292, 298, 315, 321, 327, 342, 351, 353
alcohol use 12, 137, 138, 139, 154, 168, 180, 187, 200
Alcoholics Anonymous 253, 278
alcoholism 141, 160, 184, 264, 321, 328, 336, 341, 355

alexithymea depression 193
alexithymia 71, 181
allergic responses 96
allergies 128
allergy 345
alter ego 270, 298, 329
alternative birth center 130
Ambivalence 149
ambulatory care 233
amenorrhea 155, 187, 189, 209, 220, 352
American Cancer Society 312, 313, 355
American Indians 135
amnesia 71, 72
amniocentesis 141, 229, 243
amphetamines 142, 190, 286
ampicillin 217
Anal intercourse 201
anal fissure 96
analgesia 172, 173
analgesic 54
analgesics 150
analysis of covariance 332
androgens 142, 150
anemia 121, 343
anesthesia 147, 161, 162, 164, 173
anesthetics 150, 295
anger 70, 79, 111, 178, 196, 260, 292, 313, 314, 317, 320
angina 179, 302, 345
angina pectoris 302
angiograph 119
animal fat 198
anomie 110
anorexia nervosa 187, 189
anorexia 352
anorexic 287
anovulation 139, 198, 199, 216, 219

antenatal hostility 148
antenatal care 10, 143, 160, 162, 171, 172, 176, 234
anti-hypertensives 315
anti-nausea agents 140
anti-nauseant 141
antianxiety medication 113
antibiotic therapy 223
antibiotics 199
antibody 15
anticholinergics 315
anticoagulants (coumarins) 142
antidepressants 190
antiemetics 210
antifungal agents 216
antigens 140
antihistamines 315
antihypertensives 190
anileptic drugs 141
antineoplastics 94, 142
antipruritics 218
antituberculosis 142
anxiety 13, 43, 55, 62, 68, 73, 78, 98, 128, 133, 138, 144, 146, 148, 150, 152, 154, 160, 172, 173, 176, 178, 180, 189, 190, 191, 199, 221, 229, 230, 234, 236, 251, 259, 269, 275, 278, 279, 291, 292, 299, 303, 305, 306, 309, 310, 311, 312, 314, 322, 323, 333, 342, 344
apgar scores 222, 223, 337
Apresoline 222
Archetypical AT 9 Alexithymea Test 337
arginine 220, 221
aromatic amines 211
arsenic 211
arteriosclerosis 4, 178
arthritis of pregnancy 202
arthritis 5, 244, 315, 352

Subject Index

artificial insemination 38, 184
asbestos 211
Aspirin Myocardial Infarction Study 119
aspirin 142
asthma 19
atherosclerosis 21, 102, 106, 111
atrophic vaginitis 96
atropine 300
attentiveness 65, 66
Attitude to Pregnancy Scale 336
auto accidents 278
Autonomic Perception Questionnaire 334
autonomic system 66
autopsy 93

balanitis 96
Baltimore study 53
barbiturates 315
bartholin cyst 96
basal body temperature 219
Bayley Scales of Infant Development 337
BBT 216
Beck Depression Inventory 335
bed rest 158
bedrest 248
Beford College Life Events and Difficulties Scale 334
behavior modification 248
behavioral therapy 252
benzine 211
benzodiazepam 338
bereavement 112, 113
Berle Social Support Index 336
beta endorphin 343
beta endorphins 338
bichloromethyl ether 211
biofeedback 6, 186, 247, 251, 256
biofeedback training 349

biorhythm 343
bipolar affective disorder 133
bipolar disorder 73
birth interval 138
birth intervals 136
birth order 139, 150
birth control pills 258
birth defects 97
birth induction 137
birth weight 136
bisexual 96
blackouts 286
bladder cancer 183
Blau Maternal Attitudes to Pregnancy Scale 336
blindness 72
blood pressure 101
blood pressure self-monitoring 143
blood sugar 219
blood transfusion 184
blues 322
body rhythm 155
body weight 252
bonding 130, 150
boric acid douches 216
Bortner Scale 335
BP control 253
brain 20
Braverman-Roux Postpartum Depression Scale 336
Brazelton Neonatal Behavior Assessment Scale 337
breast feeding 148
breast cancer 30, 106, 107, 113, 114, 122, 195, 208, 240, 257, 259
breast disease 233
breast feeding 9, 186, 190
breast self examinations 208
breast self-examination 5, 100, 101, 102, 104, 195, 253, 261

breasts 91, 219
breech 165
Brief Symptom Inventory 336
Briquet's syndrome 301
British Medical Journal 325
bronchitis 183
BSE 355
bulemia 287
Burnstein Pregnancy Anxiety Test 336
Buros MENTAL MEASUREMENTS YEARBOOK 332
butyrephenone 190
Byrne Sex Information Questionnaire 336
Byrnes Repression-Sensitization Scale 335

cadmium 211
Caesarean section 89
caesarean 151, 162, 163, 172, 295
caesarean delivery 160
caesarean section 131, 147, 153
caffeinated drinks 202
caffeine 142, 195, 269, 290
Caine & Foulds Hostility & Direction of Hostility Questionnaire 336
calcium intake 101, 187
California Medical Association 240, 347
California Personality Inventory 334
cancer 10, 14, 18, 21, 22, 30, 31, 32, 33, 44, 59, 102, 112, 113, 116, 122, 147, 181, 208, 211, 223, 250, 256, 259, 260, 262, 268, 279, 298, 304, 311, 312, 313, 314, 315, 319, 328
cancer of the breast 209

cancer of the cervix 208, 209
cancer of the colon 106, 107
cancer of the oral cavity 129
cancer of the rectum 106
cancer of the vulva 313
cancers 106, 120
candida 199
cannabis 121, 128, 135, 279
carcinogens 181
cardiac arrhythmias 61
cardiac disease 115, 147, 157
cardiopulmonary resuscitation 291
cardiovascular diseases 21, 103
cardiovascular 3
cardiovascular disease 22, 61, 116, 118, 209, 303, 311, 315
cardiovascular hyperresponsivity 148
cardiovascular pathology 54
cardiovascular symptoms 80
cardiovascular system 302, 344
case history 15
catacholamine 221
catecholamine 178
catecholamines 180, 221, 338
Catel 16PF Test 335
cathacholamine 221
Cattell Infant Intelligence Scale 337
central nervous system 94, 104
cerebrovascular accident 106
cerebrovascular accidents 147
cerebrovascular disease 102
cervical inflammation 202
cervical cancer 61, 95, 104, 106, 107, 196, 208, 311, 313, 341
cervical conization 216
cervical intraepithelial neoplasia 94

cervictis 216
cervix uteri 91
chancroid 93
CHD 110, 111, 118, 124, 178, 204, 205, 207, 210, 265, 274, 279, 341, 347
Checklist for Somatization Disorder (DSM III) 335
chemical waste site exposure 142
chemotherapy 258, 259, 313
chest pain 55, 93, 302
child abuse 130, 150, 151
childbirth training 171
chlamydia 54, 139, 140, 194, 202, 217, 289
chlamydia trachomitis 94
chlamydiae 91
chlorinated water 201
chocolate 202
chocolates 275
cholecystectomy 199, 318
Cholera 205
cholesterol 101, 178, 179, 181, 204, 207, 254, 274
Cholesterolemics 142
cholestyramine 204
chorioamnionities 140
Christensen Health History 336
Christian Science 34
chromium 211
chronic obstruction pulmonary 5, 21
chronic disease care 5
chronic obstructive lung disease 102, 106
chronic pain 318
CHS 120
Cigarette smoking 136, 137, 143
Cigarette use 181
cigarette 135
cigarette smoking 97

cigarettes 3, 99, 150, 207, 259, 274, 279, 285, 351
circulation 338
cirrhosis 21, 102, 106, 112
cleft palate 141
clonidine 315
CNS 67, 72, 74, 111, 315, 344
cocaine 55, 128, 135, 139, 150, 153, 275, 279, 286, 325, 342
coffee 128, 183, 198
Cohen/Hoberman Symptom Checklist 336
coital frequency 139
colostomy 6, 311, 259
Commission on Chronic Diseases 53
compliance 95, 105, 245, 247, 340, 347
complications 344
compulsions 279
computer 305, 346
condidiasis 94
condoms 139, 194, 196, 217, 223, 274, 289, 350
Condylomata acumenata 94
conjunctivitis 289
conservatism 353
constipation 155, 218
contamination 164
Continuous Performance Test 334
contraception 12, 37, 42, 91, 99, 107, 139, 144, 145, 146, 147, 184, 194, 196, 202, 209, 217, 218, 221, 223, 235, 241, 265, 274, 275, 288, 341
Cook-Medley Ho MMPI Subscale 111, 336
cord pH 223
Cornell Medical Index 336

Coronary Drug Research Project 125, 265
coronary heart disease 22, 37, 67, 110, 119, 175, 177, 258, 302
Corticosteroids 142
cortisol 168, 178, 338, 343
cortisol serum value 219
cortrosyn 219
counseling 37, 38, 149, 185, 199, 261, 264, 299, 303, 304, 305, 306, 307, 312, 313, 316, 318, 319, 320, 321, 324, 325, 329, 340, 355
cramping 216
cryocautery 217
cyclozine 142
cystic disease 201
cystic diseases 91
cystic fibrosis 243
cystitis 92, 93, 94, 96, 104, 200, 201, 289, 290
cytomegalo virus 94
cytomegalovirus 139, 142
cytotoxic drugs 142

Daily Hassles Scale 334, 336
defense mechanism 258, 276
delivery 91
demerol 150
denial 133, 146, 152, 173, 196, 236, 258, 276, 278, 313
denticator 288
Department of Agriculture 256
dependency 250, 254, 339
depression 6, 13, 18, 44, 55, 58, 59, 60, 61, 62, 68, 69, 71, 73, 77, 78, 79, 80, 82, 97, 98, 100, 104, 106, 112, 113, 114, 116, 118, 128, 129, 133, 137, 148, 170, 176, 178, 182, 185, 188, 189, 190, 191, 194, 200, 218, 220, 221, 223, 234, 243, 253, 268, 269, 275, 278, 289, 291, 292, 303, 305, 309, 310, 312, 313, 314, 315, 317, 318, 319, 321, 322, 324, 325, 333, 335, 339, 341, 343, 345, 349
Derogatis Sexual Function Inventory 336
dexamethasone 219
Di Matteo 232
diabetes 5, 18, 21, 22, 26, 54, 59, 96, 102, 104, 106, 141, 142, 179, 181, 186, 209, 221, 222, 247, 260, 266, 287, 290, 315, 327, 341
diabetics 56, 267
diagnostic reliability 171
diagnostic systems 98
diaphragm 196, 218, 201
diarrhea 21
diazepam 150, 339
diet 4, 12, 22, 76, 101, 124, 137, 144, 147, 176, 247, 256, 264, 269, 275, 298, 344
dietary salt intake 101, 180
dieting 189, 199, 352
Differential Emotion Scale 335
differential diagnosis 345
digestive system complaint 90
digestive disorder 73
dilation and curettage 89
dilation 319
diphtheria 21, 205
discriminant analysis 341, 353
diuretics 315
divorce 60, 243
Doctor Opinion Questionnaire 336

Subject Index

dogmatism 335
dopamine 190
douches 290
Down's syndrome 243
drinking 156, 230, 231, 265, 275, 278
drug abuse 1, 43, 128, 138, 184, 247, 266
drug use 4, 5, 15, 8, 12, 13, 22, 29, 88, 128, 135, 150, 151, 193, 211, 229, 262, 263, 275, 278, 279, 280, 292, 327, 339
DSM III 345
Dubowitz Assessment of Gestational Age 337
dysmenorrhea 71, 72, 80, 148, 154, 171, 190, 209, 215, 340, 344, 349
dysparenuia 217, 71, 216, 300, 317
dysphoria 229
dysplasia 217

ear ache 93
eating disorders 321
eating habits 154
ECG 302
eclampsia 6, 92, 103, 104, 131, 147, 150, 291
ectopic pregnancy 54, 103, 147, 155, 217, 218
Edwards Personal Preference Inventory 335
egalitarianism 43
Einstein Scales of Sensormotor Intelligence (Escalona & Cormon) 337
ejaculation 317
Ekankar 34
EKG 311
elderly 303, 304, 345

electromyograph 256
Elliot Eisdorfer Stressful Events Scale 334
embolism 103, 111
emotional distress 5, 44, 69, 71, 72, 77, 96, 97, 98, 133, 148, 150, 154, 155, 156, 170, 171, 189, 190, 192, 195, 200, 268, 301, 304, 309, 310, 313, 316, 323, 326
emotional drain 345
emotional support 303
emotional trauma 178
emphysema 183
endocrine disorders 94
endocrine disturbance 72
endocrine gland 219
endocrine systems 67
endocrinopathies 219
endometrial cancer 198, 240
endometriosis 96, 140
endometritis 154
endorphins 338
enteric disease 21, 94
environmental exposure 140
environmental toxin 138, 139, 140, 150
epidemiology 10, 19
epidurals 150
epilepsy 143
episiotomy 96
epithelium 216
erotophobia 146
EST 34
estrogen 150, 88, 195, 258, 198
estrogen therapy 187
Ethnic status 146
ethnicity 127, 134, 136, 138, 140, 141, 143, 147, 194
euphoria 148

examination 12, 91, 92, 184
exercise 4, 5, 12, 58, 76, 99,
    102, 109, 124, 135, 138,
    144, 155, 168, 186, 187,
    189, 191, 204, 247, 254,
    261, 267, 268, 269, 275,
    278, 280, 286, 298, 321,
    327, 350, 352, 355
exhaustion 178
exoparasitic infections 94
exposure to cold 144
Eysenck EPG 335

factor analysis 168
fad diets 135
fallopian tubes 91
false pregnancy 220
Family Environment Scale 334
Family History Diagnostic
    Criterion (Andreasen) 337
family planning 90, 98, 107, 235
fasting glucose 222
fat intake 196
fatigue 24, 50, 58, 100, 135,
    138, 153, 178, 278, 292,
    300, 307, 310, 311, 342,
    343, 344
fear 70
Feedback 249
Fels Institute 344
feminism 40
fenfluramine 252
fertility 105
fertility rates 99
fetal alcoholism syndrome 352
fetal distress 131
fetal growth retardation 131
fetal heart rate monitoring 158
fetal loss 171
fetal malformation 171, 320
fetal malfunction 320
fever-influenza 168

fiber intake 101
fibrocystic disease 196, 202,
    290
fibroids 140
field dependence 191, 337
flatus 220
Fleish formula 228
foam 217
folic acid antagonists 142
food disorders 269
forceps 165
Framingham Scale 335
Free Anxiety Subscale
frequency of coitus 144

galactorrhea 155, 195, 219
galactorrhea-amenorrhea 189
Gardinella 199
Gardnerella vaginalis 94
gastrointestinal disease 9
gastrointestinal disorder 53,
    155, 209
gastrointestinal pathology 19
gastrointestinal tract 92
General Well Being Scale 336
genetic counseling 42, 243
genital warts 196
genital candidosis 94
genital herpes 94, 107, 184
genital tract disorder 233
genital warts 61, 94
genitourinary complaint 90
genitourinary disorders 53
genitourinary system 90, 93
genotypes 141
gentian violet 216
Gesell Developmental Schedules
    337
Gessel Developmental Rating
    344
glucometer 222
glucose levels 186, 343

Subject Index

Goldstein Repression-Threat Denial 335
gonadotrophins 219
gonoccocal infection 196, 202
gonococcal salpingitis 217
gonorrhea 93, 194
Graham Behavior Test and Graham-Rosenblith Tests 337
granuloma inguinal 94
grief 243, 313, 317
Griffiths's Mental Development Scale 337
Grimm Psychology Tension Inventory 335
ground water contamination 283, 288
growth hormone 343
growth retardation 143
guilt 70, 230, 314, 317, 320
guilt-shame 149
gum inflammations 231
gums 288

Halbreich Premenstrual Assessment 337
Hamilton Rating Scale for Depression 337
hand guns 283
Harris poll 101
Hawthorne effect 259
headache 19, 53, 55, 71, 73, 93, 100, 104, 80, 194, 218, 256, 257, 221, 300, 345, 349
Health Education Council 357
Health Instrument File 333
Health Status Questionnaire 336
heart attack 55, 124, 298, 303, 347
heart disease 18, 21, 26, 59, 102, 106, 181, 203, 264
heartburn 155

Heisenberg principle 161
helplessness 278, 305, 317
hematocrit 219
hemoglobin 167, 222
hemorrhage 103, 131, 147, 157, 172, 173
hemorrhoidectomy 216
hemorrhoids 96
hepatitis B 94, 140, 141
heroin 25, 33, 121, 128, 135, 143, 150, 252, 266, 278, 286, 315, 352
herpes 31, 107, 142, 196, 202, 247, 289
high altitude 135
high risk care 134
HIP Pregnancy Questionnaire 336
HMO 17, 26, 45, 269, 271, 299, 305, 329, 357
Hodgkins disease 313
home birth 34, 38, 130, 160, 170
home pregnancy test 220
home visits 239
homicide 22, 111, 211
homosexuality 30, 33, 184, 201
hopelessness 29, 170
Hopkins Symptom Checklist SCL 90R 336
hormone 315, 343
hospital admission 15, 97, 115, 169, 184, 220
hospital births 132, 160, 169
hospitalization 113
hostility 111, 116, 119, 122, 178, 189, 243, 275, 278, 292, 310, 336
hot flashes 195
HP viruses 350
HPV 196, 208
HSV 1 and 2 139

humor 336
Hydatidiform mole 202
hydramnios 222
hygiene 9, 201, 218
hyperbilirubinemia 222
hyperemesis 71
hyperemesis gravidarium 154
hyperlipemia 210
hyperprolactinemia 155
hyperremia 19
hypertension 6, 13, 18, 19, 26, 54, 77, 80, 92, 99, 103, 106, 110, 111, 125, 128, 135, 138, 139, 141, 143, 144, 147, 153, 179, 180, 191, 198, 207, 229, 237, 238, 239, 247, 250, 264, 274, 278, 287, 290, 315, 341, 345
hypochondriasis 178, 184, 192
hypoglycemia 222
hypoglycemic drugs 142
hypothalamic function 221
hysterectomy 6, 89, 96, 195, 235, 267, 301, 318, 328
hysteria 192, 345

IgE antibodies 168
ileostomy 312
imaging 172, 251, 258, 316, 349
immune function 338
immune response 338
immune system 1, 66, 138, 343
immunization 18, 140
immunosuppression 77, 129, 142, 198
inadequate weight gain 134
incontinence 93
induced abortion 144, 154, 155
induction of labor 131, 158, 222
industrial solvents 142
infection 103, 139, 185, 216, 338, 140

Infectious exposure 142
infectious disease 31, 32, 91, 111, 112, 205
infertility 5, 83, 97, 99, 105, 198, 200, 201, 209, 218, 310, 317, 323, 327
inflammation 338
insomnia 113, 221, 302
Institute for Health Policy 260
Institute for Personality Assessment and Research 344
Institute of Medicine 210, 357
insulin 222, 251
insurance 324, 350
intelligence 64, 242, 334
intercourse 99, 317, 350
interleukin 1 168, 338, 343
interleukin 2 168, 338, 343
intracranial lesions 5, 3, 21
intrauterine growth retardation 137, 223
introversion 190
introversion-extraversion 192
Inventory of Family Feelings 334
IPAT Anxiety Scale 335
ipicac 300
ron intake 187, 287
irradiation 313
irritability 100, 150, 349
item analysis 331
IUD 139, 141, 155, 194, 223

Jenkins Activity Survey 119, 335
Job-Related Tension Index 336
John Hopkins 110
Joint Commission on the Accreditation of Hospitals 294

Karnofsky Performance Status Scale 337

Kellner Symptom Questionnaire 335, 336
ketoacidosis 222
Kielland's forceps 136

L-dopa 220
labor induction 158
lacerations 172
lactation 105
laparascopy 192
laparotomy 217
lead 150
learned helplessness 178
lesbian 96
leukoplakia 96
leutinizing hormone 220
Leverson-Miller Locus of Control 334
levothyroxine sodium 219
LH 220, 221
lice 199
lidocaine 150
Life Event Scale for Obstetrical Patients 336
Life Events Inventory 334
Life Experience Survey 334
Life Orientation Test (LOT) 335
Life Satisfaction Index Z 336
life expectancy 22
Lipid Research Project 204
lipids 178, 256
lipoproteins 178, 300
LISREL 332
literacy 356
lithium carbonate 315
Lizzie Bordon 211
Lock Wallace Marital Adjustment Scale 334
locus of control 344
loneliness 278
longevity 110

low birth weight 121, 128, 131, 137, 143, 149, 158, 167, 210, 331, 342, 357
LSD 286, 352
lubrication 221
lung cancer 22, 27, 104, 106, 107, 121, 274
lung disease 29
luteal phase 211, 278, 343
Lykken Activity Preference Questionnaire 337
lymph nodes 122, 195
lymphogranuloma venerium 93

Maastricht Myocardial Infarction Risk Questionnaire 335
MacMillan HOS 336
macrophages 168, 338, 343
magnesium 187
malaria 288
malnutrition 287
malpractice 35, 40, 43, 45, 93, 161, 233, 240, 241, 242, 294, 320, 347
mammography 274
manic-depressive disorder 133
marijuana 139, 150, 239, 285
marital status 138, 140
marital problems 95, 199
MARLIC principle 57, 58, 65, 255
Marlowe Crowne Social Desirability Scale 335
Massachusetts Health Care Panel Study 110
mastectomy 30, 96, 267, 313, 323, 327, 328
masturbation 314
McGill Pain Questionnaire 337
McReynolds Preference for Control Scale 334

meclozine 141
meconium staining 166
Medicaid 3, 357
medication 143, 147, 190, 207, 228, 238, 239, 244, 247, 252, 259, 263, 265, 258, 274, 275, 290, 292, 299, 301, 310, 315, 316, 322, 328, 339
meditation 5, 239, 257, 258, 350, 355
melanoma 182
menarche 80, 105, 134, 339
Menopausal symptoms 90, 91, 300
menopausal disorder 329
menopause 80, 105, 195, 202, 323
menorrhagia 191, 300, 301
menses 221
menstrual cycle 202, 215, 220, 221, 224
menstrual diary 219
menstrual disorder 90, 91, 104, 105, 107, 113, 133, 267, 309
menstrual mood 333
menstruation 72, 80, 201, 217, 233, 337, 343
Mental Health Inventory 335
mental disorders 98
mental health 150
mental illness 148, 149
mentation 219
mercury 142, 150
Michigan Alcoholism Screening Test 336
Middlesex Hospital 335
midwife 134
migraine 19
migration 77, 353
Mill Hill Test of Verbal Intelligence 334

Miller Social Intimacy Scale 336
minerals 256, 288
Minnesota Multiphasic Personality Inventory (MMPI) 110, 334
mirasmus 15
miscarriage rate 96
misinformation 145
mitosis 338
MMPI 111
mobiluneus 94
molloscum contagiosum 94
monilial vulvo-vaginitis 215, 222
moniliasis 92, 216
monocyte 168, 338, 343
mononucleosis 94
monorrhagia 209
mood 335, 337
mood swings 219
Moose Menstrual Distress Scale 337
morning sickness 220
morphine 129
mortality 102
mourning 320
MRFIT 264, 119
mucopurulent cervicitis 94
mugging 283
Multidimension Health Locus of Control 334
Multiple Risk Factor Intervention Trial 119, 210, 258
multiple discriminant analysis 165
multiple sclerosis 304
murder 211
Musculoskeletal complaints 90
mustard 211
mycoplasma hominis 94
myocardial infarction 4, 63, 119, 122, 301, 306, 310, 345

myoma 175, 198

Naltrexone 129, 229
narcissism 170
National Ambulatory Medical Care Survey 11
National Health Service 208
National Hospice Study 113
Nausea and vomiting 71, 154, 218, 258, 316
negative affect 73, 333
neonatal death 320
neoplasm 91, 102, 129
neoplastic disease 129
nephritis 21
nervousness 100, 194
neural tube 141
neuroendocrine system 1, 343
neuroleptics 150
neuropathy 315
neuropeptides 338
neurosis 68, 69, 92, 148, 191
neuroticism 68, 171, 185, 301, 302, 304, 333, 345
nickel 211
nicotine 254
nicotine gum 248
nightmares 291, 340
NIMH Depression Scale 335
NIMH Diagnostic Interview Schedule (DIS) for Psychiatric Disorders 335
NIMH Trait Anxiety Scale 335
NK cells 113, 129, 338
non-neoplastic breast disease 91
Nowlis Mood Adjective Checklist 335
nsurance 357
nulliparity 190
nursing home 241

nutrition 5, 15, 39, 64, 101, 105, 134, 136, 137, 138, 140, 141, 149, 153, 168, 183, 205, 256, 261, 274, 275, 280, 287, 342, 352

obesity 1, 5, 12, 13, 53, 94, 99, 101, 109, 110, 124, 134, 135, 136, 141, 144, 147, 154, 179, 180, 191, 195, 196, 198, 247, 250, 252, 254, 260, 265, 266, 274, 275, 278, 287, 327, 355
observation 91, 92, 167
Office visits 90
OHB 159
Older American Resources and Services Questionnaire 336
Ontario Perinatal Mortality Study 167
opiates 190
opium addicts 229
optimism 335
oral contraceptive 24, 144, 147, 154, 177, 179, 181, 186, 188, 190, 198, 199, 202, 223, 180, 223, 218, 315
orgasm 201, 311
orthopedic pain 92
OSHA 207
osteoporosis 54, 187, 287
ostomy 96, 193, 311, 312, 323, 327
OTC 72, 142, 154, 282, 348
outcome criteria 173, 331
ovarian cancer 106, 198, 240
ovarian cycle 343
ovarian cysts 96
ovarian mass 221
ovariectomy 96, 195
overconfidence 254

overeating 58, 275
overprescription 104
ovulation 201
oxytocin 222

pain 24, 77, 146, 157, 188, 212, 251, 277, 298, 307, 310, 312, 314, 316, 322, 324, 328, 329, 337, 340, 343, 345
Pap smear 50, 100, 197, 217, 208, 290
paralysis 72
parametrium 91
Parental Attitudes Research Inventory 336
parity 134, 136, 143, 146, 156, 163, 190, 202
Parmalee Neurological Examination 337
passivity 114
Patient Attitude Test 336
Patient Cooperativeness Test 336
Paykel Interview for Recent Life Events 337
payments system 357
PBB 150
PCB 150
PCP 121, 286
PCT
pediculosis 94
pelvic pain 191, 212
pelvic congestion 193
pelvic exenteration 311, 313, 323
pelvic inflammatory disease 94, 192, 194, 209, 217
pelvic mass 96
pelvic pain 72, 73, 75, 105, 171, 209, 309, 318, 340
pelvic peritoneum 91

penicillin 217
Pennebaker PILL 336
peptic ulcer 18, 300
perceived social support 336
perception 19
peritoneal fluid 343
permissiveness 145
Personal Assessment of Intimacy in Relationships Scale 336
personality 19, 30, 32, 33, 133
personality distress 68
personality disturbance 333
pesticide 142
pH 216
pharmacotherapy 229, 252, 269, 310
phenacetin 183
phenothiazines 155, 190
phenylketonuria, 242
Phenytoin 142
phobias 291
phthirus pubis 94
physician error 147
PID, leiomyoma 96
pills 139
PKU 207
placebo 76, 95, 188, 238, 257, 259, 265, 268, 269, 300, 302, 315, 316, 321, 342, 356
placenta previa 131, 153
plasma 343
plasma glucose 216
pluralism 354, 355
PMC 148
PMS 5, 71, 72, 76, 80
PMS 148, 171, 211, 257, 267, 268, 269, 278, 300, 309, 318, 327, 328, 329, 340, 342, 343, 344, 345, 349, 356

Subject Index

pneumonia 21, 102, 106, 183
point prevalence rate 97, 98
poisons 283
polio 288
polycyclic hydrocarbons 211
Pooling Project 203
positive feedback 250
postpartum emotional disorders 322, 336
poverty 149
powerlessness 244, 245
PPO 269, 271, 329
Pre and post operative care 90
pre-eclampsia 92, 104, 131, 143, 144, 223, 247, 268
Prechtl and Beintema Neurological Examination 337
Precursor Study Family Attitudes Scale 334
prediction error 167
preeclampsia 103, 125, 274, 344
Pregnancy Research Questionnaire 336
premature deliveries 21, 96
premenstrual mood change 148
premenstrual syndrome 52, 76, 79, 188, 209, 211, 321
prenatal care 90, 91, 92, 132, 138, 141, 160, 222
prescription drugs 138
prescription 72, 88, 89, 106, 94, 95, 141, 150, 227, 228, 239, 244, 248, 282, 307, 301, 318, 339, 340, 348
Preventive Health Care in Obstetrics-Gynecology Training 11
primary care 13, 17, 38, 39, 113, 328
primiparae 144, 255
PRL 221
probenecid 217
procoagulation 338

Profile of Mood States 335
progesterone 150, 257, 268, 269, 321
progestin 142, 217
prolactin 219, 220, 343
prolapse 91, 96
promiscuity 31, 33, 197, 217, 279, 314, 325
propanalol 315
prophylaxis 32, 184, 197, 247
prostaglandin 319, 338, 343
prostigmine 300
protein 187
proteinuria 143
Protestant ethic 352
pruritis 199, 209, 300, 340, 345
pseudocyesis 155, 220, 221
psychasthenia 192
psychiatric disorder 133
Psychiatric Epidemiology Research Interview 337
psychoactive drug use 80
psychoactive drugs 94, 98, 188
psychodrama 262
psychodynamics 270
psychoimmunology 122
psychological defenses 242
psychometric research 332
psychometrics 118
psychoneurosis 111
psychosexual dysfunction 96
Psychosocial Adjustment to Illness Scale 334
psychosomatic distress 31, 192
psychosomatic reactivity 140
psychosomatics 34, 36, 338, 347
psychotherapy 182, 259, 268, 269, 299, 304, 305, 306, 332
puberty 105

public assistance 134
puerperal disorders 53
puerperal sepsis 140
pulmonary embolism 103

quality of care 2, 35, 36, 89, 93, 104, 106, 134, 139, 150, 161, 162, 199, 209, 233, 236, 240, 241, 294, 314, 339
quality of life 203, 236

race 64, 82, 109, 118, 134, 138, 141, 146, 147, 180, 183, 187
radiation exposure 143, 211
radiation therapy 95, 235, 311, 313
radical mastectomy 258
radiography 220
rape 96, 279, 283, 289
rash 289
rationalism 352
rationalizations 254
rebellion 222
Recent Life Change Questionnaire 334
Reiter's disease 94
relaxation 251, 327, 350
REM 340
REM-sleep 343
renal disease 96
repression 190, 196, 236, 258, 278
Research Diagnostic Criteria (Spitzer) 335
resistance 325, 326, 347
resperpine 315
respiratory distress 136
respiratory failure 173
retaches 45
retinoic acid 142

retrolental fibroplasia 158
Rh problems 163
Rheumatoid arthritis 185
rhythm method 139
Rifampin 142
rigidity 335
risk prediction 132, 157, 158, 162, 164, 168, 338, 341, 345, 348, 354, 358
risk scales 167, 331
Rokeach Dogmatism Scale 335
role conflict 139
Rorschach test 110, 337
Rosenzweig Pictures Frustration Test 336
Rotter Locus of Control 334
rubella 139, 140, 142
Rubinow Visual Analog Scales 335

Salicylates 142
saline 319
saline and prostaglandin instillation 149
salpingectomy 217
salpingitis 218
salt intake 269
sanitation 9
satisfaction 294, 298
scabies 94
Schedule of Daily Experiences 334
Schedule of Recent Experiences 334
schistosomiasis 288, 300
schizophrenia 133, 139, 192, 341
Screening Test for Somatization (Othner and DeSouza) 335
screening 158, 159, 208, 305, 332

seat belt use 12, 25, 45, 99, 101, 102, 186, 254, 261, 268, 274, 275, 278, 283
SEC 64, 65, 80, 109, 118, 121, 123, 127, 136, 140, 141, 143, 144, 145, 146, 149, 156, 159, 167, 172, 176, 180, 182, 184, 209, 210, 233, 236, 282, 303, 319, 341, 352, 356
sedatives 79, 94, 158, 278, 286
sedentary life styles 99
self-blaming 148
Self-Consciousness Scale 335
self-esteem 4, 144, 145, 184, 250
self-hypnosis 258
self-image 146
self-medication 155
self-monitoring 259
Self-Transcendence Scale 335
Sense of Humor Questionnaire 336
separation 149
serum electrolytes 219
sex 150
sexism 74
sexual preference 288
sexual dysfunction 5, 95, 96, 104, 106, 155, 278, 309, 311, 312, 313, 315
sexual practices 96
sexual problems 95, 189
sexually transmitted disease 25, 29, 32, 37, 91, 93, 104, 107, 135, 137, 139, 140, 142, 155, 183, 194, 196, 199, 202, 208, 209, 265, 267, 274, 275, 278, 323, 341, 342, 350
Short Marital Adjustment Scale 334

Sickness Impact Profile 334
SID 143
side effects 258, 339
Situational Humor Response Test 336
skin cancer 182
sleep disturbance 178
sleep 12, 100, 286
sleep disorder 73, 193, 340, 343
sleeping patterns 109
sleeplessness 61, 291
smoke detector 101, 102
smoking 1, 4, 5, 8, 10, 12, 17, 23, 25, 27, 31, 67, 104, 107, 109, 110, 112, 118, 120, 123, 124, 129, 139, 141, 143, 148, 153, 154, 156, 160, 167, 168, 169, 172, 176, 177, 179, 180, 183, 187, 188, 195, 196, 197, 198, 200, 204, 230, 231, 247, 248, 250, 252, 253, 254, 255, 258, 259, 260, 261, 264, 265, 266, 269, 275, 278, 279, 280, 298, 321, 327, 328, 342, 352, 355, 356
Social Readjustment Rating Scale 334
Social Support Questionnaire 336
social support 20, 38, 62, 73, 80, 112, 113, 114, 115, 116, 122, 129, 137, 140, 148, 160, 172, 176, 178, 182, 196, 199, 205, 237, 238, 253, 255, 257, 265, 266, 276, 295, 303, 305, 314, 333, 336, 348
somatization 71, 73, 77, 105, 106, 189, 300, 305, 324, 335, 344

somatoform disorder 301
sonography 220
spectinomycin 217
Spielberger State Anxiety 335
spina bifida 158
spinal anesthesia 150
spironolactone 315
spontaneous abortion 139, 171
staff error 147
Stanford University 244
status quo 353
sterility 92
sterilization 99, 107
steroids 150, 300
stilboesterol 142
stillbirth 128, 170, 320
Stimulus Screening Scale 335
stress 1, 10, 12, 15, 18, 19, 20,
    37, 43, 44, 45, 53, 59, 60,
    61, 62, 63, 66, 73, 77, 78,
    80, 82, 100, 101, 102, 107,
    110, 114, 122, 129, 133,
    134, 137, 138, 139, 140,
    141, 144, 152, 168, 172,
    176, 180, 185, 186, 188,
    189, 198, 199, 211, 216,
    241, 247, 251, 255, 257,
    259, 260, 261, 262, 265,
    266, 275, 280, 290, 298,
    300, 302, 312, 317, 319,
    321, 322, 327, 333, 338,
    339, 340, 342, 348, 349,
    350, 356
stroke 181
sudden death syndrome 63
suggestibility 257
suicide 21, 22, 43, 77, 79, 97,
    102, 106, 111, 112, 147,
    157, 211, 268, 314, 317,
    324

support group 248, 270, 250,
    266, 267, 269, 274, 296,
    316, 317, 321, 325, 327,
    329, 324
Surgeon General 357
Surgeon General's 1979 report
    124
surgery 90, 95, 193, 312
Surtees Index of Social Support
    336
symptom diary 305
syphilis 93

T lymphocyte 168, 338
tachycardia 73, 223
talc 198
tampon 199, 201, 202
Taylor Manifest Anxiety 335
Tecumseh study 111
teeth 288
temperament 344, 349
teratogenic medications 141
tetanus 288
tetracycline 217
Tetracyline 142
thalidomide 142, 150, 210
Thematic Apperception Test 337
thiazide diuretic treatment 229
thiocynate 143
thipental 150
Three Mile Island nuclear power
    accident 116
thromboembolism 179
thrombosis 111
thyroid gland 163, 219
thyroid stimulating hormone
    219
thyroidism 219
tissue repair 338
toxemia 92, 103, 106, 147, 172
toxic shock syndrome 202
toxin exposure 150

Subject Index

toxins 129, 135
toxoplasmosis 140, 142
trait anxiety 133, 185, 333
trait hostility 111
trait hysteria 178
trait marker 121, 128, 160, 172, 338
trait/state measures 333
tranquilizer 88, 94, 186, 190, 278, 286, 315, 339
transcendence 335
transference 70, 262
trauma 96, 182, 199, 212, 221, 278, 279, 320, 328, 343
travel 288
trichinosis 54
trichomonas 199
trichomoniasis 94
trifluoperazine 141
tubal litigation 188
tubal infection 155T cell 122
tubal obstruction 201
tuberculosis 21, 30, 111, 205
tumor 19, 110, 195, 211
Type A 1, 4, 37, 67, 78, 116, 119, 122, 176, 177, 179, 206, 210, 248, 267, 274, 290, 335
Type A Structured Interview (ATBP SI) 335
Type B 206
typhoid 288

UCLA Loneliness Scale 336
ulceration 21
ulcers 33, 183, 345
ultrasound 138, 150, 231, 319
ultraviolet light 211
undernourishment 357
underreporting 104
underweight 101, 187, 195, 287
unemployment 179, 181

upper respiratory disease 21, 53, 106, 288, 289
urethral syndrome 94
urethritis 94
urinary tract infection 201
uterine contractions 138
uterine cramps 223
uterine fibroma 92
uterus 91, 343
Uzgiris and Hunt Assessment Procedure 337

vagina 91
vaginal delivery 89
vaginal discharge 199
vaginal lesions 200
vaginal infection 96, 200, 209
vaginal sprays 290
vaginismus 200, 317
vaginitis 72, 201, 217
vascular disease 179
vascular lesions 111
venereal warts 199
vibrators 201
Vickers Scale 335
vinegar 216
vinyl chloride 211
viruses 91
vitamin 256, 268, 269, 278
vitamin A 187, 288
vitamin B 187
vitamin B6 188
vitamin C 288
vitamin D 187
vitamin deficiencies 287
vulva 91
vulvar surgery 313
vulvovaginitis 94, 199, 209

Wahler Physical Symptoms Inventory 336
WAIS Verbal 334

Waring Intimacy Questionnaire 334
Ways of Coping Checklist 334
weight gain 137
weight control 4, 12, 102, 251, 267, 278
Western Collaborative Study 207
Western Electric Study 113, 259
Westinghouse studies 262
white blood count 300
withdrawal 254
Work Environment Scale 336

Yale University 110
Yeast infections 200
yoga 239, 251

ZAR Pregnancy Attitude Scale 336
zinc 188
Zung Self-Rating Anxiety Scale 335
Zung Self-Rating Depression Scale 335